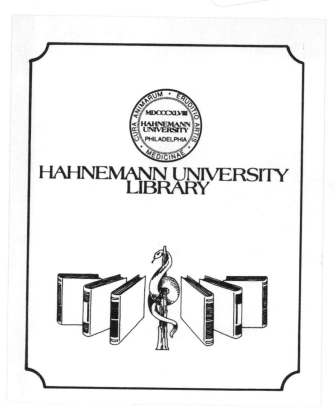

Milestones in Immunology

Milestones in Immunology

A Historical Exploration

Debra Jan Bibel

With a Foreword by Arthur M. Silverstein

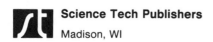

Science Tech Publishers
Madison, WI

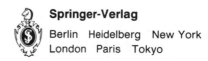

Springer-Verlag
Berlin Heidelberg New York
London Paris Tokyo

Library of Congress Cataloging-in-Publication Data

Milestones in immunology / edited by Debra Jan Bibel.
        p.   cm.
      Consists of reprints of articles from various sources.
      Includes bibliographies and index.
      ISBN 0-910239-15-0
      1. Immunology.   I. Bibel, Debra Jan.
      [DNLM: 1. Allergy and Immunology--history--collected works.   QW
11.1 M643]
QR181.5.M55 1988
616.07′9--dc19
DNLM/DLC
for Library of Congress   88-15773
                                                                        CIP

Science Tech Publishers, 701 Ridge Street
Madison, Wisconsin 53705 U.S.A.

Sole distribution rights outside of the USA, Canada, and Mexico granted
to Springer-Verlag Berlin Heidelberg New York London Paris Tokyo

ISBN 0-910239-15-0   Science Tech Publishers   Madison, WI
ISBN 3-540-19345-6   Springer-Verlag   Berlin Heidelberg New York

Design and production supervision: Science Tech Publishers
Editorial supervision: Ruth Siegel
Interior design: Thomas D. Brock
Cover design: Jerry Minnich

Printed in the United States of America

10 9 8 7 6 5 4 3 2 1

As if,
i.e., all that we apprehend is but metaphor

To Sara, in the hope that one day she will grasp the ways of science

Contents

Foreword

When a science enters a period of relatively slow growth and progress, its practitioners often find the leisure to explore the past, and to search out their conceptual and philosophical roots. When a science is making rapid and giant strides forward, as has been the case in immunology these past 25 years, there is little time to reminisce; the future seems to hold more interest and more promise than does the past. This is especially true of the young scientists, whose education has often neglected the study of the historical and cultural traditions of their discipline. Most of them act (and write the introductions to their scientific papers) as though the entire history of the field were completely contained in the last five years' issues of the principal journals. They seem unaware of the rich background that provided the bases for modern research interests, of the conceptual and technological threads that connect them to the giants of the past, and of the changing styles of and influences upon research over the years.

It is for this reason that Debra Jan Bibel's book on *Milestones in Immunology* is an important and timely contribution. It reminds us that prior to the present era of immunobiology, there were equally important eras of bacteriology (1880–1910) and of immunochemistry (1910–1960), when Pasteur, Koch, Metchnikoff, Bordet, Ehrlich, Landsteiner, and many others laid the foundations of our modern science. But these workers did more—they showed that science could be pursued with style and flair; that controversy can be a useful stimulus to progress; and that even now-outmoded concepts are worthy of study as important stepping stones towards today's received wisdoms. Santayana's statement that "Those who cannot remember the past are condemned to repeat it" may be something of an overstatement as applied to science, but surely those who disregard the past suffer a loss of that broad cultural influence to which they are entitled.

As Dr. Bibel points out, the choice of significant historical "milestones" in any discipline is a highly personal matter, but all will agree that she has chosen most of the papers that appear on anyone's list. But it is her treatment of these significant immunologic papers that renders this volume especially useful, both to the expert and to the amateur. In the comment before each paper she has set the contemporary scene in which the work was done, providing not only a brief biography of the scientists, but a summary of the environment that caused a question to be asked, and that influenced the interpretations made. She has, further, reduced the scientific report itself to its essentials, so that the reader might be spared extraneous background material and unnecessary technical detail, to permit immediate focus upon the heart of the matter. In addition, she has made available for the first time a number of communications that might otherwise have remained inaccessible to those not fluent in French or German, as they have never been translated into English before.

Arthur M. Silverstein
Immunology Laboratories
Johns Hopkins University School of Medicine

Preface

Whenever a new discovery is reported to the scientific world, they say first, "It is probably not true." Thereafter, when the truth of the new proposition has been demonstrated beyond question, they say, "Yes, it may be true, but it is not important." Finally, when sufficient time has elapsed to fully evidence its importance, they say, "Yes, surely it is important, but it is no longer new." —Michel de Montaigne

The farther one pursues knowledge, the less one knows. —Lao Tzu

---

This book is a guided historical exploration of immunology that focuses on the classic contributions to this ever developing science. Preparatory discussions of these milestones are organized into three levels of detail to help the reader navigate the complex network of immunological structures and functions. The first level is the general introduction that follows this preface. It provides a broad overview of the science and of the nine convenient categories under which the milestones are arranged: immunotheraphy; allergy; hypersensitivity and immunopathology; immunochemistry; cells and interactions; theories; agents and adjuncts; immunogenetics; technology; and systems. As the reader approaches each group of papers, a more particular introduction is encountered that examines the given topic in relation to the previous material. A yet more specific discussion, including biographical sketches of the authors, precedes each featured paper. Finally, the book closes with a philosophical epilogue that returns the reader to the heights for a fresh perspective of the territory and the interconnective paths of the journey.

Immunology is a peculiarly pivotal and relatively recent formal science. Derived from the Latin word for exemption in reference to military and tax obligations, immunology emerged in the late nineteenth century as a narrow study of innate and acquired resistance to poisons and microorganisms. Although it developed in tandem with medical microbiology, and many academic departments still encompass both titles, immunology has expanded beyond the realm of infectious disease and has become a true multidisciplinary field of inquiry. Immunochemistry, immunogenetics, immunopharmacology, psychoneuroimmunology, transplantation, serology, allergy, and tumor immunology are some of its interactive divisions. These fusions of once separate scientific areas have forced the redefinition of immunology in more fundamental terms: the physiological process of biochemical specificity and memory in self-nonself discrimination. Traditional immunology is restricted to the classical humoral and cellular arms of the reticuloendothelial system; however, under its umbrella is also the more microbiologically related field of medical microbial ecology, which concerns host-parasite interactions.

This book will not focus on the myriad innate selective factors that help determine host resistance to infectious disease, but I should mention their wide scope in passing: A microorganism landing on host tissue will be ecologically disadvantaged, compared to normal host flora, if unable to bind to specific cellular receptors; the process is called microbial adherence. The nutrient content of tissues and metabolic regulators, such as transferrin, can restrict invasion by fastidious bacteria. Especially selective are the environmental features of pH, temperature, humidity, salinity, and local levels of oxygen and carbon dioxide. Microorganisms that are able to establish themselves may hold their niche against competitors through the production of antagonistic secretions, such as antibiotics and bacteriocins. Lysozyme and platelet beta-lysin, which reach high levels in inflamed tissue, can be lethal for some microorganisms. Also able to retard invasion is the flow of saliva, sweat, intestinal juices, tears, and in the respiratory system, mucus and air. The respiratory tract includes back-sweeping cilia, and the size of passages exerts an influence on flow dynamics. Since these and similar factors are largely nonspecific, nontransferable, and relatively static in their cumulative and synergistic activity, they have provided less distinct and reproducible data and yet no significant therapy or other medical application. Still, these general environmental barriers provide the host with efficient and comprehensive protection against many infectious microorganisms. The outcome of contact with many other pathogenic microbes, particularly those introduced into underlying tissues, is often determined by the development of specific host resistance factors, the immunological response.

So rapidly and extensively has immunology evolved over the last 25 years that we have not only been unable to comfortably digest the advances made even yesterday, but we have not had an opportunity to look back from where we came. Despite the many annals of research now placed on the laboratory shelf, is this the proper time to reflect on the roots that have led to the Brave New World of genetically engineered monoclonal antibodies, immunotoxin "magic bullets," and the first immunological plague, AIDS? The foreseeable future may be too exciting for present day investigators to look over their shoulder, and some students seem to focus only on the hot research areas that lead to their own careers. Nevertheless, most students are curious about the origins of their science.

I argue that a historical anchor is beneficial to both the science and the scientist. At the core of any formal discipline within or outside of science is the quest to determine exactly and completely what we are, including the functional relationships with our surroundings. To examine a science in isolation and out of the broader and deeper context is like inspecting a specimen with a stereoscopic microscope while keeping one eye closed. History provides a formal linkage of science and technology with the humanities. Although some may regard history of science as only a series of key advances and the biographies of their authors, i.e., archival knowledge, the subject is much broader, including large measures of philosophy, economics, politics, and psychology. Immunology, an extraordinarily complex body of knowledge, presently rests on the premise that the immune system functions to bio-chemically differentiate "self" and "other." Modern immunology, therefore, taps our deepest concerns, addressing the question of individuality. The matter, however, is not as simple and self-evident as it might seem, as will be shown in this work. Immunologists, if so inclined, can join those nuclear physicists, cosmologists, and psychobiologists who are interested in probing directly the epistemological questions of existence—the relationship of self and the universe; the reality of elemental matter, consciousness, and cognition; and the governing of organization and process. History is one of the proven paths of such philosophical pondering and transcendence, but it has some immediate practical advantages as well.

To start, history helps to maintain the newly gained structure and independent identity of immunological science. These take on importance when organizing and budgeting academic departments, establishing research institutes, and funding research grants. Science, after all, is grounded in the interacting world of scientists, government, and economics, and a historical perspective can aid policy decisions. Furthermore, immunologists are not immune to the need, common and natural to all people, to create traditions and myths through chronicles that help bring order to their lives. Also in a sociological context, a sizeable number of those who entered the field at the start of its renaissance are now middle-aged, the normal time for taking stock and reassessment.

A vigorous academic defense of history, however, need not be mustered, for historical pursuits can be edifying and inspiring in themselves as well as a source of enjoyment and pride. History is a splendid, stimulating intellectual exercise. It has also served as a warning. Students and researchers on the immunological path might be surprised to find instead of an eight-lane highway, a meandering river system with many tributaries, rapids and eddies, dry gulches and, thanks to immunological technology being adopted in many other scientific and industrial applications, a wide delta. They may also be amused to learn that the mainstream and ancient splits in the river have frequently merged. Science is filled with examples of rediscovery, and I recall my own astonishment when as a graduate student examining a certain phenomenon, I found on a dusty shelf of the library a 40-year-old, long-forgotten report describing the same manifestation.

Although immunology has a 100-year-old tradition, there are no books solely dedicated to its history, except for some accounts of antimicrobial vaccines. The present book is not a formal history of immunology, but neither is it merely an anthology of the classics. A reading of scientific milestones is a traditional method of science education, but intact reprints are filled with obsolete and insignificant information. Also forewords to most such collections are as cold and lifeless as their featured articles, offering only a keyhole perspective along orthodox lines. I have pruned the extraneous, often tedious material of introductions, methodology, footnotes, detailed case histories, and references so that focus can be directed at the heart of each opus. Each of the nine parts of this work as well as each article is prefaced by my comments which are intended to give both scientific and historic perspectives. As such, the book is directed primarily to the student apprentice and the working scientist rather than the professional historian. The commentaries include my personal insights and interpretations. The reader is advised that such views are not carved in stone; since stones eventually erode to dust.

As I observed in preparing this book, the path along the milestones presents the reader with a remarkable overview of the science and its conduct. "Science" may mean knowledge, but it is more than a coherent assemblage of facts. Scientific investigation is an adventure with risks to career and reputation as well as rewards of satisfaction, thrills, and peer and perhaps even societal recognition. For the student, especially, the examples of experimental design, insight, and logic may instill a sense of the investigative art, which may later be of service. Between the lines can also be found the influences— on one hand of personality, rivalry, and politics, and on the other, a thirst for understanding and the simple joy of discovery—be the study a treatment for a grave disease or some seemingly minor fact of cellular function. The excitement and apprehension of Pasteur in his paper on rabies contrasts with his utter confidence and expertise in public relations during his demonstration of the anthrax vaccine at Pouilly-le-Fort. The careful, stepwise, technical precision of Bordet in his research on complement is countered with the bold, creative approach of the theoreticians Ehrlich, Metchnikoff, and Jerne. We also can appreciate the wonder of the pioneer immunogeneticists struggling in the molecular and mechanistic void of the period preceding the clarification of the DNA helix.

Most of the early reports were in German or French, as these countries were then the scientific centers of the world. I have attempted to maintain the literary style of these accounts in their translations, of which I am directly responsible for the French. Some of these abridged papers are presented in English for the first time. In contrast with the bland, partitioned, and quasi-objective approach of present day works, which beginning students often find incomprehensible by their organization and terminology, these first milestones have a far more relaxed, personal flavor. The reader may even discern a British or French style. The studies are also chronological and continuous in presentation, offering a more realistic rendering of the experimental method.

Which then among the countless pages of research are the immunological milestones? The choice will surely vary with each investigator, although some papers are so outstanding as to be included on any such list. While all articles in the present collection are keenly significant, the criteria for selection vary. Most of the papers included are the first major article on a discovery or theory. Some selections from a pioneer's large body of similar studies were chosen as either representative or as an influential summation. Others are the crowning of an approach previously developed by diverse authors. Some milestones are brilliant failures deemed historically important by the research they engendered. At times a discovery is made independently by two or more investigators; unless their approaches are sufficiently unique, only one is featured here. Because the scientific path is rarely straight, a few milestones were not immediately hailed. Instead, they languished for a while in a peripheral, almost forgotten corner. I grant that the historical significance of all but a few of the recent reports in the research literature can not be fairly assessed, since they may eventually lead away from the thrust of the field or perhaps be reinterpreted and relegated to mere footnotes. For this reason I have not considered any article published within the last ten years, and only three of those selected have appeared within the last fifteen years.

I wish to thank Arthur Silverstein and Thomas Brock for their helpful suggestions, Ruth Siegel for the final polish in editing, and my friends and immunological colleagues Joyce Yamada, Larry Lambert, and Leslie Tobler for their critical discussions and support. Special mention goes to Dorothy Whitcomb, historical librarian of the University of Wisconsin School of Medicine at Madison, for locating obscure biographical data. Some of the commentaries are based on my series of columns "Rummagings Along the Dusty Shelf," appearing in the newsletter of the Northern California branch of the American Society for Microbiology. An appreciative salute goes to Bob Metcalf, who as editor helped me to initiate these historical notes. I also thank Esther Sammann for providing the basic translations of most of the German articles, a difficult and tedious task.

I apologize to those researchers who may find errors within my sketch of their career. My sources, unless otherwise cited, generally were the standard biographical anthologies, whose listings are usually provided and reviewed by the concerned party.

Introduction

*"Life is very strange," said Jeremy. "Compared to what?" replied the
spider.*   —Anonymous

*Science can not exist without some small portion of
metaphysics.*   —Max Planck

Microbiology is one of the few sciences that has a distinct origin: It arose
together with the microscope. Its grandfather was the cloth merchant and
amateur microscopist Antony van Leeuwenhoek (1632–1723), who was the
first person to unquestionably observe bacteria. Thanks to these tangible
microbes and the subsequent discoveries of their ability to cause fermentation
of organic fluids and putrefaction of tissues, the abstract, nebulous concept
of contagion eventually led to the germ theory of disease.

The beginning of immunology, at least as a scientific principle, is not so
precise. It arose in those murky mists of ancient civilizations when priest-
physicians, shamans, or other healers observed that some individuals escaped
the sufferings of plagues or, if so affected and survived, were able to remain
alive and often free of disease on recurrence of the given pestilence. Because
immunology is not confined to infectious disease, I should also mention the
empirical approach in the first century B.C. of King Mithridates VI of Pontus,
a nation bordering the Black Sea. Like so many illustrative tales, it is based
on irony. To protect himself against a possible assassin's poison, he daily
consumed a small dose of the presumed toxin. He lived to old age and when
he desired to end his life by poisoning, he, of course, failed.

As will soon be described, attempts to acquire resistance to lethal poisons—
and not Edward Jenner's smallpox vaccine of 1798—were the door to modern
molecular immunology. In the history of immunology the studies of Jenner
played the same pioneering role as those of Leeuwenhoek did in microbiology. Through outstanding powers of observation and rough, but never-

theless effective, experimentation, the naturalist Leeuwenhoek and the physician Jenner laid a solid foundation for the long-delayed development of their respective sciences. Thus, the first group of milestones on immunotherapy begins with reports by Henry Sewall and by the team of Emil von Behring and Shibasaburo Kitasato on the acquisition of specific immunity to animal and bacterial toxins. Jenner's work is then formally introduced.

The father of microbiology is also the father of immunology, and that would be Louis Pasteur. Three key representatives of his voluminous works will be presented in this section. Pasteur belongs to the pantheon of humanity, and among all those in this collection only his name will be recognized by the laity. A brilliant physical chemist, he found himself serving as a troubleshooter in the fermentation industry. Soon he was thinking in medical terms: the "diseases" of wine and beer. Everything he touched turned to gold as he examined the natural history and origins of the infusoria. Once a mere curiosity and viewed as passive creatures, microorganisms became a central scientific focus when found to actually do something. Their active association with infectious disease, as established by Agostino Bassi and especially Robert Koch, was a particularly significant something. However, despite all of his microbiological discoveries, including pasteurization, Pasteur is best known for his vaccines against the economically significant anthrax bacillus and the terrifying rabies virus. Many other scientists have subsequently picked up the banner of vaccination, since on principle it is better to prevent a disease than attempt to cure it, and this section concludes with three such pioneering efforts by American and English research teams. Because antibiotics are generally useless against viral diseases and chemotherapy is fraught with difficulties of low efficacy and serious side effects, immunological approaches remain the first choice for treatment and prevention of many diseases.

This is not to say that immunological reactions are without risk. The second group of milestones, covering a variety of phenomena, show that the inflammatory physiological cascade following the immune trigger can be a real nuisance (as any hay fever or other allergy sufferer can aver). The immune response can also be lethal. In addition, hypersensitivity phenomena, like all characteristic immune activities, are directed to foreign substances, and the discomfort is a secondary effect. When the immune system directly attacks particular tissues of the organism, i.e., itself, autoimmune disease ensues. The recognition of these rare disorders challenged any remaining teleological notions of the immune system.

The discoveries presented in this section on immunopathology came mainly to clear-eyed and curious clinicians, but others sought answers by exploring immunology at the molecular level. Biochemistry was insufficiently developed at the time for Pasteur to take on its complexities; still, his fascination with molecular dissymmetry never ceased, especially with the selectivity of biological systems for particular light-rotating stereoisomers. The foundation of immunochemistry would be left to Paul Ehrlich, a physician only by diploma. His love from the very start was the laboratory. Ehrlich's work appropriately leads the selection of milestones concerning the chemistry of antibodies and their corresponding antigens. It soon became apparent that the actively or passively acquired antitoxic property of blood and lymph was due to antitoxic substances. Ehrlich soon found that these antibodies were a heterogeneous population with diverse biological and chemical properties. In coupling to target antigens, for instance, they varied in specificity and degree of avidity. They were also sensitive to denaturation. Quantitation by simple weight measurements or dilution titers was not practical. Ehrlich, being responsible for antisera standardization, developed suitable methods for quality assurance based on his astounding insight about the spatial and functional relationships of atomic groups. Those who followed Ehrlich's approach concentrated their studies on the composition of antigens, the specificity of the antibody receptor, the physical arrangement of antigen-antibody complexes, and the existence and structural composition of the various antibody classes. Major papers on these immunochemical subjects are featured.

The study of antibodies has until recently dominated immunology. Humoral immunity, however, is only one wing of the immune response. The next group of milestones presents the cellular components and their interactions. The honor of first demonstrating cellular immunity belongs to a Russian invertebrate zoologist, Elie Metchnikoff. Intently witnessing through his microscope the combat of microbe and defending phagocyte, this disciple of Darwin sought the phylogenic origins of immunity in humans. In phagocytosis Metchnikoff found a mechanism whose sophistication and variation depended on the principles of evolution and which seemed to explain all the host-parasite interactions, except acquired immunity. The cellular approach, which eventually lost favor against the steamroller of antibody studies, was resurrected after some 50 years with the work of Karl Landsteiner, the great serologist and immunochemist, and his student Merrill W. Chase. However, the cells that excited researchers were not the phagocytes, their now somewhat tedious old friends, but the mysterious lymphocytes. At first these cells, or their derivative plasma cells, were linked with antibody formation. Next, a subset was associated with nonantibody-related phenomena, such as delayed hypersensitivity and transplantation immunity. Then, synergistic, cooperative, and other regulatory interactions among the various lymphocytes and phagocytes were recognized, uniting all the components into a vast system.

The fifth series of papers concerns the theoretical development of immunology from Pasteur, Ehrlich, and Metchnikoff to the immunological ontogenist Sir Macfarlane Burnet and the systems analyst Niels Jerne. Theories provide the scaffold of all scientific investigations. Although dependent on laboratory experimentation or field investigations, theorization is an armchair, midnight oil activity. It is the most creative element of science; it is the least successful. It is also the exercise by which scientists holding a Ph.D., a doctor of philosophy degree, who typically have never taken a course in philosophy, tap into their ancient roots. A working hypothesis, the very cornerstone of research, may serve to challenge or support the current model of reality. Some of these milestones are narrow in scope, such as Sir Almroth Wright and Stewart Douglas's attempt to reconcile the cellular and humoral theories of immunity. They proposed the existence of soluble opsonins, which way tire chains provide traction on icy roads. Other papers are revolutionary, causing great numbers of unexplained phenomena across the whole field to fall into place.

Immune responses involve numerous nonspecific adjuncts and inflammatory agents. The sixth group of milestones concerns these factors. Most noteworthy is complement, which is actually a cascading series of structural and enzymic proteins. These substances were first detected through studies on Pfeiffer's phenomenon, whereby cholera vibrio are destroyed solely by fluids. The investigations of complement by Jules Bordet, a student of Metchnikoff, were able to unify the bactericidal and hemolytic effects of serum and help settle much confusion in immunological specificity and function. However, much more was left open until fairly recent chemical studies on complement pathways, receptors, and mechanisms of action. Histamine, discovered by Sir Henry Dale and Sir Patrick Laidlaw, is the most familiar inflammatory agent, it being responsible for the misery of the common cold and allergic rhinitis. The physiological response of inflammation is meshed with immunity through an elaborate trigger mechanism that typically involves the attachment of at least two IgE antibodies to a tissue mast cell or blood basophil. The signal for cellular degranulation occurs when the immunoglobulins are bridged by their corresponding antigen. Papers in this part continue with the discovery of interferon, a protein produced by virus-infected cells that indirectly confers resistance to surrounding tissues. Interferon has long been a candidate for viral chemotherapy. The last milestone of the section introduces the lymphokines, secreted mediators that regulate the immune response. John R. David and Barry R. Bloom described the first of many such agents, migration inhibitory factor, by which activated lymphocytes affect the movement of surrounding macrophages.

Immunology has been described as the science of self and nonself discrimination and the defense of individual integrity. Immunogenetics is at the heart of this definition, and is the subject of the next series of milestones. This specialty took form with attempts to explain the rejection of blood transfusions and skin grafts not only from donors of different species, which might be expected, but even within the same species. These related phenomena are much more dramatic and specific indicators of individuality than the subtle and aggregate variation of morphology, physiology, or resistance to diseases. That self could be correlated with distinct antigenic differences among common tissues, especially that ancient hereditary metaphor, blood, gave these investigations an importance beyond the practice of surgery, and today histocompatibility genes, so important in tissue transplantation, are markers associated with a variety of nonimmunological disorders and characteristics. While any consideration of individual consciousness and the apparently imperative origin of ego, a psychological and philosophical quagmire, is outside our particular interest, multipersonality disorder and the consequential ego-dependent flux of physiology, including immune responses, challenge complacency.

Another set of milestones within this section demonstrated that antigenic specificity also extends into another biological level: Antibodies of a given class and subclass are not only antigenically different among individuals of the same species, they differ antigenically even within the individual. Introduced foreign matter initiates the formation of antibodies, which in turn are recognized by other antibodies, which serve as antigens for a third set of antibodies, and so forth. A peculiar characteristic of this system of idiotypes is that the spatial configuration of the antigen-combining site of the anti-antibody mimics the original antigen. This internal image was predicted by Jerne's network theory, and offers new approaches to immunotherapy. Somatic recombination and mutation were eventually determined to share responsibility for this antibody diversity. What does this do to the structural definition of immunology given above? Does self originate simply from the sequences of genes or through the interactions of environment and the developing body? What about autoimmune diseases? It seems that the material recognized by the individual as foreign or nonself is reduced to a three-dimensional arrangement of atomic groups, the external shape rather than the elemental composition, that paradoxically operates as an integral part of the organism. Germane is a proposal, based on experimental data, that for a peptide to be antigenic in a given individual, it must resemble a region of the histocompatibility molecule. This domain serves as an internal ligand, a combining site, for the peptide receptor formed by other domains of the molecule. According to the model, the peptide and the ligand are operationally compared. Self thereby is not a static form, but the unique ephemeral pattern of the dynamic, fluctuating system itself.

The next group of milestones covers the development of immunological tools now utilized by scientists of all biomedical disciplines. Modern science is dependent on both phenomenon and measurement, and these papers present either the discoveries or the first quantitative investigations of agglutination, precipitation, complement-fixation, immunofluorescent staining, and so forth. Three of these technological works, the development of inbred congenic animal strains for immunogenetic histocompatibility studies, radioimmunoassays, and the engineered fusion of myeloma and plasma cells (hybridomas) to secrete almost any given monoclonal antibody, led their authors to Stockholm and the Nobel Prize.

The last milestone in this book, a radical work by Serge Metalnikov, is a paradigm shatterer, for it is a founding work in the field of psychoneuroimmunology. This fusion of scientific disciplines transcends materialism, linking mind, consciousness, and nervous tissue with the community of immune cells. What is a paradigm? The word refers to a model or pattern, but it has become a catchword of deeper significance. Paradigms have been described as moods, metaphors, and myths, underlying frameworks describing our perspective of life and the universe, that are shared by social groups usually across various disciplines. Concepts and beliefs, including scientific ones, change over time, and many observers find the current paradigms of science and society undergoing a profound shift, indeed a reversal: (1) from the parts to the whole—properties of parts can be understood only from the dynamics of the whole; (2) from structure to process—structures are manifestations of process; (3) from objective to epistemic science—scientific descriptions are not independent of the observer; (4) from edifice to network as the metaphor of knowledge; and (5) from truth to approximate descriptions. Immunology with its recent emphasis on network and process has become a leading science contributing to the formation of a new paradigm, a new world view. This book, hence, traces the evolution of an immunological-process metaphysics from its Cartesian reductive and compartmentalized origins.

   While taking this raft expedition along the waterways of history to survey the field, the reader may want to consult some general textbooks and other publications on immunology and its development. The references given below are particularly worthy. Other recommended readings will follow each commentary. These may include articles or books specific to the respective milestone or its authors, or the commentary itself. Have a good journey, and watch out for rapids!

For further information:

Fleck, L. 1979 (1935). *Genesis and Development of a Scientific Fact.* (T. J. Trenn and R. K. Merton, editors; F. Bradley and T. J. Trenn, translators). University of Chicago Press, Chicago. 203 p.

Foster, W. D. 1970. *A History of Medical Bacteriology and Immunology.* William Heinemann Medical Books, London. 232 p.

Klein, J. 1982. *Immunology. The Science of Self-Nonself Discrimination.* John Wiley & Sons, New York. 687 p.

Latour, B. 1987. *Science in Action.* Harvard University Press, Cambridge, MA. 274 p.

Lewin, R. 1974. *In Defense of the Body. An Introduction to the New Immunology.* Anchor Books, Garden City, NY. 146 p.

Roitt, I. M., J. Brostoff, and D. K. Male. 1985. *Immunology.* C. V. Mosby Company, St. Louis. [unnumbered pages]

Ziman, J. 1984. *An Introduction to Science Studies. The philosophical and social aspects of science and technology.* Cambridge University Press, Cambridge. 203 p.

Part 1
Immunotherapy

And with some sweet oblivious antidote
Cleanse the stuff'd bosom of that perilous
stuff. —William Shakespeare, *Macbeth*

The physician of the future will be an
immunisator. —Sir Almroth E. Wright, 1909

Nearly all historical reviews of immunology begin with a discussion of small-pox and Edward Jenner's vaccine against it, and then proceed chronologically through the work of Louis Pasteur followed by Emil von Behring's discovery of diphtheria antitoxin. For the following reasons, I choose instead to commence with Henry Sewall's little known but important pioneering study of snake antitoxins: It was probably poisoning from reptile or arachnid bites or the consumption of toxic plants, rather than contagious diseases that was first encountered and recognized by our Neolithic ancestors at the dawn of civilization. In addition, plant and animal toxins have historically been treated separately in immunological and microbiological textbooks; they were considered tangental to the main question of resistance to invasive microorganisms. However, it was his study of these chemical agents and their corresponding antibodies, not intact, complex bacteria or viruses, that provided Paul Ehrlich with his insightful molecular understanding of immunological responses. In contemporary immunology the flags of molecular biology and biochemistry are paramount. Hence, the first report on experimentally acquired resistance to snake venom is an appropriate pier from which to launch the expedition.

While the investigation of antitoxins—this time initiated in response to bacteria—is continued in the paper of Shibasaburo Kitasato and Behring, their milestone article also introduced the use of serum as therapy. Until this demonstration, immunity was considered as either innate and nonspecific or acquired by previous contact with the particular living or chemical agent.

7

Kitasato and Behring showed that this quality could be transferred. Unfortunately, such passive resistance is incomplete and transitory. The hope of serum therapy soon faded but has not completely disappeared. It is still utilized in instances when lasting immunity is unnecessary; when, as in an emergency, vaccination is not possible; when it is used as a supplement to a vaccine; and when a particular vaccine has not been developed. The inoculation of concentrated and pooled gamma-globulin from convalescent patients is a form of serum therapy when neither a specific antiserum or vaccine is available.

The milestone by Jenner is presented as the lead to a series of papers covering vaccines based on attenuated microorganisms. The vaccinia virus may have been a naturally attenuated strain of the smallpox virus. Jenner did not engineer; he merely took advantage of an existing strain of pox virus. Pasteur and his colleagues, however, discovered that the virulence of both visible and unseen infectious agents can be increased as well as reduced. They purposefully attenuated these microorganisms in developing vaccines, first to fowl cholera, later to anthrax, and finally to rabies. It was later determined that the rabies virus itself was not actually attenuated; the preparations varied in their proportion of active and inactivated viral units.

Attenuated vaccines have been the preferred approach, since they permit stimulation of the various local and systemic immune responses. Infections with such live vaccines are subclinical, i.e., without serious symptoms. Attenuation, however, may occasionally reverse through mutation. This risk can be eliminated with a microbial preparation that has been killed or, with respect to viruses, inactivated. The concomitant question was whether such vaccines are effective, and whether they are still immunogenic. The report of Daniel Salmon and Theobald Smith answered the question in the affirmative, although their experiment was designed for another purpose. Their hypothesis, which focused on the possible immunogenicity of bacterial secretions, was inadequately tested.

The next milestone in this section had no ambiguity. Sir Almroth Wright and Sir David Semple developed one of the more successful killed bacterial vaccines against typhoid fever. Its impetus, as for many advances in medicine, science, and technology, was war. First tested during the Boer War, its worth was proven during the rigors and infectious opportunities of World War I. The second world war brought forth an inactivated viral vaccine to influenza. Unfortunately, few of the killed vaccines were as effective as their attenuated counterparts. The relative merits and disadvantages of the live poliomyelitis vaccine of Albert Sabin and the inactivated vaccine of Jonas Salk still are argued in the corridors of research centers and governmental agencies.

Michael Heidelberger's team produced the last paper of this section. Their data clearly established the first of the modern approaches to immunization. Their method was similar in principle to the injection of toxin or of its derived and inactive toxoid, and they demonstrated that immunity can be achieved by introducing just the key antigenic, structural component of the infectious organism. No hazard due to inadequate killing or loss of attenuation, nor of side effects from either other microbial constituents or growth media exists when a purified inert molecule or molecular complex is the vaccine. This milestone concerns the capsule (a virulence factor) of the streptococcus responsible for pneumonia. Antibodies directed merely against this external layer can render the host immune.

To find, isolate, and purify the immunogen of a microorganism is not easy. It took another 25 years after the Heidelberger report before the capsular vaccine for bacterial meningitis was licensed. Entirely novel techniques, however, promise to provide safe and efficient vaccines that are also economically practical. If the physicians of the future will be immunizers, as Wright wishfully predicted, then it will be thanks to biological engineers.

Currently under development are agents that are attenuated by deleting from their chromosomes genes associated with virulence factors. A variation using recombinant DNA technology is to transfer the genes responsible for the immunogenic antigen to a benign microorganism, typically one indigenous to the host. Several such chromosomal segments from different infectious agents may be incorporated, producing a polyvaccine. Antigens do not even need to be harvested from microorganisms; they may be synthesized in vitro. Amino acids are assembled into a peptide chain whose steric configuration, as analyzed by a computer, resembles the given microbial antigen. Hazard-free, mass production of ultrapure vaccines, which this approach offers, is also possible with the extraordinary antigen-free technique that uses anti-idiotype monoclonal antibodies. These in essence are anti-antibodies normally produced by the host to its own immunoglobulins. The antigen recognition site of the primary antibody is like a casting mold for a sculpture; its pattern in turn is antigenic. The antigen recognition site of the secondary antibody directed to the mold will mimic the sculpture, i.e., the foreign antigen. These secondary antibodies, produced by hybridoma technology, are used as the vaccine.

New approaches to serum therapy are also forthcoming. By coupling ultraspecific monoclonal antibodies with lethal radioisotopes, toxins, or enzymes, Paul Ehrlich's "magic bullets" may be achieved at last. These immunotoxins can react against microorganisms, tumors, or the particular host lymphocytes responsible for autoimmune disease. From the explosion of technology coupled with new theoretical frameworks, we can expect within a short time the planting of several more milestones in immunotherapy.

For further information:

Chase, A. 1982. *Magic Shots.* William Morrow and Company, New York. 576 p.

Parish, H. J. 1965. *A History of Immunization.* E. and S. Livingstone, Edinburgh. 356 p.

Roitt, I. M. 1984. *Immune Intervention 1: New Trends in Vaccines.* Academic Press, New York. 160 p.

Wilson, Sir G. S. 1967. *The Hazards of Immunization.* Athlone Press, London. 324 p.

Experiments on the preventive inoculation of rattlesnake venom

1887 • Henry Sewall

Comment

Snakes. Immunology owes much to these mysterious creatures, as befitting their legendary and symbolic association with health. Although the first proof that the body can produce protective antitoxins is by tradition ascribed to Emil von Behring and Shibasaburo Kitasato for their studies of tetanus and diphtheria, it actually stems from experiments on snake venom by Henry Sewall (1855–1936). His innovative work is one of America's earliest and more fruitful contributions to the science.

Sewall began his undergraduate education in 1871 at Wesleyan University, which had just instituted a science curriculum. He was the first student to receive its diploma of Bachelor of Science. Sewall next entered the doctorial program in physiology at Johns Hopkins University in 1876. Again it was a first, since the university had just opened its doors that autumn, and the medical school was still several years away. In 1879, with Ph.D. in hand, he traveled to the laboratories of Sir Michael Foster, Carl Ludwig, and Willy Kuhne in England and Germany while on a fellowship for further training in physiology. Upon his return to Johns Hopkins the following year, Sewall was appointed Assistant, and applied his newly gained experience to the teaching of several courses. Two years later, he was elected to the faculty at the University of Michigan.

Louis Pasteur by this time had stirred the world with his vaccines to fowl-cholera and anthrax. The young American recognized the inherent hazard of using living, although attenuated microorganisms for immunization. Because of his biochemical orientation, Sewall hypothesized that since microorganisms injure their hosts through their secretions, protection might be achieved by regulated inoculations of such products. However, he did not immediately put this to test, since he lacked bacteriological training. Instead, an analogous approach occurred to him after he read Weir Mitchell and Edward T. Reichert's treatise on snake venoms, and he began research in this area in autumn 1887. A professor of zoology supplied Sewall with six small rattlesnakes. After several hazardous episodes of escaped serpents within his tiny laboratory, and of unsteady, nervous handling while harvesting venom, he was finally ready to test his long-incubated idea. The result follows in the paper presented below.

Illness prevented Sewall from continuing his work, but his discoveries, although uncelebrated, were not ignored by American and European colleagues. Their follow-up, however, was delayed and indirect. In 1893 Charles Ewing, an assistant to William Henry Welch at Johns Hopkins University, determined that rattlesnake venom could block the bactericidal activity of normal serum against anthrax and common colon bacilli. Beginning in 1901, Hideyo Noguchi, that tragic character of microbiology, examined the pathology and serology of venoms with Weir Mitchell and later with Simon Flexner. Among other advances, they concluded that the venom-sensitive serum factor was a new component (still not entirely identified today) of complement.

Albert Calmette, the famous attenuator of the tubercle bacillus (the BCG strain), also became interested in snakes, particularly in cobras, while organizing a branch of the Pasteur Institute in Saigon in 1891. A flood of the Mekong delta had caused rodents, and then predatory serpents, to seek shelter in village dwellings, much to the distress of the native population. Calmette was able to attenuate cobra venom with calcium hypochloride and thereby produce antitoxin in horses for serum therapy. Later, in 1908, Calmette and some other French scientists made a pilgrimage to Ann Arbor to visit Sewall's old laboratory. It was short-sleeve weather, but they wore formal cutaway coats and silk hats and carried canes. They were disappointed that the laboratory building had been recently gutted by a fire, but the edifice still stood, site of a milestone along the immunological waterway.

For further information:

Gelinas, J. A. 1973. Albert Calmette. The Saigon Years 1891–1893: a historical review. *Military Medicine* 138:730–733.

Harvey, A. M. 1978. Snake venom and medical research—some contributions related to the Johns Hopkins University School of Medicine. *Johns Hopkins Medical Journal* 142:47–60.

Plesset, I. R. 1980. *Noguchi and His Patrons.* Fairleigh Dickinson University Press, New Jersey. 314 p.

Webb, G. B. and D. Powell. 1946. *Henry Sewall. Physiology and Physician.* Johns Hopkins Press, Baltimore. 191 p.

The Paper*

The following work was undertaken with the hope that it might form a worthy contribution to the theory of Prophylaxis, and the results obtained during the first stage of its progress are put forward at this time because of the impression that, perhaps, at least their practical significance may induce investigators more fortunately situated for the performance of such experiments to take up the same line of observation. I have assumed an analogy between the venom of the poisonous serpent and the ptomaines produced under the influence of bacterial organisms. Both are the outcome of the activity of living protoplasm although chemically widely distinct, the ptomaines belonging to the group of alkaloids, while the active principles of the venom . . . are of proteid nature.

If immunity from the fatal effects of snake-bite can be secured in an animal by means of repeated inoculation with doses of the poison too small to produce ill effects, we may suspect that the same sort of resistance against germ-disease might follow the inoculation of the appropriate ptomaine, provided that it is through the products of their metabolism that bacteria produce their fatal effects. . . .

It is a matter of common experience that with the repeated exhibition of various kinds of poisons in the therapeutic doses, more and more of the substance must be employed to produce its physiological action, and, finally, ordinarily fatal doses may be given with impunity. And yet there is reason to believe that this resistance may result from either of two opposite conditions impressed upon the living parts of the body, a pathological or a physiological.

In the first case the sum total energy of the protoplasm is diminished; its irritability is lowered as well as its efficiency as a machine. In the second case the total energy of the protoplasm is not diminished but, perhaps, is even increased as the effect of the inexplicable tendency of living matter to adjust itself to its environment; such a physiological resistance is shown by the secretory cell which does not digest itself, and by the unicellular animals which dissolve ingested matter but spare their own substance. . . .

The venom used in these experiments was obtained from three specimens of the Massasauga, *Crotalophorus tergeminus,* one of the smallest of the rattlesnakes. . . . In order to obtain the poison the snake was allowed to bite the side of a porcelain dish while being held round the neck by a loop fastened to the end of a stick. The number and variety of the experiments performed were narrowly limited by the small amount of venom obtained. . . .

The total amount of venom obtained was estimated to be about six small drops, though as part of it dried after extraction an accurate measure was impossible. The six drops of venom were dissolved in about 88 drops of glycerine, as recommended by Weir Mitchell, so that each drop of the glycerine-venom contained .068 drop of the pure venom. The venom was clear and greenish-yellow in color and decidedly acid in reaction. In preparing for an inoculation, the requisite number of drops of glycerine-venom were allowed to fall into a porcelain capsule and diluted with distilled water to such an extent that each animal should receive 15 minims of the mixture.

Mitchell and others have found that pigeons are peculiarly sensitive to the influence of rattlesnake

---

*Sewall, H. 1887. Experiments on the preventive inoculation of rattlesnake venom. *Journal of Physiology* 8:203–210.

poison, and these birds were therefore uniformly used in the experiments. The inoculations were made under the skin of the back by means of a hypodermic syringe. . . .

The first symptom of the action of the poison was invariably a weakness in the legs, inducing the pigeon to sit down or to move with a tottering gait when forced to rise. Complete paralysis of the legs follows a larger dose of the venom. The general health and appetite of the bird may remain apparently unaffected while the legs are nearly completely paralyzed. Another symptom of the poisoning is the apparently excessive lachrymal secretion. When a fatal dose of poison is given, the paralysis extends from the legs to the wings; the head rests upon the floor; the mouth is open and the respiration gasping, and, after a longer or shorter period of clonic convulsions, the pigeon dies. . . .

[R]attlesnake venom preserved in glycerine undergoes a gradual deterioration in its power. . . . November 7 the fatal dose of glycerine-venom was 2/5 drop; on December 2 it had risen to 2/3 drop; and on May 19 nearly 1 drop was injected into a pigeon without producing death. . . .

There appeared to be a maximal dose of venom which produced death as quickly as any greater amount. . . .

Thinking that the fatal effects of the poison might be due to some sort of ferment action of the venom, half a dozen drops of the blood from [a venom-killed pigeon] were injected into each of two fresh birds. The result was negative.

A number of inoculations were made upon various pigeons to determine the minimal fatal dose of the glycerine-venom mixture, and then it was sought to discover whether repeated inoculations with subminimal but continually increasing doses of the poison would produce immunity against the fatal effects of unlimited amounts of the [agent] and whether such immunity might be merely transient or persistent in its character. The action of the poison in the early stages of a series of observations was to some extent cumulative; for a dose too small to alone produce death could become fatal if given to a pigeon which had not yet recovered from a previous inoculation. . . .

The experiments were carried out on seven pigeons. . . .

From time to time control experiments were made on fresh pigeons. . . .

[R]epeated inoculation of pigeons with sub-lethal doses of rattlesnake venom produces a continually increasing resistance towards the injurious effects of the poison without apparent influence on the general health of the animals. On December 3, when the fatal dose of glycerine-venom is less than 2/3 drop, 4 1/2 drops, or about 7 times the fatal dose, were injected without the least effect into pigeon I. The efficiency of resistance against the venom gradually fails in absence of fresh inoculation, as is witnessed in the case of pigeon I which is perceptibly weakened by the inoculation on January 6 of 3 drops of glycerine-venom, a little more than one month after 4 1/2 drops had been injected without effect. Also on April 29, nearly five months after the next preceding inoculation of 2 drops of the poison, III and IV were killed by inoculation, the one with 3 and other with 2 drops of the poison. That the prophylactic effect of the repeated inoculations is persistent over the interval of five months is shown by the example of pigeon II, which on May 6 is uninjured by a fatal dose of the poison, and thereafter rapidly recovers its powers of resistance against the ill effects of inoculation with doses of venom much in excess of the fatal amount.

On the mechanism of immunity to diphtheria and tetanus in animals

1890 • Emil von Behring and Shibasaburo Kitasato

Comment

Sewall's report, although published in a major journal, seems to have been overlooked by the researchers of Robert Koch's laboratory in the Institute of Hygiene at the University of Berlin. Three years later an investigative team there conducted an independent frontal attack on the question of resistance to microbial toxins. The work on diphtheria toxin and antitoxin developed at a rapid rate after the causal organism of this dread childhood disease was discovered in 1884 by Friedrich Loeffler in Koch's laboratory: Emile Roux and Alexandre Yersin at the Pasteur Institute in 1888 beat Loeffler in the race to discover and efficiently recover the exotoxin of the diphtheria bacillus, whose existence was predicted by Loeffler when he first isolated the organism. In 1889 Shibasaburo Kitasato (1852–1931), working in Koch's laboratory, developed anaerobic methods of cultivation that allowed him to successfully isolate the tetanus bacillus. In the same year, Knud Faber, a Danish physician, showed that like diphtheria, the secreted tetanus toxin rather than the bacterium itself seemed responsible for the disease. Now in 1890, as French and other researchers began to exploit the isolation of bacterial toxins, the Berlin group of Kitasato, Behring, and Carl Fraenkel pressed forward with a well-coordinated plan. Science does not have political borders, but scientists do, and friendly nationalistic rivalry still has an influence on the conduct of experiments and the pursuit of knowledge.

Kitasato came to Koch's laboratory in 1886 after completing his medical education at the Tokyo Medical School and serving with honor in the Japanese Central Sanitary Bureau. After fulfilling a series of research and training assignments, Emil von Behring (1854–1917), an army physician, arrived at Koch's research facility in 1889. He had graduated from the Friedrich Wilhelm Institute, the army medical school, as did Koch's other famous assistants, Loeffler, Richard Pfeiffer, and Georg Gaffky. Kitasato, acclaimed for his talents in bacteriological technology, joined Behring in his endeavor to develop a means of protecting first, animals, and then people against diphtheria. Carl Fraenkel was the third member of Koch's diphtheria task force, but his approach for immunization was based on the inoculation of heated broth cultures.

In December 1890, Fraenkel, Kitasato, and Behring published their respective or joint researches. The possibility of serum therapy or immunization against tetanus, and especially against diphtheria, created a great upsurge of hope. Tetanus and diphtheria were common, lethal diseases, and young children were particularly susceptible to epidemics of diphtheria. Pasteur's vaccines for livestock were certainly appreciated, but a cure for such human diseases was much more exciting. The actual trial of serum therapy on an infected child came on Christmas night the following year; it led to Behring's receipt of a title (the von in his name) in 1896, and also of the very first Nobel Prize, in 1901.

The main reason that Fraenkel's vaccine of heated broth cultures could not be consistently produced was because, as we now know, not all strains of the bacterium produce toxin. The genes responsible for toxin production are carried by a virus, a bacteriophage, and under certain circumstances these genes are incorporated into the bacterial chromosome. Another source of inconsistency was the use of sterilizing heat during vaccine production, which denatured the toxin.

Kitasato and Behring's milestone is unique in two key ways: First, it showed that resistance to microbial diseases can occur through the power of serum. A few years earlier the bactericidal property of serum had been established in vitro, but this did not necessarily correlate with immunity. Second, it demonstrated passive immunity—the ability to acquire resistance to a pathological agent by transfer of the property from an actively immunized donor. These scientists first regarded passive immunity as a permanent condition. It proved not to be so, because it fades as the antibodies are slowly broken down, or neutralized by the recipient's own immune response. Today, only in the case of bites by spider or snake or of botulism, does the injection of a specific antiserum remain the standard therapy. However, Kitasato and Behring's inoculation of neutralized toxin offered an opportunity for active immunization by the gradual dissociation of the toxin and its antibody. Such an approach, despite its hazard and practical difficulties, was applied, beginning in 1902, among others, by Alexander Besredka and Elie Metchnikoff at the Pasteur Institute with a living typhoid vaccine.

Kitasato and Behring could speak only of a specific antitoxic property of serum. The existence of a substance, a salt-precipitated globulin, was discovered in 1891 by the Italian specialists in tetanus toxin, Guido Tizzoni and Guiseppina Cattani, who coined the term antitoxin (antitossina in Italian).

Kitasato returned to Japan in 1892 after he became the first foreign scientist to receive the honorary title of Professor from the German government. Two years later he and Alexandre Yersin independenty discovered the plague bacillus. Kitasato subsequently acquired his own research institute, in whose ₁ᵤuseum are artefacts of Robert Koch and Kitasato, including some of Koch's hair that previously was housed in a shrine. Behring and Koch did not share such a close relationship, and after many heated disputes the former resigned from Koch's institute in 1894, eventually founding a research institute of his own and, in 1904, a diagnostic and pharmaceutical manufacturing company, Behring-Werke.

For further information:

Fox, H. 1934. Baron Shibasaburo Kitasato. *Annals of Medical History* Series II. 6:491–499.

Nuttall, G. H. F. 1924/1925. Biographical notes bearing on Koch, Ehrlich, Behring, and Loeffler, with their portraits and letters from three of them. *Parasitology* 16:214–238.

Nuttall, G. H. F. and G. S. Graham-Smith (ed.). 1908. *The Bacteriology of Diphtheria*. Cambridge University Press, Cambridge. 718 p.

The Paper*

In the studies which we have been carrying out for some time on diphtheria (Behring) and tetanus (Kitasato), we have also considered questions of therapy and immunization. In both infectious diseases, we have been able to cure infected animals, as well as to pretreat healthy animals so that later they will not succumb to diphtheria or tetanus.

In what way the therapy and immunization have been obtained will only be stated here in enough detail to demonstrate the truth of the following sentence: "The immunity of rabbits and mice, which have been immunized against tetanus, depends on the ability of the cell-free blood fluid to render harmless the toxic substance that the tetanus bacillus produces."

This explanation of immunity has not been considered in any of the works on the immunity question that have appeared in recent years.

Aside from the studies on phagocytosis, which seek to explain immunity in terms of the vital activities of the cells, others have considered the bactericidal action of the blood and the adaptation of the animal body to the toxin.

When one of these explanations has been found unacceptable, then it has been believed that the exclusion of one is an argument for the other. Thus Bouchard . . . stated: "Let us no longer speak of the action of the leucocytes or the adaptation of the nerve cells to the bacterial toxin: this is pure rhetoric," and "It is actually the bactericidal action that is responsible for vaccination or acquired immunity. . . ."

However, one of us (Behring) could determine in his studies on rats immune to diphtheria and on immunized guinea pigs, that none of the theories mentioned above could explain the immunity of these animals, and he realized that it was necessary to look for another principle to explain these phenomena. After many negative experiments, it was discovered that the blood of immune animals had the ability to neutralize the diphtheria toxin, and this discovery revealed the reason for the insensitivity of these animals to diphtheria. But it was only by applying this concept to tetanus that we were able to achieve results, which, so far as we can tell, are completely conclusive.

The experiments to be outlined below show:

*Behring, E. and S. Kitasato. 1890. Ueber das Zustandekommen der Diphtherie-Immunität und der Tetanus-Immunität bei Thieren. *Deutsche Medizinische Wochenschrift* 16:1113–1114. [With permission of Georg Thieme Verlag.]

1. The blood of rabbits immune to tetanus has the ability to neutralize or destroy the tetanus toxin.
2. This property exists also in extravascular blood and in cell-free serum.
3. This property is so stable that it remains effective even in the body of other animals, so that it is possible, through blood or serum transfusions, to achieve an outstanding therapeutic effect.
4. The property that destroys tetanus toxin does not exist in the blood of animals that are not immune to tetanus, and when one incorporates tetanus toxin into nonimmune animals, the toxin can be still demonstrated in the blood and other body fluids of the animal, even after its death.

As proof of these statements, we present the following extensive series of experiments:

A rabbit was immunized against tetanus by a method which will be reported in detail later. The degree of immunity of this animal was such that it would stand a dose of 10 cc of a bacteria-containing culture of virulent tetanus bacilli, while a normal rabbit would always die from a dose of 0.5 cc. Every rabbit remained completely healthy after this injection.

This was not only true of the infection with living tetanus bacilli, but also by injection with tetanus toxin, for each immune rabbit would tolerate without symptoms a dose of toxin 20 times that which would kill normal rabbits.

Carotid blood was removed from these rabbits.

Before coagulation, 0.2 cc of the fluid blood was injected into the abdominal cavity of one mouse, and 0.5 cc into another. After 24 hours, these two mice were inoculated along with two control mice with virulent tetanus bacilli. The inoculation was so strong that the control mice became sick after 20 hours and died after 36 hours. However, both treated mice remained perfectly healthy.

Most of the blood from the immunized rabbits was allowed to stand until it had coagulated and the serum had formed.

The abdominal cavity of six mice was injected with 0.2 cc of this serum. After 24 hours the infection had no effect on these animals, while the control mice died from tetanus after 48 hours.

The serum could also be used for therapeutic treatment whereby the mice were first infected and then injected intraperitoneally with the serum.

We have further experimented with the serum, showing its enormous toxin-destroying activity.

A ten-day old tetanus culture, filtered to render it free of bacteria, was sufficiently lethal that 0.00005 cc would kill mice after 4–6 days; 0.00001 cc caused death after less than 2 days.

Now we mixed 5 cc of serum from rabbits that were immune to tetanus with 1 cc of this toxin-containing culture, and allowed the serum to act on the toxin for 24 hours. We injected 0.2 cc of this mixture into each of four mice. This corresponded to 0.033 cc of culture fluid, or more than 300 times the lethal dose for mice. All four mice remained perfectly healthy. The control mice, however, died 36 hours after an injection of 0.0001 cc of culture.

The mice from all of the experiments that had received either serum alone or serum with toxin were rendered permanently immune, as far as one can tell. Repeated injections at a later time with virulent tetanus bacilli caused not a trace of illness in them. . . .

Naturally we have performed every experiment with control blood and serum from nonimmune rabbits. Such blood and serum are neither therapeutic nor active against tetanus toxin.

The same is true of serum from cows, calves, horses, and sheep. . . .

In earlier times, blood transfusions were considered to be effective . . . methods for the treatment of diseases. Recently it has been believed that physiological saline can exert the same effects. The results of our experiments remind us forcibly of these words: "Blut ist ein ganz besonderer Saft," ["Blood is a very unusual fluid."]

An inquiry into the causes and effects of the variolae vaccine

1798 • Edward Jenner

Comment

Once it became established that people and livestock can acquire immunity by surviving an epidemic (or epizootic) or a bite by a poisonous reptile, healers and other people with adventurous minds sought means to artificially confer such resistance. The major problems were the result of the poor differentiation of diseases and the lack of clues to disease origin and mechanism of spread. Of all the acute infectious diseases, one of the most prevalent and easily recognized was smallpox. Its skin lesions (pustules and subsequent scabs) made diagnosis simple; the resultant scars were a sign of immunity. Even in the absence of a germ theory of disease, the healer could easily associate the power of contagion with these lesions.

The first to develop relatively safe means of transferring this infection to susceptible people while causing the least harm, and thereby confer immunity, were probably the wandering Taoist healers of Szechuan at the end of the tenth century. The Chinese traditionally held preventive medicine in higher regard than treatment of a manifested disease. The process, variolation, was first documented in 1549 during the Ming period. The Chinese had developed a procedure for attenuating the disease by, as we know today, reducing the population of active viruses in dried lymph in much the way Louis Pasteur would later develop his rabies vaccine. Scabs of particular size and shape were collected from a subpassaged series of children who probably suffered with variola minor. The healer carried the harvested scabs, sealed in a dated bottle and protected from sunlight and strong heat, on his body for 2 to 5 weeks depending on the season, for the warmth of summer would hasten inactivation.

The pulverized scabs were then blown into the nose of the susceptible patient.

Through their travels across caravan and sea routes to China, Arab and Turkish merchants and scholars learned the art of variolation and carried it back first to their nations and then to Africa. By the seventeenth century other procedures had been found. One common way was to make a small cut in the skin and then with a needle introduce the infectious powder made from scabs. Europeans stationed in Asian outposts reported such immunizations to the Royal Society beginning in 1700 as did Cotton Mather of Boston, who advocated the procedure after noting its use in African slaves.

The foremost promoter of variolation, however, is Lady Mary Wortley Montague, the wife of the British Ambassador to Constantinople. She was keenly interested in variolation as a result of her own scarring bout with smallpox years earlier, and she wrote to a friend in 1717, "I am patriot enough to take pains to bring this useful invention into fashion in England; and I should not fail to write to some of our doctors very particularly about it, if I knew anyone of them that I thought had virtue enough to destroy such a considerable branch of their revenue for the good of mankind." This noble woman of wit and independence had her son variolated on 18 March 1718 and, after returning to England, her daughter in 1721. Her campaign gained the support of some physicians but also the wrath of some clergy, who deemed it interference with God's will. Despite the inoculation of many of the upper classes and the grandchildren of George I, interest soon waned. Variolation could be lethal, and the subjects themselves proved to be a source of contagion until they healed.

Such is the immunological background of Edward Jenner (1749–1823), the son of a clergyman, whose milestone is featured next. A friend of the noted English surgeon and anatomist John Hunter, Jenner shared an interest in natural history, and his study on cuckoos earned him election to the Royal Society. After Jenner received his medical degree from St. Andrews in Scotland in 1792, he left general practice to become a successful consultant. Although his observation that cowpox would offer protection against smallpox may not have been original, Jenner was first to test and publish the idea. His opus was not met with universal cheer. The image of being given a disease of cows fueled the imagination of skeptics and caricaturists. Improper inoculations and infections by contaminants, the common thorn of immunizers and therapists, hindered acceptance. However, when the value of smallpox vaccination was finally appreciated, Jenner was duly honored and rewarded.

Vaccines are usually developed from inactivated or attenuated agents or from their immunogenic components. The deep significance of the Jenner vaccine is that immunity was uniquely achieved by cross-reactivity to a similar but distinct agent. Changes have occurred since Jenner's time, as the present vaccinia strains do not behave like either cowpox or smallpox viruses. The contemporary vaccinia virus has no natural reservoir. After over one hundred years of evolution, manipulation, and possible contamination and recombination, we simply do not know what agent Jenner tested nor what its origin was. Yet the principle remains.

Thanks chiefly to Edward Jenner's vaccine, natural smallpox was finally expunged from our planet, as the World Health Organization officially declared on May 8, 1980. Two and one-half years previously, on 26 October 1977, Ali Maow Maalin of Merka in Somalia was the last person diagnosed with epidemic smallpox. Thus, the histories of immunity and smallpox are intrinsically linked in one of the longest, yet best, success stories of medicine.

For further information:

Baxby, D. 1981. *Jenner's Smallpox Vaccine. The Riddle of Vaccinia Virus and Its Origin.* Heinemann Educational Books, London. 214 p.

Le Fanu, W. R. 1973. Edward Jenner. *Proceedings of the Royal Society of Medicine* 66:28–32.

Needham, J. 1980. China and the origins of immunology. *Eastern Horizon* 19(1):6–12.

Shurkin, J. N. 1979. *The Invisible Fire. The Story of Mankind's Victory Over the Ancient Scourge of Smallpox.* G. P. Putnam's Sons, New York. 447 p.

Silverstein, A. M. and G. Miller. 1981. The royal experiment on immunity: 1721–1722. *Cellular Immunology* 61:437–447.

The Paper*

The deviation of man from the state in which he was originally placed by nature seems to have proved to him a prolific source of diseases. From the love of splendor, from the indulgence of luxury, and from his fondness for amusement he has familiarized himself with a great number of animals, which may not originally have been intended for his associates. . . .

There is a disease to which the horse, from his state of domestication, is frequently subject. The farriers have termed it the Grease. It is an inflammation and swelling in the heel, from which issues matter possessing properties of a very peculiar kind, which seems capable of generating a disease in the human body (after it has undergone the modification which I shall presently speak of), which bears so strong a resemblance to the Small Pox, that I think it highly probable it may be the source of that disease.

In this dairy country a great number of cows are kept, and the office of milking is performed indiscriminately by men and maid servants. One of the former having been appointed to apply dressings to the heels of a horse affected with the Grease, and

---

*Jenner, E. 1798. *An Inquiry into the Causes and Effects of the Variolae Vaccinae, a Disease Discovered in Some of the Western Counties of England, Particularly Gloucestershire, and Known by the Name of The Cow Pox.* London, Sampson Low. 75 p.

not paying due attention to cleanliness, incautiously bears his part in milking the cows, with some particles of the infectious matter adhering to his fingers. When this is the case, it commonly happens that a disease is communicated to the cows, and from the cows to the dairymaids, which spreads through the farm until most of the cattle and domestics feel its unpleasant consequences. This disease has obtained the name of the Cow Pox. It appears on the nipples of the cows in the form of irregular pustules. . . . The animals become indisposed, and the secretion of milk is much lessened. Inflamed spots now begin to appear on different parts of the hands of the domestics employed in milking, and sometimes on the wrists, which quickly run on to suppuration. . . .

Thus the disease makes its progress from the horse to the nipple of the cows, and from the cow to the human subject.

Morbid matter of various kinds, when absorbed into the system, may produce effects in some degree similar; but what renders the Cow-pox virus so extremely singular is that the person who has been thus affected is forever after secure from the infection of the Small Pox; neither exposure to the variolous effluvia, nor the insertion of the matter into the skin, producing this distemper.

In support of so extraordinary a fact, I shall lay before my reader a great number of instances.

Case I. Joseph Merret, now an Under Gardener to the Earl of Berkeley, lived as a servant with a farmer near this place in the year 1770, and occasionally assisted in milking his master's cows. Several horses belonging to the farm began to have sore heels, which Merret frequently attended. The cows soon became affected with the Cow Pox, and soon after several sores appeared on his hands . . . previously to the appearance of the distemper among the cows there was no fresh cow brought into the farm, nor any servant employed who was affected with the Cow Pox.

In April, 1795, a general Inoculation [variolation] taking place here, Merret was inoculated with his family; so that a period of twenty-five years had elapsed from his having the Cow Pox to this time. However, though the variolous matter was repeatedly inserted into his arm, I found it impracticable to infect him with it; and efflorescence only, taking on an erysipelatous look about the center, appearing on the skin near the punctured parts. During the whole time that his family had the Small Pox, one of whom had it very fully, he remained in the house with them, but received no injury from exposure to the contagion.

It is necessary to observe, that the utmost care was taken to ascertain, with the most scrupulous precision, that no one whose case is here adduced had gone through the Small Pox previous to these attempts to produce that disease. . . .

Case XVII. The more accurately to observe the progress of the infection, I selected a healthy boy, about eight years old, for the purpose of inoculation for the Cow Pox. The matter was taken from a sore on the hand of a dairymaid, who was infected by her master's cows, and it was inserted, on the 14th of May, 1796, into the arm of the boy by means of two superficial incisions, barely penetrating the cutis, each about half an inch long.

On the seventh day he complained of uneasiness in the axilla, and on the ninth he became a little chilly, lost his appetite, and had a slight headache. During the whole of this day he was perceptibly indisposed, and spent the night with some degree of restlessness, but on the day following he was perfectly well.

The appearance of the incisions in their progress to a state of maturation were much the same as when produced in a similar manner by variolous matter. The only difference which I perceived was, in the state of the limpid fluid arising from the action of the virus, which assumed rather a darker hue. . . .

In order to ascertain whether the boy, after feeling so slight an affection of the system from the Cow-pox virus, was secure from the contagion of the Small-pox, he was inoculated on the 1st of July following with various matter, immediately taken from a pustule. Several slight punctures and incisions were made on both his arms, and the matter was carefully inserted, but no disease followed. The same appearances were observable on the arms as we commonly see when a patient has had variolous matter applied, after having either the Cow-pox or the Small-pox. Several months afterwards, he was again inoculated with variolous matter, but no sensible effect was produced on the constitution. . . .

These experiments afforded me much satisfaction, they proved that the matter in passing from one human subject to another, through five gradations, lost none of its original properties, J. Barge being the fifth who received the infection successively from William Summers, the boy to whom it was communicated from the cow.

I shall now conclude this Inquiry with some general observations on the subject and on some others which are interwoven with it. . . .

Those who are not in the habit of conducting experiments may not be aware of the coincidence of circumstances necessary for their being managed so as to prove perfectly decisive; nor how often men engaged in professional pursuits are liable to interruptions which disappoint them almost at the instant of their being accomplished: however, I feel no room for hesitation respecting the common origin of the diseases, being well convinced that it never appears among the cows (except it can be traced to a cow introduced among the general herd which had been previously infected, or to an infected servant), unless they have been milked by someone who, at the same time, has the care of a horse affected with diseased heels. . . .

The active quality of the virus from the horses' heels is greatly increased after it has acted on the nipples of the cow, as it rarely happens that the horse affects his dresser with sores, and as rarely that a milk-maid escapes the infection when she milks infected cows. . . .

It is singular to observe that the Cow-pox virus, although it renders the constitution unsusceptible of the variolous, should, nevertheless, leave it unchanged with respect to its own action. I have already produced an instance to point out this, and shall now corroborate it with another.

Elizabeth Wynne, who had the Cow-pox in the year 1759, was inoculated with variolous matter, without effect, in the year 1797, and again caught the Cow-pox in the year 1798. . . .

Should it be asked whether this investigation is a matter of mere curiosity, or whether it tends to any beneficial purpose? I should answer, that not withstanding the happy effects of Inoculation [variolation], with all the improvements which the practice has received since its first introduction into this country, it not very unfrequently produces deformity of the skin, and sometimes, under the best management, proves fatal.

These circumstances must naturally create in every instance some degree of painful solicitude for its consequences. But as I have never known fatal effects arise from the Cow-pox, even when impressed in the most unfavorable manner . . . and as it clearly appears that this disease leaves the constitution in a state of perfect security from the infection of the Small-pox, may we not infer that a mode of Inoculation may be introduced preferable to that at present adopted, especially among those families, which, for previous circumstances we may judge to be predisposed to have the disease unfavorably? . . .

Thus far have I proceeded in an inquiry, founded, as it must appear, on the basis of experiment; in which, however, conjecture has been occasionally admitted in order to present to persons well situated for such discussions, objects for a more minute investigation. In the mean time I shall myself continue to prosecute this inquiry, encouraged by the hope of its becoming essentially beneficial to mankind.

The attenuation of the causal agent of fowl cholera

1880 • Louis Pasteur

Comment

Eighty years lapsed after Jenner's vaccine work before another significant advance in immunotherapy took place. In the intervening period the science of microbiology evolved largely from the diverse research of Louis Pasteur (1822–1895). Pasteur aided the distillers in preventing contamination and improving fermentation and he helped the silkworm industry to control disease among its insects. Thus, in 1879 when an epizootic of fowl cholera spread across the French countryside, it was natural for the veterinarian Henry Toussaint to ask Pasteur for his expert assistance. Toussaint had discovered the bacterium of this disease (now named *Pasteurella multocida*), but Pasteur was the first to culture it in isolation and ascertain its specificity.

The following report, concerning Pasteur's development of a vaccine against fowl cholera—the first of three successive milestones by him presented in this section—is experimentally powerful. It laid the foundation for all selective approaches for both attenuation and enhancement of virulence. Alas, this fine study has also been the focus of a romantic fiction, a scientific fable apparently created by his colleague Emile Duclaux, the truth of which is only now emerging.

The tale first appeared in 1896, a year after Pasteur's death. Duclaux, who had become the new director of the Pasteur Institute, published the account in his book analyzing his mentor's research. All biographies of Pasteur since that year present as fact that while Pasteur had gone on vacation in the summer of 1879, the laboratory was unattended and the cultures of fowl cholera bacilli were set aside without subculturing. On his return in autumn, he inoculated some chickens in the hope of invigorating any surviving organisms. The animals survived, indicating that the agent was either dead or no longer pathogenic. But as he began to discard these old flasks as useless, Pasteur had the intuitive insight of inoculating these same chickens and also some new ones with a fresh, active culture of the bacillus. The controls died but the first series of chickens again survived. A vaccine was discovered; prolonged exposure to oxygen was deemed the cause; chance had favored the prepared mind of Pasteur. This was a wonderful story, but apparently the vaccine was not developed that way. The legend was not even close to the truth.

In 1979 the family of Pasteur at last made available his laboratory notebooks and personal notes. These documents, along with other supporting evidence, show that Pasteur's assistant Emile Roux was independently continuing the study while Pasteur was at his summer residence in Arbois. Roux had begun experiments to attenuate the bacterium by seeking an optimum combination of broth acidity and duration of exposure. (Roux's method of hastening acidification by directing a current of oxygen over the cultures, which confused Pasteur, was also applied in Roux's later research on rabies.) Up to a year afterwards, Pasteur did not understand the method of attenuation or the role of oxygen. The challenge inoculation of chickens with virulent bacilli was also Roux's doing. Nevertheless, Pasteur made no reference to Roux's studies in the publications on fowl cholera.

The acquisition of another's work as one's own without appropriate credit is rare but not unknown among scientists; aspects of authorship will be discussed later in this section. Roux was simultaneously an accomplished independent researcher and a loyal team member. A scientific or ethical dispute with Pasteur could cause Roux to absent himself from a project, but an unwarranted attack on Pasteur by the press or other colleagues would bring him back to his director's defense. The apparent snub of his contributions in the investigation of fowl cholera was put aside when Roux, along with Pasteur's other assistant, Charles Chamberland, received authorship in the subsequent studies on anthrax. However, Roux was hurt again when Pasteur seized his method for attenuating rabid rabbit spinal cords. Roux was also honored, together with Alexandre Yersin, for discovering and isolating the diphtheria toxin, for improving methods for the production of diphtheria antitoxin in horses, for developing with Elie Metchnikoff a primate model for syphilis, and for demonstrating with Metchnikoff the fact that syphilis could be prevented by application of calomel, mercurous chloride. In 1904 Roux succeeded Duclaux as director of the Pasteur Institute.

Two matters of terminology within this report should be addressed. First, except in the French title, I have substituted the word "agent" for "virus." The term "virus" has undergone considerable change in meaning since Pasteur's day. Referring first to a toxic principle, the term almost became equivalent to "germ" before the infectious agent was morphologically and genetically characterized. Another word that has changed in meaning is "attenuation," as coined here by Pasteur. He had spent many years establishing the uniqueness, specificity, and stability of microorganisms, and he once believed that variation in virulence was due to a mixture of different bacterial species. This was closer to the truth than his view presented here that the virulence of the individual bacterium is slowly altered according to its surroundings. Pasteur, being trained as a chemist, did not have a sufficient grasp of Darwinian variation and selection in host as well as parasite characteristics, one of the reasons why he later so readily invited the biologist Metchnikoff to his laboratory. Attenuation is today a procedural term referring to the selection and isolation, or at least enrichment, of a mutant or genetic recombinant having a lower virulence than its parent. The acidification of the cultures of fowl cholera bacilli rather than oxygen per se apparently favored the growth and, on subculture, the selective enrichment of weakly virulent bacilli.

For further information:

Cadeddu, A. 1985. Pasteur et le choléra des poules: révision critique d'un récit historique. *History and Philosophy of the Life Sciences* 7:87–104.

Duclaux, E. 1920. *Pasteur. The History of a Mind.* (E. F. Smith and F. Hedges, translators.) W. B. Saunders Company, Philadelphia. 363 p.

Vallery-Radot, R. 1885. *Louis Pasteur. His Life and Labours.* (Lady Claud Hamilton, translator.) Longmans, Green, and Company, London. 300 p. [French title: *Histoire d'un Savant par un Ignorant.*]

Vallery-Radot, R. 1902. *The Life of Pasteur.* (R. L. Devonshire, translator.) Archibald Constable, London. 629 p.

The Paper*

Among the various facts which I have had the honor of communicating to the Academy regarding the disease commonly called fowl cholera, I take the liberty of recapitulating the following:

1. Fowl cholera is a virulent disease of the first order.
2. The agent consists of a microscopic parasite that multiplies readily in culture away from the body of those animals that can be affected by the disease. From this it is possible to obtain the virus in a state of perfect purity and to demonstrate irrefutably that it is the sole cause of the disease and death.
3. The agent may vary in its virulence. Sometimes the disease is followed by death; at other times, after causing morbid symptoms of variable intensity, recovery ensues.
4. The differences in the virulence of the agent are not merely the result of natural variations: the experimenter can produce them at will.
5. As is generally the case for all virulent diseases, fowl cholera does not recur, or rather the recurrence is of such a degree that it is inverse in intensity with that of the earlier infection, and it is always possible to extend the resistance that inoculation with most virulent agent does not produce any effect.
6. Without wishing at this time to assert any relationship between the viruses of smallpox and cowpox, it seems from the preceding facts that in fowl cholera there exists a state of the virus, relative to the most virulent virus, which functions the same way as cowpox virus in relation to smallpox virus. Cowpox virus, properly stated, brings about a benign illness, cowpox, which protects against a more serious illness, smallpox. In the same way, the fowl cholera agent can occur in such a state of attenuated virulence that it induces the disease but not death, and in such a way that after recovery, the animal can withstand an inoculation with the most virulent agent. Nevertheless, in certain respects the difference between the two orders of facts is considerable, and it is not amiss to remark with respect to knowledge of facts and principles, a course of studies on fowl cholera will probably be more helpful. Whereas there is still a dispute about the relationships between smallpox and cowpox, we know for certain that the attenuated agent of fowl cholera is derived directly from the most virulent agent of this disease, so that their natures are fundamentally the same.

The time has come for me to explain the main assertion, which is the basis of most of the preceding propositions, namely, that there are variable degrees of virulence in fowl cholera. This is assuredly a strange result when one thinks of the agent of this disease as a microscopic organism which can be handled in a state of perfect purity, in the same way as the yeast of beer or the mycoderma of vinegar. And further, if one calmly considers this mysterious idea of var-

---

*Pasteur, L. 1880. De l'attenuation du virus du choléra des poules. *Comptes rendus de l'Academie des Sciences* 91:673–680. [With permission.]

iation in virulence, one can quickly acknowledge that this phenomenon is probably common to the diverse species of organisms causing infectious diseases. But where is the common factor in this group? To cite only one example, do we not see epidemics of very severe smallpox side by side with others almost benign, without being able to attribute the difference to environmental conditions, of climate or to the health of the individuals attacked? Is it not equally seen that major epidemics gradually die out, then reappear, and die out again?

The idea of the existence of variable degrees of virulence of the same virus is not made merely to surprise the physician or layman, but because it may be of tremendous importance if it could be established scientifically. In the present case, the mystery especially involves the fact that the agent, being a microscopic parasite, reveals variation in its virulence that is at the control of the observer. It is this point that I would like to establish rigorously.

Let us begin with the agent of fowl cholera in a very virulent state, the most virulent possible, if I may so say. Previously I revealed a curious method for obtaining an agent with this property. This was done by collecting the virus from a chicken that was about to die, not from an acute but from a chronic infection. I have observed that the cholera occurs occasionally in this latter form. These cases are rare, but it is not difficult to encounter some examples. In such cases, the chicken, after becoming very ill, grows more and more emaciated but resists death for weeks and months. When it perishes, it is because up to this time the parasite, localized in certain organs, passes into the blood and reproduces there. One can then observe that the virulence of the agent cultured from the blood of an animal that has taken a long time to die is considerably higher than the virulence of the agent that was used to inoculate this animal, so that it is able to kill ten times in ten, twenty times in twenty.

This being granted, let us make successive cultures of this agent, in a pure state, in a broth made from chicken muscles, by taking the inoculum for each culture from the preceding culture, and then assaying each culture for its virulence. Observations demonstrate that this virulence does not change significantly. In other words, if we agree that two virulences are identical when, upon injecting the same number and species of animals under the same conditions, and the proportion that die in the same length of time is the same, then we have ascertained that the virulence of our successive cultures is identical.

In what I have said above, I did not mention the length of time between one culture and the next, or to be accurate, the length of time from one inoculation to the next, and its possible influence on the successive degrees of virulence. Let us now turn our attention to this point, however minor its importance seems. An interval from one to eight days does not affect the virulence of the successive cultures. An interval of 15 days gives the same results. With an interval of one month, six weeks, or two months, one does not observe any change in virulence. Nevertheless, as the interval is increased, certain signs of seemingly little value can be noted, suggesting a weakening of the inoculating agent. For example, the rapidity of death, if not the proportion of deaths, reduces. In the various series of inoculations, one sees chickens that languish, are very ill, and often very lame, because the parasite in its multiplication has passed into the muscles and has attacked those of the legs; pericarditis is prolonged; abscesses appear around the eyes; in short, the agent has lost, so to say, its fulminating character. Let us then go to longer intervals than these, before we again transfer the culture. Let us prolong the intervals to three, four, five, eight months, or more before the virulence of the new microscopic beings is examined. This time the picture is considerably changed. Differences in virulence, which were previously insignificant or only equivocal, are considerable.

With such intervals between inoculations, one finds on testing the cultures that instead of identical virulence, that is to say a mortality of ten chickens in ten inoculated, the virulence decreases, so that nine, eight, seven, six, five, four, three, two, or one out of ten die, and at times not a one dies, that is to say, the disease develops in all the subjects, but they all recover. In other words, by a simple change in the way the parasite is cultured, merely by lengthening the time between transfers, we have obtained a method for progressively decreasing virulence until finally we have a true vaccine agent, which does not kill, but induces a benign illness that immunizes against a fatal illness.

It would not be expected that in all these attenuations results occur with reproducible and mathematical regularity. Some cultures which have not been transferred in five or six months always show a considerable virulence, while others of the same origin may already be very attenuated after three or four months. We will later explain these anomalies, which are only apparent. Often there is an abrupt jump from great virulence down to the death of the microscopic parasite, and this may take place in a very short interval. In passing from one culture to the next, one is surprised by the absence of growth: the parasite is dead. Death of the parasite is, furthermore, a common and constant occurrence whenever a sufficient length of time passes between inoculations. . . .

It is appropriate to say that if one takes cultures at each level of virulence for starting new cultures and transferring them successively at short intervals, the virulence of each culture is maintained at its original level. For example, an attenuated agent that kills only one out of ten maintains this virulence in successive cultures, if the interval of transfer is not increased. An equally interesting fact, one which is in accord with the preceding observations, is that an interval between transfers that is sufficient to bring about the death of an attenuated agent may not necessarily kill a more virulent agent, although it may attenuate it.

At this point of our report an important question arises: what is the cause of the decrease in virulence?

The cultures of the parasite are necessarily kept in contact with air, because our agent is an aerobic creature and it cannot grow in the absence of air. It is therefore natural to ask at the outset if contact with oxygen of the air would not be the influence that weakens virulence. Would it not be possible that the tiny organism which constitutes the agent, being left exposed to oxygen of pure air present in the culture medium where it multiplies, undergoes some modifications that appear to be permanent when the organism is removed from the modifying influence? One could ask, truly, if there be some principle in the atmosphere, other than oxygen, some chemical or fluid, which might not mediate the production of a phenomenon so strange that it justifies any supposition.

It is easy to understand that the solution of this problem in the case raised by our first hypothesis, that is, some influence of the oxygen in the air, can easily be put to test: If oxygen in the air truly is the modifying agent of virulence, we could probably prove it by observing the effect of its removal.

To this end, cultures were made in the following manner. A convenient quantity of chicken broth was inoculated with our most virulent virus, and glass tubes were filled to two-thirds of their volume, three-fourths, and so forth. Then the tubes were sealed under a flame. Thanks to the small amount of air remaining in the tubes, the infectious agent began to grow, as observed by the growing turbidity of the liquid. All of the oxygen in the tube gradually disappeared with the growth of the culture. Then the turbid material fell to the bottom, the agent was deposited on the tube wall, and the liquid became clear. It took two or three days for this to occur. The tiny organisms are thereafter protected from contact with oxygen and they will remain in this state for as long as the tube is not opened. What has happened to their virulence? In order to be more certain in our studies, we prepared a large number of parallel tubes, and at the same time an equal number of flasks of the same culture, but freely exposed to contact with pure air. We have already stated what will happen to cultures that are exposed to air; we learned that they undergo a progressive attenuation of their virulence. Let us speak only of cultures in the closed tubes, those without contact with air. Let us open one after a period of one month and after having transferred a portion of its contents, we test its virulence; open another after an interval of two months, and so on for three, four, five, six, seven, eight, nine, and ten months. . . . Remarkably, as the experiment shows, virulence is always the same as that of the agent used to prepare the original closed tubes. As for the cultures exposed to air, they are either dead or are less virulent.

Our question has been resolved: it is oxygen in the air that weakens and destroys virulence.

Truly, there is more here than an isolated fact: We are in possession of a principle. One may hope that there may be an action inherent in atmospheric oxygen, a natural force always present, that will be efficacious with other viruses. In any case, we have a situation worthy of interest for the possible great generality regarding a method for the attenuation of virulence, which may derive from some influence of the cosmic order. May we not presume henceforth that the limitation of the great epidemics, in the present as in the past, can be attributed to this influence? . . .

Summary report of the experiments performed at Pouilly-le-Fort, near Melun, on anthrax vaccination

1881 • Louis Pasteur, Charles Chamberland, and Emile Roux

Comment

No better example can be found to illustrate the importance of public relations and marketing in applied immunology than the public trial of Louis Pasteur's anthrax vaccine at a farm in Pouilly-le-Fort. Political and economic considerations are as much a part of science as the acquisition of a special apparatus. Basic scientists are not immune to these influences; their requests for research grants are often phrased to link their true motivation of curiosity about an arcane phenomenon with some future practical use. Science and technology, i.e., knowledge and application, are inseparable in practice.

Pasteur was a master of drama. His vivid demonstrations of experiments before the French Academy of Sciences, his tireless power of debate, his keen political sense, and his regard for the press all served to boost the impact of his cold inert scientific facts. His brilliant series of successes over some 25 years, which had greatly enhanced French industry and French pride, made Pasteur a renowned scientist among his fellow citizens. His reputation was not as well established in medical and veterinary circles, where the germ theory of disease was still resisted. Although other scientists in France and England were developing vaccines to anthrax, only Pasteur had the financial and moral backing of the French government.

The following milestone reads as if the field test was merely an ordinary, straightforward extension of a long series of laboratory experiments, one whose results would only confirm an established truth. Pasteur had confidence in his vaccine, otherwise he would not have accepted the challenge of a public trial, but as any experimenter knows, a miscalculation, an oversight, or some unforeseen external factor could have brought failure. The experiment at Pouilly-le-Fort was a gamble even with the odds well in his favor: It could have either provided acceptance of his particular vaccine or a major setback with a blow to his reputation. Furthermore, Pasteur recognized that the results had to be clear and complete to convince skeptical farmers and veterinarians.

The Society of Agriculture of Melun, a town 15 miles southeast of Paris, did not seek out Pasteur on their own. A Monsieur H. Rossignol, who offered his farm in the nearby village of Pouilly-le-Fort for the trial, was an editor of *Veterinary Press,* a popular French newspaper for farmers. A critic of Pasteur, he was responsible for the idea, and through his newspaper he helped raise a subscription for a public demonstration of the vaccine. Word quickly spread around the world. Newspapers, including the *London Times,* sent representatives to cover the story. Veterinarians, physicians, politicians, villagers, and the curious gathered at the farm. After the first inoculations, Pasteur went to a nearby hall to deliver a brief lecture on the design of the experiment and what was to be expected. This information intensified the suspense and public interest.

According to his published accounts, which apparently differ from his notebook records, Pasteur had attenuated the anthrax bacillus through a process of heating, aging, and selection. The bacillus stops growing at 45°C, but at 42° to 43°C, only sporulation is blocked. From such heated old cultures Pasteur and his colleagues claimed to have isolated a progressively weakened organism that on passage in vitro could again sporulate yet maintain its reduced virulence. They could subsequently reverse the process by subculturing the bacterium in guinea pigs until they obtained a highly virulent strain.

When it came time to inoculate the challenge culture into the test animals, Pasteur's opponents literally took matters into their own hands. A local veterinarian, following the suggestion of one of Pasteur's academic foes who cynically asserted that the liquid was in two layers, the top layer containing inactive bacteria and the lower virulent ones, grabbed the flask out of Pasteur's hands and shook it vigorously. Then new conditions were imposed. Triple doses were to be given, alternating between control and vaccinated animals. This actually worked in Pasteur's favor. First, it strengthened the results by allowing his critics to help in the experimental design; second, it overcame the variation in host resistance that might have permitted some control animals to survive the challenge and hence weaken the final statistics.

Reports of fever and malaise among the vaccinated animals began to worry Pasteur as he awaited the morning 2 days after the last inoculation to return to the farm. When he arrived, he was greeted with hesitant applause and then cheers. Twenty-three of the control sheep had already died; by 2 PM another fell to the disease; the last perished at 4 PM. Even though critics among the observers reported the success of the trial, final acceptance did not come until the experiment (with slight modification) was repeated in other regions. In addition, certain technical details and misunderstandings in large-scale vaccine production had to be clarified, but in a relatively short time the vaccine was being used throughout Europe to the profit of all.

Pasteur could have achieved his goal in due time without the challenge at Pouilly-le-Fort;

with it, however, he hastened the approval of the vaccine by governments and professional societies, established favorable relationships with the lay populace, and won over many of his scientific and medical opponents. By his willingness to leave the laboratory and meet the public, Pasteur seized the heavy double-edged sword of publicity to further his pursuits.

Scientists, being a component of society, should not disregard the power of the public to thwart, retard, or support research. The public through subscriptions can erect research institutes, as they did for Pasteur after he developed the rabies vaccine, and can stimulate complacent and sluggish governing bodies to increase research funding for a particular disease. Certain segments of the population can also sabotage experiments. The press and the pubic can, at least for a while, increase the prestige and influence of a researcher over a competitor whatever the scientific merits of a researcher's work may be.

For further information:

Brandt, A. M. 1978. Polio, politics, publicity, and duplicity: ethical aspects in the development of the Salk vaccine. *International Journal of Health Services* 8:257–270.

Dubos, R. J. 1950. *Louis Pasteur. Free Lance of Science.* Little, Brown and Company, Boston. 418 p.

Farley, J. 1978. The social, political, and religious background to the work of Louis Pasteur. *Annual Review of Microbiology* 32:143–154.

Vallery-Radot, R. 1902. *The Life of Pasteur.* (R. L. Devonshire, translator.) Archibald Constable, London. 629 p.

The Paper*

Each year France loses so many millions to anthrax that it would be highly desirable to provide protec-

---

*Pasteur, L., C. Chamberland, and E. Roux. 1881. Compte rendu sommaire des expériences faites à Pouilly-le-Fort, près Melun, sur la vaccination charbonneuse. *Comptes rendus de l'Academie des Sciences* 92:1378–1383. [With permission.]

tion to sheeps, cows, and horses. The opportunity to apply the vaccination method of which I speak was offered to us almost immediately, without our having had to wait for the period in which sheep are penned.

Last April, the Society of Agriculture of Melun, through its president Baron Rochette, proposed that I ascertain its effectiveness by a decisive experiment, whose results I came to the Academy to announce. I eagerly accepted, and on April 28 the following was agreed to and affirmed:

1. The Society of Agriculture of Melun offered Pasteur 60 sheep.

2. Ten of these sheep would not undergo any treatment.

3. Twenty-five of these sheep would undergo two vaccinal inoculations, at an interval of 12 to 15 days, of two unequally attenuated anthrax agents.

4. These 25 sheep, simultaneously with the remaining 25, would be inoculated with very virulent anthrax bacilli after another interval of 12 or 15 days.

    The non-vaccinated 25 sheep would all perish; the vaccinated 25 would be resistant, and afterwards would be compared with the 10 sheep reserved as above, in order to show that vaccination does not prevent sheep from returning to a normal state.

5. After the general inoculation of the very virulent agent to the two lots of 25 vaccinated and non-vaccinated sheep, the 50 sheep would be reunited in the same stable. The two series would be distinguished by forming a hole in the ear of 25 vaccinated sheep with a punch.

6. All the sheep which died from anthrax would be buried individually in distinct trenches, adjacent to each other and situated in a fenced enclosure.

7. In May 1882, 25 new sheep, having never served in these experiments, would be penned up in the above enclosure in order to prove that new sheep would spontaneously become infected by anthrax germs that will have been restored to the surface of soil by earthworms.

8. Another 25 new sheep would be penned up together near the preceding enclosure, some meters away, where animals with anthrax had never been buried, in order to demonstrate that none among them would die of anthrax.

The president of the Society of Agriculture of Melun had expressed the desire that these experiments be extended to cows. I responded that we would adapt them to do so, warning the Society, however, that presently, the evidence of vaccination in cows was not as advanced as that of sheep, so that consequently the results would not be as clearly convincing as in sheep. In any case, I expressed my gratitude to the Society of Melun for their placing ten cows at our disposal, six to be vaccinated and four not vaccinated. After vaccination, the ten cows would receive simultaneously with the fifty sheep the inoculation of the very virulent agent. I noted in addition that the six vaccinated cows would not be ill, while all or some of the four nonvaccinated would perish, or at least all would be very ill. . . .

The experiments commenced on May 5 in the community of Pouilly-le-Fort, near Melun, on a farm belonging to Mr. Rossignol.

According to the desire of the Society of Agriculture which had initiated the studies, we agreed to replace two sheep with two goats, and, as any condition whatsoever of age or race had not been fixed by us, the 58 sheep were of different age, race and sex. For the ten animals of bovine species, there were eight cows, an ox, and a bull.

May 5, 1881, we inoculated by means of a Pravaz syringe 24 sheep, a goat, and six cows, each animal receiving five minims of a culture of attenuated anthrax agent. May 17, we reinoculated these animals with a second, also attenuated anthrax virus, but more virulent than the preceding.

May 31, we proceeded to the very virulent inoculation which would determine the efficacy of the preventive inoculations of May 5 and 17. To this effect, we inoculated the 31 vaccinated animals and, in addition, 24 sheep, a goat, and four cows. Each of the latter animals had not undergone the previous treatment.

The very virulent agent used on May 31 was grown from anthrax spores maintained in my laboratory since March 21, 1877.

In order to render the experiments more comparative, we alternately inoculated the vaccinated and nonvaccinated animals. The operation carried out, a meeting was set by all persons present for Thursday, June 2, only 48 hours after the general virulent inoculation.

When the examiners arrived on June 2, the results astonished the audience. The 24 sheep and the goat which had received the attenuated agent, besides the six cows, had all the appearances of health; in contrast, 21 sheep and the goat which were not vaccinated were already dead of anthrax; two other nonvaccinated sheep died before the eyes of the spectators, and the last of the series expired at the end of the day.

The nonvaccinated cows were not dead. We had

already shown before that cows were less subject than sheep to death by anthrax, but all had voluminous edema at the point of inoculation, behind the shoulder. . . . The temperature of these cows was elevated up to 3°C. The vaccinated cows showed neither increase of temperature, nor tumor, nor loss of appetite, thereby rendering the demonstration successful in all accounts for cows as for sheep.

With the arrival of June 3, one of the vaccinated ewes had died. The autopsy was made the same day by Rossignol and Garrouste, a military veterinarian. The ewe was found to have been pregnant, at term, and the lamb dead in the womb already for 12 to 15 days. The opinion of these veterinarians is that the death of this ewe was attributed to the death of the fetus. . . .

A method for preventing rabies after a bite

1885 • Louis Pasteur

Comment

With the vast open frontier of infectious disease inviting, enticing them onward, Louis Pasteur and his associates could not be satisfied with successive projects. While in the midst of the Pouilly-le-Fort field trial, Pasteur, Emile Roux, Charles Chamberland, and Louis Thuillier were advancing in their study of rabies. They established that the agent could be experimentally transferred among dogs, after trephining, by inoculation of the cerebral surface with infected brain tissue. The terrifying image of rabies-crazed, foaming-at-the-mouth dogs furiously attacking humans and beasts began to fade.

Pasteur's remembrance of his childhood encounter with a rabid dog may have stirred him to accept the difficult problem of preventing the disease when, in 1880, a hopeful veterinarian brought him two caged rabid dogs. At that time rabies was an infrequent disease and there were few clues to its origin and pathology; Pasteur could just have easily focused his attention on any of the more important and accessible infections, such as typhoid, pneumonia, or tuberculosis. In addition, the incidence of rabies in animals could be minimized by quarantining strays.

The year before, Victor Galtier, a veterinarian, had found that the agent existed in the saliva of rabid animals, that it seemed to grow in nervous tissue, and that it could be transferred to rabbits. This investigator used subcutaneous injections of saliva for inoculations, but results were irregular in morbidity and in incubation period (three to eight weeks). Pasteur and Roux's direct procedure shortened the incubation time (eventually to seven days) and produced consistent infections. Further studies ascertained that the diverse appearances of rabies stemmed from the same agent and were probably correlated with the location and degree of damage to nervous tissue. Pasteur also learned that the incubation period varied with the distance of the wound to the brain, and that the mysterious agent was not always present in the cerebrospinal fluid. He was unable to see any microorganism under his light microscope to grow the agent in artificial media.

Prophylaxis was the goal, since it was believed that the disease was invariably fatal once major symptoms appear. Neither Pasteur nor anyone else knew whether acquired immunity was really possible. This question was solved in 1881 when the one survivor of three experimentally infected dogs, which had suffered only early, minor symptoms, proved resistant to subsequent inoculations even after trephining. Intravenous injections of infectious saliva did not produce immunity. Pasteur then tried to attenuate the agent by subpassaging it in various animals. However, such weakening via monkeys also increased the incubation period and decreased the antigenicity. Taking a lesson from his work on anthrax, Pasteur then increased its virulence through passage in guinea pigs until it was even stronger than that found among rabid street dogs. The next step was to reduce its pathogenic power by aging and exposure.

Here Roux set the stage. Pasteur's assistant was determining the survival time of the agent in incubated spinal cords that were hung from a stopper in flasks. When Pasteur saw this arrangement, he quickly realized that he had found the way to attenuate the agent. The agent of potassium hydroxide helped to preserve and desiccate the material. He used the most virulent agent to inoculate a different rabbit each day. After removal, the spinal cord was aged in the vessel. A series of cords of decreasing age was organized. Beginning with the oldest cord and proceeding every other day toward freshly isolated tissue, a piece was cut off and suspended in broth for subcutaneous injections of the test dog. The dog survived both treatment and challenge.

The paper that follows related Pasteur's first treatment of humans. Roux among others felt that testing the vaccine on humans was premature and refused to participate in further studies on rabies, but Pasteur forged ahead. As word of Pasteur's success spread, scores of bitten people from as far away as Russia and the United States flocked to Pasteur's laboratory. By January 1886 some 350 people had been treated; at the end of the year the figure rose to 2500. The time between exposure and immunization is crucial, and even under the best of circumstances some failures occurred. Pasteur was openly criticized and even accused of murder by his foes. His statistics were interpreted in various ways, since besides treatment failures, not everyone who was bitten by a rabid animal would have necessarily contracted the disease. However, opposition eventually abated, and Pasteur, whose long scientific road took him from physical chemistry to the foundation of microbiology and now to the prevention of disease in humans, was heralded around the world as a secular saint.

Since then the rabies vaccine has undergone further developments: In 1911 phenol-inactivation replaced aging of infected tissue. The use of spinal cords, eventually shown to pose a hazard of autoimmune reactions to the patient's own nervous tissue, was discarded in 1956 in favor of embryonated duck eggs. Today viruses inactivated with beta-propiolactone are harvested from human tissue culture. This new, highly immunogenic vaccine requires only six injections, and additional improvements are likely with advances in technology. Passive serum therapy, first developed in 1889 by Victor Babes and M. Lepp, has been used to supplement vaccine treatment.

History documents to date only three people who survived rabies after developing symptoms. The first, in 1970, was a six-year-old boy. After previously receiving the usual series of inoculations, he was saved by a heroic effort in regulating his neurological and physiological condition until immunity developed. Another historical footnote is that Pasteur's first patient, Joseph Meister, later became the gatekeeper of the Pasteur Institute and committed suicide when German troops arrived in Paris during World War II, fearing that he would be forced to open the crypt of his savior.

For further information:

Koprowski, H. and S. A. Plotkin (ed.). 1985. *World's Debt to Pasteur. Proceedings of a centennial symposium commemorating the first rabies vaccination.* Alan R. Liss, New York. 342 p.

Nicolle, J. 1961. *Louis Pasteur. The Story of His Major Discoveries.* Basic Books, New York. 252 p.

The Paper*

The prophylaxis of rabies, such that I have revealed in the preceding papers under my name and the names of my associates, assuredly constitute real progress in the study of this disease, progress, however, more of scientific use than practical. Accidents were apt to occur in its application. Of 20 dogs treated, I was not able to protect more than 15 or 16 against rabies.

It was useful, furthermore, to conclude the treatment with a very virulent final inoculation—an inoculation of the control virus—in order to confirm and reinforce the immune state. In addition, prudence demanded that the dogs be kept under observation longer than the incubation period of the disease produced by the direct inoculation of this last virus. Hence, it was sometimes necessary to wait at least a period of three to four months to be certain of their immunity to rabies. The application of this method would have been greatly limited by these requirements.

Finally, the method would not easily lend itself for the immediate action necessitated by the accidental and unforeseen ways rabid bites are produced.

It thereby became necessary, if possible, to find a more rapid method capable of giving, I dare say, perfect security to dogs.

And how, moreover, could one dare to permit any experiment on humans before this progress was attained?

After countless experiments, I have discovered a prophylactic method, both practical and rapid, whose results in the dog already has been sufficiently numerous, certain and successful that I have confidence in its general application to all animals and even to man himself.

This method depends essentially on the following facts:

The inoculation under the dura mater, by trephination, of the infective spinal cord of a dog with ordinary rabies always produce rabies in this animal after a mean incubation period of about fifteen days.

With passage of the virus from the first rabbit to the second, from this to a third, and so forth in succession by the preceding manner of inoculation, a more and more pronounced tendency toward the reduction of the incubation period of rabies is soon apparent in successively inoculated rabbits.

After 20 to 25 passages from rabbit to rabbit, one encounters an incubation period of eight days, which is maintained over a new period of 20 to 25 passages. Then an incubation period of seven days is attained, which one finds again with striking regularity during a new series of passages extending until the ninetieth. This is at least the figure which I have reached at the present, and only a slight tendency is manifested toward an incubation period of a little less than seven days.

This kind of experiment, commenced in November 1882 (already three years in duration) has never had an interruption in the series, neither has it ever required recourse to another virus other than that from rabbits successively dead from rabies. Consequently, nothing is easier than having constantly at our disposal throughout the considerable intervals of time a perfectly pure rabies virus always or very nearly identical. This is the practical core of the method. . . .

If sections of a few centimeters are removed from the spinal cords with every possible precaution to maintain purity, and that one suspends them in dry air, virulence in these spinal cords slowly disappears until it is gone entirely. The lapse of time for extinguishing virulence varies somewhat with the thickness of the pieces of spinal cord, but mainly with the external temperature. The lower is the temperature the longer is the preservation of virulence. These results constitute the scientific point of the method.

These facts being established, here follows the means by which a dog is rendered resistant to rabies in a relatively short time.

In a series of flasks, whose air is maintained in a dry state by fragments of potash deposited at the bottom of the flask, one suspends each day a bit of rabid spinal cord fresh from a rabbit dead of rabies developed after seven days of incubation. Also every day a dog is inoculated under the skin with a Pravaz syringe filled with sterile broth, in which one has mixed a small fragment of one of these desiccated spinal cords, beginning with a spinal cord so distant in passage from the day of the operation that it was certain not to be at all virulent. . . . On the following days, one operates the same way with more recent spinal cords, separated from each other by an interval of two days, until one comes to the last, most virulent cord, placed only a day or two in the flask.

The dog is then rendered resistant to rabies. One could inoculate the rabies virus under the skin or even, by trephination, the surface of the brain without demonstration of rabies.

By the application of this method, I soon acquired fifty dogs of all ages and every race resistant to rabies, without having encountered a single failure, when unexpectedly three people from Alsace came to my laboratory on Monday, last July 6:

---

*Pasteur, L. 1885. Méthode pour prevenir la rage après morsure. *Comptes rendus de l'Academie des Sciences* 101:765–773. [With permission.]

Theodore Vone, grocer of Meissengott, near Schlestadt, bitten on the arm on July 4 by his own dog, which became rabid;

Joseph Meister, nine years of age, also bitten July 4 at eight o'clock in the morning by the same dog. This child, knocked down by the dog, showed numerous bites on the hand, legs, and thighs, some of which was so deep to make walking difficult. The principal bites were cauterized only 12 hours after the accident with phenic acid by Dr. Weber of Ville.

The third person, who was not bitten, was the mother of little Joseph Meister.

At the autopsy of the dog killed by his master, the stomach was found filled with hay, straw, and scraps of wood. The dog certainly had been rabid. Joseph Meister was pulled from underneath it covered with foam and blood.

Mr. Vone had some severe contusions on the arm, but he assured me that his shirt had not been pierced by the fangs. As he had nothing to fear, I told him that he could return to Alsace the same day, which he did. But I kept with me little Meister and his mother.

The weekly meeting of the Academy of Sciences took place on July 6; there I met our colleague Dr. Vulpian, to whom I recounted what had occurred. Vulpian, also Dr. Grancher, professor in the faculty of medicine, had the kindness to see little Joseph Meister immediately and verify the state and number of lesions. There were no less than 14.

The opinion of our learned colleague and Dr. Grancher was that by the severity and number of bites, Joseph Meister was almost certain to succumb to rabies. Then I communicated to Vulpian and Grancher the new results that I had obtained. . . .

The death of the child appearing to be inevitable, I decided, not without lively and cruel anxiety, as one could imagine, to attempt on Joseph Meister the method which for me was constantly successful with dogs. . . .

Consequently, on July 6 at eight o'clock in the evening, 60 hours after the bites of July 4, and in the presence of Drs. Vulpian and Grancher, little Meister was inoculated under a fold of skin in the right hypochondrium with a half-full Pravaz syringe of spinal cord from a rabbit dead of rabies taken June 21 and preserved since then in a dry air flask, that is to say, fifteen days.

New inoculations were made the following days. . . . I thus delivered 13 inoculations in 10 days of treatment. . . . In order to follow the level of virulence of these spinal cords, two new rabbits were inoculated by trephination with the various cords employed.

Observation of rabbits permitted us to ascertain that the cords of July 6, 7, 8, 9, and 10 were not

virulent, as they did not render the rabbits rabid. The cords of July 11, 12, 14, 15, and 16 were all virulent, and the virulent material was detected in larger and larger proportion. Rabies appeared after seven days of incubation in the rabbits of July 15 and 16; after eight days in those of the 12th and 14th; and after fifteen days in those of July 11. . . .

Joseph Meister, therefore, escaped not only the rabies that would have developed from his bites, but that which I had inoculated in order to check the immunity produced by the treatment, rabies more virulent than ordinary canine rabies.

The final, very virulent inoculation had, in addition, the advantage of limiting the apprehension that could have ensued from the bites. If rabies could occur, it would appear more quickly with a more virulent virus than that from the bites. Since the middle of August, I have looked forward with confidence to the future good health of Joseph Meister. Again at the present time, after three months and three weeks had passed since the accident, his health leaves nothing to be desired.

What interpretation can be given to the new method that I have introduced for preventing rabies after bites? . . . In referring to the methods for the progressive attenuation of lethal virus and the prophylaxis which one could derive, given, in part, the influence of air in attenuation, the first idea that comes to mind for accounting completely for the effects of the method, is that the continuance of rabbit spinal cords in contact with dry air progressively diminishes the degree of virulence in these cords until it is rendered absent.

It would, hence, lead us to believe that the prophylactic method, which I have described depends on the employment of a virus at first without appreciable activity, then weakly and gradually more virulent.

I will subsequently show that facts do not agree with this view. I will prove that the increase in the incubation period of rabies imparted each day to rabbits, as I have mentioned frequently, in order to determine the state of virulence of our spinal chords desiccation on contact with air, is an effect of the decrease in the quantity of rabies virus contained in these cords and not an effect of its reduction in virulence.

Can it be admitted that the inoculation of a virus, always of identical virulence, would be capable of initiating the refractory state to rabies, when it is employed in very small but daily increasing quantities? I am focusing my experimental studies on this interpretation of the facts.

One can give the new method yet another interpretation, an interpretation surely very strange at first sight, but which merits every consideration, since it is in harmony with certain data already known from the phenomena of life in some lower organisms, notably in various pathogenic microbes.

Many microbes appear to synthesize in their cultures substances that have the property of interfering with their proper development.

Since the year 1880, I have instituted researches in order to establish whether the microbe of fowl cholera produces a sort of poison for itself. I have not succeeded in finding evidence for the presence of such material, but I think now that this study ought to be resumed. . . .

Can it be that the rabies virus is formed of two distinct substances and besides that, which is living and capable of multiplying in the nervous system, there is another, not living but having the faculty, when it is in suitable proportion, of arresting the development of the first? In a future communication, I will examine experimentally with all the attention that it merits this third interpretation of the method of prophylaxis of rabies.

I do not need to state in conclusion that the most significant question to be solved at this moment is perhaps that of the interval permitted between the time of the bites and that of the commencement of treatment. This interval for Joseph Meister has been two and a half days. But it must be expected that this may often be much longer. . . .

A new method of producing immunity from contagious disease

1886 • Daniel E. Salmon and Theobald Smith

Comment

The following classic, in addition to its significant experimental content—whose discussion is momentarily deferred—offers a lesson in the conduct of science that is not found in the usual university curriculum. It concerns ego, recognition and its rewards, and personal relationships; it concerns authorship.

The article lists as authors Daniel E. Salmon (1850–1914) and Theobald Smith (1859–1934). The reader may logically suppose from the order in which their names are presented that Salmon was either the primary investigator— the person who designed the experiment or discovered and explored the phenomenon—or an equal contributor, with sequence perhaps dependent on the alphabet. However, neither supposition is correct, for Salmon did not participate in any way in this experiment! The inclusion of his name was the result of a political situation. As many experienced investigators are aware, particularly those associated with medical departments, the honor of authorship is frequently conferred to the department chairman, an administrative mentor, or a senior colleague who provides financial support. Their name by custom may be attached toward the end of the list. What is the background to this anomaly of Salmon and Smith?

Theobald Smith received his M.D. at Albany Medical School in New York. He never practiced medicine, but instead in December 1883 accepted appointment as director of the pathology laboratory of the United States Bureau of Animal Industry in Washington, D.C. His boss was Daniel Salmon, a veterinarian trained at Cornell University. Salmon earlier that year had established the veterinary division of the Department of Agriculture, and in 1884 became Bureau Chief. After Smith had suffered three years of Salmon's continuing injustices and usurpation of credit due to him, Smith's regard to his supervisor soured so much that he vowed never again to publish jointly with him. Indeed, the inappropriate naming in 1900 of the bacterial genus *Salmonella* reflects Salmon's control of publicity, presentations, and publications rather than his few laboratory accomplishments.

In this report on acquired immunity, Smith was clearly interested in the metabolic products of the bacillus that he mistakenly linked with hog cholera. He believed that the disease is a result of poisoning by bacterial secretions. Such toxins were still hypothetical; the isolation of the diphtheria toxin was another two years away. Even Henry Sewall's snake venom model would not be published until the following year. Exploring his toxin hypothesis, Smith killed the bacteria in his test culture by heating in order to exclude any direct invasive effect or cellular activity. However, he injected the dead bacterial suspension; he did not separate the fluids from the cells. For this reason, his paper is considered and honored as the first example of the use of a killed whole cell vaccine. His conclusion that immunity to this bacterium is associated with the secreted growth products, however, was inappropriate and wrong.

We may well wonder why Smith had not tested the fluid portion alone. How could he be certain that living bacteria were entirely absent? Unfortunately, the hand-driven, gear-operated centrifuge was not commercially available until 1893. Filtration was not feasible. Pasteur's crude, clumsy, and inconsistent Plaster of Paris filter had been introduced in 1877, but was little used. Charles Chamberland's famous unglazed porcelain candle filter was only developed in 1884 with further improvements the next year. In 1886 the only commercial filters were of paper, and these did not hold back bacterial cells. Of course, Smith could have at least allowed the bacteria to settle in the culture tube and then withdrawn the top layer with a pipette, but he gave no indication that he was even aware of any need to remove the bacteria.

Smith left the U.S. Department of Agriculture in 1895, becoming a professor of comparative pathology at Harvard and Director of the Massachusetts Antitoxin and Vaccine Laboratory. Later he joined the Rockefeller Insti-

tute at Princeton. He made two other contributions to immunology. In 1903 he and A. L. Reigh demonstrated that flagellar and cell wall agglutinins against the bacillus of hog cholera were distinct, and in 1909 he successfully applied toxin-antitoxin mixtures for immunization against diphtheria. However, Smith is best known for establishing the role of arthropod vectors in disease in his experiments with ticks carrying Texas cattle fever.

For further information:

Dolman, C. E. 1969. Theobald Smith, 1859–1934. Life and work. *New York State Journal of Medicine* 69:2801–2816.

Dolman, C. E. 1969. Texas cattle fever. A commemorative tribute to Theobald Smith. *Clio Medica* 4:1–31.

The Paper*

More than four years ago one of us, in the study of the subject of insusceptibility to contagious diseases, reached the conclusion that, in those diseases in which one attack protects from the effects of the contagion of the future, the germs of such maladies were only able to multiply in the body of the individual attacked because of a poisonous principle or substance which was produced during the multiplication of those germs. And also that, after being exposed for a certain time to the influence of this poison, the animal bioplasm was no longer sufficiently affected by it to produce that profound depression and modification of the vital activity which alone allowed the growth of the pathogenic germs and the consequent development of the processes of disease. After several series of experiments, made at that time with only negative results, it became necessary to suspend these investigations until points connected with them, and which were then obscure, should be cleared up, and until it should become possible to repeat the experiments under more favorable conditions. Our expectations in regard to this important subject have

---

*Salmon, D. E. and T. Smith. 1886. On a new method of producing immunity from contagious diseases. *Proceedings of the Biological Society,* (Washington, D.C.) 3:29–33.

at last been realized by the results of experiments recently made in the laboratory of the Bureau of Animal Industry.

The bacterium, which we lately discovered and which we believe to be the cause of swine plague, is killed in liquid cultures by an exposure to 58°C for about ten minutes.

This method of destroying the bacterium in liquid cultures was resorted to in studying the effects on pigeons of the chemical products (ptomaines?) formed by the bacteria in their vegetative state, and which are probably dissolved in the culture liquid. The heated cultures used in these experiments were always tested by ioculating fresh tubes therefrom, and, if no growth followed this inoculation, the death of the microbes was considered established.

It has been previously determined that the subcutaneous injection of 0.75 cc of a liquid culture of the swine plague bacterium containing 1% of peptone was invariably fatal, in the majority of pigeons within 24 hours. One half of this dose was fatal to a few only.

As a preliminary experiment, four pigeons were inoculated December 24, 1885, with a liquid culture that had been heated for 2 hours at 58–60°C. Three of these received subcutaneously 0.4, 0.8, and 1.5 cc of the heated culture, respectively. The fourth received 1.5 cc of the pure culture liquid, into which no microbes had been introduced. The one which had received the largest dose was evidently sick the next day, but slowly recovered. The others did not show any symptoms of illness.

January 11, the one which had received a hypodermic injection of the simple culture liquid, and the one which had received the largest dose of heated virus, received subcutaneously about 0.75 cc each of a liquid culture five days old, which had been prepared from a potato culture 15 days old. It is probable that this virus was not so strong, therefore, as a more recent culture from the pig would have been. Both pigeons were sick on the following day. [The control pigeon] died seven days after inoculation. The bacterium of swine plague was found abundantly in the pectoral muscle and in the spleen, kidneys, and liver in moderate numbers. The other pigeon slowly recovered, but had lost the use of its legs. It seemed perfectly well when killed, 15 days after inoculation. It was quite fat, the crop filled with food. In the pectoral were found imbedded two elongated masses of dead tissue or sequestra about 2 cm long and 1 cm in diameter, entirely separated from the surrounding tissue by a dense, smooth membrane. In this animal the multiplication of the pathogenic bacteria was purely local, the resistance of the tissues being sufficiently powerful to confine, and finally destroy, the bacteria. . . . A liquid culture,

inoculated with blood from the heart, remained sterile.

This experiment pointed evidently to an immunity obtained from the chemical products of the bacterium of swine plague. To confirm this view another experiment was made.

January 21, three pigeons received hypodermically 1.5 cc of heated culture liquid in which the bacterium of swine plague had multiplied for two weeks, and was then destroyed by exposure to 58–60°C for several hours. A fourth pigeon was kept as a check. [Another], which had received 0.4 cc of heated virus December 24, now received a second dose, this time of 1.5 cc. For the following three or four days all were somewhat ill, and remained rather quiet, with feathers slightly ruffled.

January 29, when all seemed well, three of four received hypodermically another dose of 1.5 cc of heated culture liquid. The other had been fiercely attacked by its fellows, and its head was so injured that it was thought best not give it an injection at this time, and it was placed in a spacious coop alone. None of the birds seemed much affected by this dose.

February 6, a final injection was practiced upon the four. . . . The dose was, as before, 1.5 cc. All seemed well a few days later.

February 13, one week after the last injection, these birds were inoculated with strong virus, the quantity injected being 0.75 cc, which had hitherto proved invariably fatal, with the single exception of the bird that had been previously treated with heated virus. Those inoculated were [pigeons] which had received the heated virus, also . . . the check pigeon, which had not been touched, and [one] which had received a small quantity, 0.8 cc of heated virus, December 24, over 50 days before.

On the following day the check pigeon was found dead; the one which had received the smaller dose was very ill and died before the next day. The other pigeons were perfectly well. The effect of this dose of strong virus, so remarkable on the unprotected pigeons, was even more evanescent than that of the heated virus in which all life had been destroyed. . . .

In the birds that died, the pectoral muscles at the place of injection were pale and friable. Necrosis was already at hand. The internal organs were not macroscopically altered, excepting the spleen of [one] which was enlarged and dark. The presence of the bacterium of swine plague in the blood from the heart was demonstrated by liquid cultures, which, inoculated with a minimum quantity of blood, were turbid with this specific microbe on the following day.

The conclusions to be drawn from this experiment we believe are of superlative importance to a correct understanding of the phenomena of contagious diseases, and the methods by which these diseases are to be combated. They probably apply to all bacterial plagues of men and animals in which one attack confers immunity from the effects of that particular virus in the future. These conclusions are:

1. Immunity is the result of the exposure of the bioplasm of the animal body to the chemical products of the growth of the specific microbes which constitute the virus of contagious fevers.

2. These particular chemical products are produced by the growth of the microbes in suitable culture liquids in the laboratory, as well as in the liquids and tissues of the body.

3. Immunity may be produced by introducing into the animal body such chemical products that have been produced in the laboratory.

Vaccination against typhoid fever

1897 • Sir Almroth E. Wright and Sir David Semple

Comment

Sir Almroth Wright. Wags would later dub him "Sir Almost Right," but his development and perseverance in instituting the vaccine of killed *Salmonella typhi* to prevent typhoid fever was one achievement few would deny. Almroth E. Wright (1861–1947) completed a dual education in literature and medicine at Trinity College in Dublin, and after a series of career changes, including law and civil service, settled in 1892 into a professorship in pathology at the Army Medical School in the Royal Victoria Hospital at Netley. Since Malta fever (brucellosis) was one of the chief diseases affecting British solders at various foreign installations, Wright chose this disease as his first target for a vaccine. His preliminary research, using monkeys and both attenuated and heat-killed microorganisms, was so encouraging that he inoculated himself and then challenged his presumed resistance with a living, virulent inoculum. Wright was following the audacious precedent of Waldemar Haffkine at the Pasteur Institute, who began the tradition among vaccinators of self-inoculation with the first and successful human test of his newly developed cholera vaccine. Wright, however, contracted severe but nonlethal brucellosis: Unfortu-

nately, not all vaccine stories have happy endings.

Wright's pursuit of a typhoid vaccine followed a logical thread: Specific agglutinins to the typhoid bacillus were known to form in serum during the course of the disease, and Richard Pfeiffer at Robert Koch's institute in Berlin had observed that agglutinins also occur when animals receive injections of heat-killed typhoid bacilli. Although Haffkine preferred his stronger vaccine of attenuated cholera vibrio over the killed preparation, Wright believed that the evidence with agglutinins indicated the adequacy of the unorthodox approach for a typhoid vaccine. Furthermore, it had the clear advantage of being safe. However, when Wright began his work no one had demonstrated that a killed vaccine could be clinically effective.

The following milestone by Wright and one of his military medical associates, later Sir David Semple, provides further historical background, establishes priority, and describes the vaccine in detail. What ensued offers us another lesson on an obstacle facing a scientist whose research directly affects humans: bureaucracy.

The first studies occurred during a small epidemic among the staff of an asylum for the mentally ill. Although far from conclusive, the data were nevertheless favorable. Wright next needed to test his vaccine on soldiers who would be exposed to typhoid. Those being sent to India were prime candidates.

Statistical analysis and field studies were poorly appreciated at this time. The practical aspects of supervision, standardization, laboratory confirmation, and appropriate record keeping had not been fully recognized. The importance and statistical advantage of a placebo and double-blind testing were unknown. Instead, Wright and others had to grope with the experimental design under less than supportive administrative circumstances: Solders could not be immunized unless they individually volunteered, and no organized means of information and recruitment existed.

Thus, in 1898 while Wright was in India participating on a plague commission, he made speeches at every opportunity in order to recruit volunteers. Some 4500 soldiers agreed to be immunized. Again, the comparison of the incidence of typhoid between vaccinated and unvaccinated soldiers did show some protection, but there were too many variables for the experiments to be convincing. Also the problem of side effects became evident. Word spread that participation in Wright's experiment could result in fever, soreness, and weakness, and this turned away potential volunteers. For this reason, Wright also lost the support of military physicians and commanders. Wright's excessive concern with the reduction of cross-reacting agglutinins in the blood and supposed increased susceptibility to typhoid during this "negative" period did not help matters.

Wright's next opportunity arose during the South African, or Boer War of 1899–1902. Over 14,000 troops volunteered for the vaccine through the network of Wright's former students, and mortality was reduced by a third. On the basis of this success, Wright sought final approval for routine immunization from the Medical Advisory Board, which set medical policy for the Army. However, the Board not only refused, it suspended further production of the vaccine until interviews and analysis were complete, estimated to take three years.

Wright, who had no opportunity to present his case, resigned his position and appealed to the Secretary of War, who passed the matter to the Royal Society, which passed it to the Royal College of Physicians, which recommended continuation of field testing. The Medical Advisory Board in 1904 formed a committee of officers and civilian consultants, including Wright. This body also agreed to the resumption of testing. However, the addition of certain stipulations by the Board resulted in Wright's and a colleague's resignation. The *London Times* and the *British Medical Journal* picked up the story, and a polemic ensued between Wright and a noted British statistician, Karl Pearson. Wright did not understand the statistical analysis; Pearson did not appreciate the practical situation. Finally, with Sir William Leishman in charge, a field study with soldiers sent to India between 1904 and 1909 produced unequivocally positive data. This study also found that killing the bacilli at 53°C instead of 60°C preserved greater antigenicity and thereby yielded better protection. The immunity induced waned within two years. To give Wright some weight in his dealings with authorities Lord Haldane, the new Minister of War, recommended his knighthood, which was awarded in 1906.

Meanwhile, the U.S. Army made inoculation compulsory in 1901, as did the French Army in 1913 after their own tests. When World War I began, neither Germany nor England had instituted mandatory vaccination, but this quickly was remedied, particularly after Wright's impassioned letter in the *London Times* and a meeting with Lord Kitchener. Of two million British troops in the conflict, 20,000 contracted typhoid, and of this population, only 1100 died. Wright had won his war.

For further information:

Colebrook, L. 1954. *Almroth Wright. Provocative Doctor and Thinker.* William Heinemann Medical Books. 286 p.

Cope, Z. 1966. *Almroth Wright. Founder of Modern Vaccine-therapy*. Nelson, London. 184 p.

Gröschel, D. H. M. and R. B. Hornick. 1981. Who introduced typhoid vaccination: Almroth Wright or Richard Pfeiffer? *Reviews of Infectious Diseases* 3:1251–1254.

Wright, A. E. 1904. *A Short Treatise on Anti-typhoid Inoculation*. Archibald Constable & Company, London. 76 p.

The Paper*

Mr. Haffkine suggested rather more than twelve months ago to one of us that the method of vaccination which has proved so effectual in combating cholera epidemics in India might, *mutatis mutandis,* be applied also to the prophylaxis of typhoid fever. Since that time, the question has been constantly engaging our attention, and we have gradually elaborated the method of antityphoid vaccination, which is to be briefly described in this paper.

Our first vaccinations against typhoid were undertaken in the months of July and August of last year. These vaccinations were put on record by one of us in the *Lancet* on September 19th, 1896, in a paper which dealt primarily with the question of serious hemorrhage. A reprint of this paper was sent among others to Professor Pfeiffer.

Nearly two months after the data of this paper Professor Pfeiffer published in conjunction with Dr. Kolle, a paper on Two Cases of Typhoid Vaccination. The method of inoculation which these authors have adopted, is exactly similar to the one that we had previously adopted. Like our own method, it was based upon the methods which have been so successfully employed by Mr. Haffkine in his anticholera inoculations.

After this historical discursus, we may without further prologue proceed to consider, first, the general principles upon which these typhoid vaccinations are based; secondly, the methods which are adopted in preparing the vaccines; thirdly, the dosage and the strength of the vaccines; fourthly, the clinical symptoms which supervene upon the inoculation of those vaccines; fifthly, the method of gauging the effect of these vaccinations; lastly, we shall consider certain questions with reference to the probable duration

of the immunity and in connection with the application of these vaccines.

The object of all vaccination processes is, first, to achieve a degree of immunity which shall be equal or greater to that which accrues to a patient who undergoes and recovers from an actual attack of the disease; and, secondly, to achieve that immunity without any risk to life or health.

The first of these objects can, as far as is known, only be satisfactorily achieved by inoculating the patient with the micro-organisms (or the products of the micro-organisms) of the particular disease. The second object can be achieved in several ways. We may either, as in the Jennerian vaccination against smallpox, inoculate the patient with micro-organisms which have lost their virulence for man by being passed through a whole series of appropriately chosen animals. Or we may, as in the Pasteurian method of vaccinating against anthrax, employ in our inoculations artificially attenuated micro-organisms. Or, lastly, we may inoculate the patient with measured quantities of dead, but still poisonous, micro-organisms.

It is this last method which we have adopted in the case of our typhoid vaccinations. The advantages which are associated with the use of such dead vaccines are, first, that there is absolutely no risk of producing actual typhoid fever by our inoculations; secondly, that the vaccines may be handled and distributed through the post without incurring any risk of disseminating the germs of the disease; thirdly, that dead vaccines are probably less subject to undergo alteration in their strength than living vaccines.

These vaccines are made from agar cultures of typhoid bacilli which have grown for twenty-four hours at blood heat. The cultures which are thus obtained are emulsified by the addition of measured quantities of sterile broth. The resulting emulsion is then drawn up into a series of sterile and duly calibrated glass pipettes. The capillary end of these pipettes are then sealed up in the flame so as to form vaccine capsules. These capsules are then placed in a beaker of cold water, which is then brought to a temperature of 60°C, and is kept at that temperature for five minutes. The sterility of the vaccines is then controlled by allowing a drop of their contents to run out on to the surface of an agar tube, which is subsequently incubated. If, as in our experience always occurs, the contents of the vaccine capsules are now found to be absolutely sterile, the vaccine is ready for use.

In proceeding to the inoculation of these vaccines, the capsule is first thoroughly shaken so as to distribute the bacteria throughout the fluid. The contents are then drawn up aseptically into the syringe. . . . The vaccines are inoculated into the flank.

---

*Wright, A. E. and D. Semple. 1897. Remarks on vaccination against typhoid fever. *British Medical Journal* i:256–259. [With permission.]

The strength of a typhoid vaccine will obviously be determined (1) by the number of bacilli which it contains, (2) by the virulence of these bacilli. We have in all our later experiments employed a typhoid culture of such strength that one-fourth tube of a twenty-four hour culture constituted a lethal dose for a guinea pig of 350 to 400 grams when hypodermically inoculated. The quantities of the culture which we have employed for our antityphoid vaccinations have varied from one-twentieth to one-fourth of a tube. . . .

When the smaller doses (one-twentieth to one-sixth of tube) are employed, the symptoms are comparatively slight. The local symptoms consist in a little local tenderness; the constitutional symptoms in a subjective feeling of chilliness, which comes on about two to three hours after the inoculation of the vaccine; further, in a very slight rise of temperature, and a little restlessness at night. The symptoms have quite passed off in twenty-four hours.

With larger doses . . . all the symptoms are more severe. . . .

[W]henever the micro-organisms which are causally associated with a specific fever are brought in contact with the serum or plasma of an animal or a patient who is undergoing, or who has undergone, an attack of the specific fever in question, the following succession of phenomena manifests itself: (a) The bacteria become agglutinated together, (b) the bacteria lose their motility, (c) the clumps of agglutinated bacteria sink to the bottom, and the culture fluid which was previously evenly turbid, becomes clarified, (d) the bacteria shrink up into the form of minute spherules, (e) lastly, the bacteria are definitely devitalized.

For the purposes of serum diagnosis, it is not essential that this whole train of phenomena should come under observation. It suffices if any one of this series of phenomena comes distinctly under observation, provided always that we keep in view the fact that the subject matter of our observations is no longer the actual bactericidal effect of the particular serum, but either its agglutinating, immobilizing, sedimenting, or spherulating effect. . . . [T]he effect which is most accessible to observation is the agglomeration and the sedimentation of the bacteria. This effect can readily be appreciated by the unaided vision. . . .

Having thus settled that the sedimentation of the bacteria is the phenomenon which will best serve as a criterion of the specific power of a serum, it will be obvious that we shall be able readily to determine in what measure the serum possesses this specific power if we make a series of successive dilutions of the serum, and determine how far the blood may be diluted without forfeiting its sedimenting powers.

The quantitative results which are obtained by this method of successive dilutions may be conveniently expressed in terms of "sedimentation units," or, if the term shall afterward appear to be justified, in terms of "preventive units." We may, for instance, speak of a blood which manifests this power of sedimentation in tenfold dilution as a blood which contains one "sedimentation" or "preventive unit." Similarly we may speak of blood which exhibits this sedimenting power in a hundredfold dilution as blood which contains ten "sedimentation" or "preventive units." . . . [T]he next question we have to consider is the question as to whether we may legitimately conclude that a person who possesses a sedimenting power—say of twenty units—is absolutely protected against typhoid by the poisonous properties which have been imparted to his blood. Experiment shows that this is not so.

We find that undiluted blood which contains 20 sedimentation units fails to kill typhoid bacilli, even when these bacilli are exposed to its influence for as long a period as forty-eight hours. It will be obvious from this fact that we cannot rely upon the blood of a vaccinated person being sufficiently poisonous to kill off such typhoid bacilli as may chance to effect an entrance into his system.

This matter having become clear, we may next proceed to consider whether we have any warranty for inferring that the vaccinated patient's blood will, short of killing the bacilli of typhoid fever, yet exert such a deleterious influence on them as will result in the effectual protection of the patient against typhoid.

Everything that we know seems to show that this inference is perfectly warranted. We know, for instance, that guinea pigs, upon whom this sedimenting power had been conferred by vaccination processes, are extremely resistant to infection by the specific micro-organisms, with respect to which they possess this sedimenting power. . . . Again, in our first case of typhoid vaccination we had proof of the association of this sedimenting power with a condition of "bacteria-proofness." For our patient, who, on September 25th, 1896, possessed a sedimentation power of 20 units, suffered no ill effects from an inoculation of one-sixth tube of living virulent typhoid bacilli, which was made upon him on that day.

Finally, we have the fact that, so far as we know, every convalescent from typhoid or Malta fever . . . shows a notable sedimentation reaction. It appears to us that the only conclusion that can be reasonably deduced from this series of facts is the conclusion that the sedimentation power of the blood is a trustworthy criterion of the immunity of the patient who furnishes it.

The conclusion cannot, however, be regarded as absolutely assured until we are in a position satisfactorily to account for the fact that the typhoid fever patients and Malta fever monkeys who succumb to these diseases show the specific sedimentation reaction in exactly the same way as the typhoid fever patients and Malta fever monkeys who recover from these diseases. . . .

The sedimenting power of a patient, who afterwards succumbs to the disease, would thus appear to indicate only the degree of immunity which has been acquired at the particular moment at which blood was drawn off. And our experience of infective disease in general tells us that a degree of immunity which would, if already attained on the first day of the disease, amply suffice to ward off a fatal issue, will be of no avail if it is acquired later on in the course of the attack. . . .

We may reasonably surmise that this condition of bacteria proofness, inasmuch as it does not depend upon the presence of any absolutely bactericidal power in the blood, depends in large measure at least upon the fact that the typhoid bacilli which have been exposed to the poisonous influence of the blood fluids are likely to fall an easy prey to the phagocytes. . . .

It is obvious that a vaccination process has little chance of being widely adopted unless immunity of a more or less durable character can be conferred. A person who submits himself to a vaccination process will always desire to have some guarantee that he will not require to be constantly reinoculated. . . . Now . . . that we are in possession of the method of serum diagnosis, it will probably be possible to ascertain the duration of an immunity by a series of successive blood examinations. As yet we have no facts to base definite conclusion upon. In the meantime, if it is legitimate to judge from the extremely slow disappearance of the perfectly comparable sedimentation power, which is acquired by undergoing an attack of typhoid, we see every reason to hope that the immunity which is conferred by these vaccinations may persist for a considerable number of years. . . .

Prevention of pneumococcal pneumonia by immunization with specific capsular polysaccharides

1945 • *Colin M. MacLeod, Richard G. Hodges, Michael Heidelberger, and William G. Bernhard*

Comment

In contrast with the previous immunological milestones, the following report is not distinguished as the first vaccine to a particular microorganism, nor is it the first test of a new approach to immunization. It is rather the culmination to an extraordinarily fruitful line of research whose application commenced in 1911 with Sir Almroth Wright.

Pneumococcal pneumonia has long been recognized as a relatively gentle yet fatal disease of the elderly and infirm, but it took on epidemic proportions when many robust young native men fell victim in the rapidly expanding South African gold and diamond mines. Such respiratory infections were also associated with military training centers. Wright's study of a heat-killed vaccine again suffered from lack of standardization and preliminary determination of optimal conditions. Dosage, number of injections, and proportions of nonimmunized control subjects varied. The antigenic types of the streptococci used in his vaccine or prevalent among the miners were unknown, but were apparently different from his laboratory strains.

Nevertheless, Wright claimed success, and subsequent independent statistical analysis did find some short-term protection among the 50,000 inoculated workers.

At the time of Wright's pioneering trials, Michael Heidelberger was completing his Ph.D. in chemistry at Columbia University. Born in 1888, this remarkable immunochemist is still actively contributing to the science. He joined the Rockefeller Institute in 1912, where he became involved with the pneumococcal research led by Oswald Avery. His tenure there begot several outstanding advances that went far beyond the problem of pneumonia; two will be presented later as other milestones. Heidelberger carried his interest in antigenicity, a lifelong project, to the College of Physicians and Surgeons of Columbia University in 1928, where he continued collaborative investigations with the Rockefeller staff.

By the later 1920s he had established that rabbit antibodies can couple with the polysaccharide capsule of *Streptococcus pneumoniae*. This external cell wall layer was found to vary antigenically among strains of the bacteria, and could be categorized into "types." Currently, 84 types are recognized. Immunity to pneumococcal infection is type-specific, explaining some of the difficulties encountered in early vaccine trials. In 1930 Thomas Francis, Jr. and William S. Tillet discovered that the capsular polysaccharide was antigenic in humans without the need for any protein carrier. This fortuitous event occurred when they had sought to induce a cutaneous allergic reaction by injecting homologous and different types of the sugar complex intradermally in convalescing patients. This was important, since humans, being the natural host, might have reacted differently than laboratory animals, e.g., the formation of capsular antibodies might have required the presence of other bacterial components. Additional studies on laboratory animals, patients, and over 100,000 healthy volunteers confirmed the potential of a purified polysaccharide vaccine.

World War II provided the opportunity and need for a definitive field trial. Colin M. MacLeod (1909–1972), who left the Rockefeller Institute in 1941 for New York University, had been appointed Director of the Commission on Pneumonia of the Army Epidemiological Board. He was responsible for administratively organizing and monitoring the experiment. In 1944 he joined Oswald Avery and Maclyn McCarty in publishing another powerful study: the determination that DNA is responsible for transforming a strain of avirulent, noncapsulated pneumococci to the typical virulent, capsulated form. The remaining authors of the vaccine report, Richard Hodges and William Bernhard, were senior military physicians. This study accomplished its goal, with the dividend of confirming the contribution of herd immunity, which reduces the opportunity in a given population for exposure to an infectious agent. Sir Spencer Lister had discovered this effect in 1916 in his analysis of a field study among South African miners that tested a pneumococcal vaccine directed against four prevalent serological types of the bacterium.

World War II brought forth another measure against pneumonia: penicillin. This and other antibiotics seemed to make the pneumococcal vaccine obsolete, and the commercial manufacturer of the vaccine eventually took the product off the market from lack of interest. Antibiotics, however, were not always effective, particularly among the elderly. In addition, pneumococcal bacteremia often resisted antibiotic therapy. The pneumococcus is indigenous to humans, and continually poses a hazard among certain occupational and age segments of the population. Thus, through the efforts of Robert Austrian and others, the pneumococcus vaccine was resurrected, modified, retested, and finally licensed in the United States in 1977. Adjusted in formula to cover current and regional prevalent types, the vaccine is reactive to 14 unique capsular polysaccharides. Its efficacy is good but not outstanding, in one trial protecting 78.5 percent of volunteers against pneumonia and 82.3 percent against bacteremia. However, prophylaxis coupled with the ready reserve of antibiotics has minimized incidence and mortality to this infectious agent, which Sir William Osler once characterized as "captain of the men of death."

An investigative team led by Malcolm S. Artenstein at the Walter Reed Army Institute of Research successfully carried on the defined chemical approach to vaccines. Their target was *Neisseria meningitidis,* the meningococcus. This microorganism, unrelated to the pneumococcus, also possesses a capsular carbohydrate of several antigenic types, is also often carried benignly as part of the normal flora of the upper respiratory tract, and also has been the common cause of epidemics among military recruits, as well as sporadic incidences among civilian populations. The vaccine, licensed in 1975 after massive international testing, has met the standard of excellence provided by the work of Heidelberger and MacLeod.

For further information:

Austrian, R., 1973. Colin Munro MacLeod, 1909–1972. *Journal of Infectious Diseases* 127:211–214.

Austrian, R. 1985. *Life with the Pneumococcus. Notes from the Bedside, Laboratory and Library.* University of Pennsylvania Press, Philadelphia. 168 p.

Heidelberger, M. 1979. A "pure" organic chemist's downward path: Chapter 2—the years at P. and S. *Annual Review of Biochemistry* 48:1–21.

The Paper*

Many studies on prophylactic immunization against pneumococcal pneumonia have been made, using a number of different antigenic preparations. Almost

*MacLeod, C. M., R. G. Hodges, M. Heidelberger, and W. G. Bernhard. 1945. Prevention of pneumococcal pneumonia by immunization with specific capsular polysaccharides. *Journal of Experimental Medicine* 82:445–465. [By copyright permission of the Rockefeller University Press.]

all investigators have concluded that immunization exerts a beneficial effect. In most of the studies, however, certain variables have clouded interpretation of the results. . . .

It has been demonstrated repeatedly that animals can be protected against infection by virulent pneumococci by means of antibodies directed against the specific capsular polysaccharides. Antibodies to the somatic portion of the cell are of considerably less importance in this respect. Francis and Tillett showed originally that the purified capsular polysaccharides of pneumococci are antigenic for man when injected intracutaneously in a single dose as small as 0.01 mg.

There are various reasons why the purified capsular polysaccharides should be advantageous immunizing agents for man as compared with whole bacterial vaccines. Not only should it be possible to avoid the local abscess formation associated not infrequently with whole pneumococcal vaccines, but in addition a stable, water-clear solution of known composition can be used. It becomes possible also to standardize the dose of antigen on a weight basis. It is of theoretical and practical importance for each of the various pneumococcal types that a single, purified antigen relatively free from heterogeneous somatic constituents can be used. Therefore, the injection of several purified capsular polysaccharides in a single dose probably involves fewer antigens than when a whole bacterial vaccine of a single serological type is used, since the whole bacterial vaccine contains numerous unrelated protein and carbohydrate antigens in addition to the specific capsular polysaccharide. . . .

The present paper deals with the immunization of man with the polysaccharides of pneumococcus types I, II, V, and VII. It has been demonstrated that a single subcutaneous prophylactic injection of 0.03 to 0.06 mg of each of these polysaccharides greatly diminished the incidence of pneumonia caused by pneumococci of the same type in immunized individuals. Moreover, evidence will be presented that the incidence of pneumonia caused by types I, II, V, and VII in the non-immunized controls who were thoroughly mingled with the immunized was also reduced. . . .

The experiment was carried out in an Army Air Force Technical School. There was much to recommend the choice of this population. First, there was the unusually high pneumococcal pneumonia rate which had prevailed in the School during the preceding two winters. . . . Furthermore, much information was available concerning the types of pneumococci responsible for these high disease rates. . . .

Thorough epidemiological study of the respiratory disease experience of the preceding 2 years brought out another advantage.... It was found that for each of the disease investigated pneumococcal pneumonia, streptococcal sore throat, epidemic influenza, and common respiratory disease, the School reacted as a whole and not by its individual, component groups or units....

From yet another epidemiological aspect the population was highly satisfactory. It is known that many factors such as seasoning and environment exert a large effect on the incidence of respiratory disease. In the study of the Technical School several of these factors could be eliminated. The living conditions, duties, and even the recreation were identical for all the men in the School....

Men passing down one side of the barrack received the polysaccharide solution subcutaneously; those passing down the other side received an injection of 1 cc of sterile isotonic saline containing 0.5 percent phenol.... In all, 8586 men were injected with the polysaccharides and 8449 with saline.... Calculation of man-days of exposure gives approximately equal figures for immunized and non-immunized, 745,997 and 772,898 respectively....

During the 7 months period of observation following the beginning of the immunization program, 4 cases of pneumonia caused by types I, II, V, or VII occurred in the immunized group as opposed to 26 cases among the non-immunized subjects. This difference is highly significant. When the individual types are considered, it is apparent that the one to fourteen difference for type II is also highly significant and definitely establishes the value of immunization with the polysaccharide of this type. The number of cases for types I, V, and VII were too small to permit definite statistical conclusions, although the zero to six difference in type VII would be due to chance only once in about 400 times. Despite the inconclusiveness of the results for these three types, there is no reason for believing that polysaccharides of types I, V, and VII should differ in their immunizing capacity from the polysaccharide of type II....

The distribution between the immunized and non-immunized groups of pneumonia due to types other than I, II, V, and VII adds validity to the differences noted in the distribution of the types against which immunization was practiced. For type XII ... 21 cases occurred in the immunized group and 25 cases among the controls. Type IV ... caused eight cases of pneumonia in the immunized and six in the non-immunized group....

The four immunized men who developed pneumonia all did so within the first 2 weeks following the immunizing injection.... [T]his distribution is contrasted with that of non-immunized men developing type I, II, V, or VII pneumonia and with im-

munized and non-immunized men who develop pneumonia due to other types.... [These] cases were scattered throughout the period in which the men were under observation....

[I]mmunity to pneumococci types I, II, V, and VII developed between 6 and 9 days after injection of the polysaccharides as estimated by the appearance in the serum of antibodies protective for mice. All subjects showed antibodies for all of the polysaccharides within a 9-day period following injection....

An upper limit for the duration of immunity could not be determined in the present study.... On the basis of previous studies in human volunteers it seems probable that immunity as indicated by the presence of antibodies should endure for a period of at least 1 year, since antibody levels of 1/3 to 1/2 the original maximum level were still present after a period of 1 to 2 years in most subjects.

Determination of pneumococcal carrier rates was made continuously throughout the course of the study.... Pneumococci of more than one type were encountered in a considerable proportion of cultures....

Thirty-two men in the [healthy] immunized group and 59 in the [healthy] non-immunized carried pneumococcus types I, II, V, or VII, or 1.79 and 3.26 percent respectively. This is a significant difference ($\chi^2 = 9.0$). The total carrier incidence for

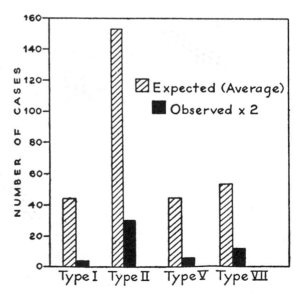

Figure 3 Expected and observed incidence of pneumococcal pneumonia caused by types I, II, V, and VII for 1944–45. The observed incidence for 1944–45 has been multiplied by two since the nonimmunes comprised only one-half the population.

these types [including pneumococcal cases] was 36 and in the non-immunized 85 ($\chi^2 = 27.0$). From these data it may be concluded that the carrier rate of pneumococci of types I, II, V, and VII was significantly lowered in the immunized group, in all likelihood as a consequence of immunization.

It is probable that the carrier rates for types I, II, V, and VII were reduced not only in the immunized but in the non-immunized group as well [epidemiologically based on the expected incidence of cases from previous years]. . . . The observed incidence of pneumonia due to types I, II, V, and VII in the non-immunized men during 1944–45 was 17.6 percent of the expected incidence. . . .

Furthermore, the almost identical reduction in the incidence of pneumonia caused by each of the four types among the non-immunes, affords very strong evidence that immunization with the capsular polysaccharides of types I, V, and VII was just as effective as the more easily visualized protection given by the polysaccharide of type II. . . .

Two possible explanations may be suggested to account for the protection afforded the non-immune half of the population. In the first place, elimination of type I, II, V, and VII pneumonia in half the population produced a corresponding reduction in case-contact carriers and thus lowered the carrier rate of the whole population. This assumes that the principal focus for dissemination was from subjects just developing pneumonia or recently recovered. . . .

A second possibility is that the immunization directly affected the carrier rate. . . . It is probable that the truth lies in a combination of the two explanations. With the thorough mixing of the immunized and non-immunized subjects in the population, the chances would be that in every other one of its transfers from man to man, the pneumococci would fall on infertile ground, either because the subject was prevented from developing pneumonia or because his ability to carry pneumococci was lessened by the immunization. . . .

The reduction of disease in the non-immune portion of a partially immunized population is not a new finding. Similar observations have been made following immunization against diphtheria. . . .

Part 2
Allergy, Hypersensitivity, and Immunopathology

You raise up your head and you ask, Is this where it is?
And somebody points to you and says, It's his.
And you say, What's mine?
And somebody else says, Where what is?
And you say, Oh my God am I here all alone?
Because something is happening here, but you don't know what it is, do
  you, Mr. Jones?   —Bob Dylan, *Ballad of a Thin Man*

Whether in the course of infection or poisoning or through the medical intervention of vaccine prophylaxis or serum therapy, the immune response at first appeared to be of flawless benefit, providing protection and maintaining the integrity of the individual. Soon, however, researchers were encountering, to their puzzlement, breaches in this defense of self, inefficiencies in the immunological process, and even the occasional sedition. We can imagine their initial astonishment at such anomalies, but in retrospect, after scrutinizing the immune interactions of cells, chemicals, and consciousness, surely one of the most complex organizations conceived, adverse effects should have been expected.

It is the nature of Nature to be perfectly imperfect, at least from the perspective of human ideals. A search for Euclidean straight lines and precise circles among planetary matter and life forms will fail. Existence is defined by change and process, and we find Utopian order but a seductive, treacherous nightmare. As often stated, the only changeless condition in this universe is change itself. However, natural variation of form and activity is not chaotic, but is of a sophisticated order described by higher mathematics and biophysical laws.

Too much of a good thing, for instance, can lead to injury. Antibiotics can destroy the defensive normal flora as well as the target pathogenic bacterium. A similar effect occurs with allergy and hypersensitivity. These once distinct terms have become interchangeable. Observing the contradiction of "immunity," which connotes resistance to disease, and "hypersensitivity," which seems to refer to the condition of being hair-trigger reactive but instead implies the pathogenic activity of the immune response, Clemens von Pirquet coined the word "allergy." The term relates to a change from normal behavior or the original state to an abnormal, altered state, a very inclusive concept. An allergen not only induces antibodies, it triggers other inflammatory agents as well. Hence, antigens are a subset of allergens. Pirquet restricted immunity to the absence of clinical symptoms. However, with time allergy itself was limited in definition, and among the public it is now associated with such immunological defects as hay fever and hives. Allergy frequently does not include the delayed hypersensitivity of tuberculin skin tests, but may encompass such reactions as serum sickness and contact dermatitis to metallic jewelry. It is worth noting that allergy is a medical specialty, and that the major agency for funding research in immunology in the United States is the National Institute of Allergy and Infectious Disease.

The present section begins with the classic papers that are the root cause of the confusion in differentiating immunopathogenic responses. Some of the described phenomena are primarily laboratory-induced; others are commonly observed results of cellular defects in individuals. Although the biological mechanisms may be significantly different, the clinical picture is often similar.

Delayed hypersensitivity, one of Robert Koch's fundamental discoveries, is an exception. The response time, the typical hard, reddish appearance from an intradermal injection or its natural analog of the mosquito bite, and the key mononuclear cell infiltration distinguish delayed hypersensitivity from other immunological processes. Thymus-derived lymphocytes (T cells) and their mediators, not antibodies, are the stars of this reaction. At the turn of the century when Paul Portier and Charles Richet were struck by the immediate, systemic, and sometimes lethal effects that occurred after reinjecting an antigen into a sensitized animal, they at first thought that the reaction was due to a loss of immunity and called it anaphylaxis. On the contrary, it was soon shown to be an immunological response itself. Antibodies of the IgE class and of those living drug storehouses, the blood-borne basophils and tissue-associated mast cells, combined to produce a virulent cascade of inflammation. A somewhat more subdued anaphylactic response is that due to sensitivity to house dust. The local necrotizing reaction of Maurice Arthus and systemic serum sickness as described by von Pirquet and Bela Schick are caused by immune complexes of antigen and antibody and the activation of the complement cascade. Food allergy, atopy, and the development of a passive skin test for anaphylactic sensitivity are the topics of the milestone by Carl Prausnitz and Heinz Küstner.

The opposite of hypersensitivity could be termed hyposensitivity, but this condition is actually known as immunodeficiency, a refreshingly apt term. Immunodeficiencies, which can be the result of almost any defect in immunity—generally involving T cells, B cells, phagocytes, or complement—is represented here by the very first report of such a defect. In 1952 Colonel Ogden C. Bruton solved the mystery behind his patient's recurrent bacterial infections: the boy lacked practically all antibodies. Bruton called this unique immunological disease agammaglobulinemia. Immunodeficiency can exist at birth or arise later from somatic mutation. It is one of the hazards of radiation. Recently it has been dramatically and tragically linked to a highly virulent, typically lethal viral infection of helper T lymphocytes.

The last three papers in this section tackle autoimmunity. *Horror autotoxicus,* fear of self-poisoning, is how Paul Ehrlich in 1900 described the vigilance of the body in maintaining tolerance to its own molecular constituents. Immune-mediated suicide seemed unthinkable; however, four years after Ehrlich's 1900 paper, Julius Donath and Karl Landsteiner gave evidence for this especially intriguing class of immunological diseases. By 1957 autoimmunity and the breaking of tolerance were the prime research endeavors of immunological pioneers Ernest Witebsky, Noel R. Rose, Deborah Doniach, Ivan M. Roitt, and others. The entire immunological apparatus, if we accept the conventional functional definition, is brought to bear to ensure individuality and separation of self and nonself. How then can self act against itself? Metaphors can be useful, but such a teleology is, of course, wrong at heart; the immune system is essentially neutral.

Autoimmunity may be induced by various mechanisms. Certain "privileged sites," such as the brain and the cornea of the eye, are normally hidden from lymphocyte circulation. Tolerance here is due to a physical barrier. Even in immunologically approachable vascular tissues, antigens can lie within protective niches. However, physical or chemical trauma can break the barrier, exposing the structures to immunologically primed cells. The subsequent immune and inflammatory responses exacerbate the problem and unmask more antigenic cells. As some keys can enter a lock without necessarily engaging all the tumblers, certain host molecular configurations can couple with antibodies produced against alien antigens, such as microorganisms, heterologous tissue, or the host's own degenerated tissue. (Less-than-perfect self is nonself.) The condition is termed cross-reactivity. These unions typically are less avid than those with the intended foreign antigen; however, they may still initiate the complement cascade or other agents to effect damage or a disease. A somatic mutation or a congenital defect of regulating suppressor T cells, a flux in the governing network of idiotypic antibodies, or the non-specific activation of antibody-producing B cells—as may occur with bacterial endotoxins—can also initiate autoimmune antibodies. The cellular machinery against one's self exists and is active.

In short, the immune system is subject to disease and irregularity as any other organization of body-mind. As for the question of material self versus other, it mechanistically reduces to a shift in a local dynamic equilibrium. Hypersensitivity is merely sensitivity: autoimmunity is nothing but immunity. Corporeal self and nonself are hence extrapolative concepts of body-mind.

For further information:

Buisseret, P. D. 1982. Allergy. *Scientific American* 247(2):86–95.

Burnet, M. 1972. *Auto-immunity and Auto-immune Disease. A survey for physician or biologist.* F. A. Davis Company, Philadelphia. 243 p.

Good, R. A. 1971. Historical aspects of immunologic deficiency diseases. In: *Immunologic Incompetence* (B. M. Kagan and E. R. Stiehm, editors). Year Book Medical Publishers, Chicago. pp. 149–177.

Patterson, R. (editor) 1985. *Allergic Diseases. Diagnosis and Management.* 3rd edition. J. P. Lippincott Company, Philadelphia. 855 p.

Turk, J. L. 1980. *Delayed Hypersensitivity.* 3rd edition. North-Holland Publishing Company, Amsterdam. 295 p.

A remedy for tuberculosis

1891 • Robert Koch

Comment

Louis Pasteur had a scientific rival. This co-founder of modern microbiology and the dean of bacteriological technology was Robert Koch (1843–1910). Pasteur and Koch were so different in personality, temperament, and approaches to science that they were inexorably opposed. Koch detested Pasteur's pageantry; Pasteur deplored Koch's arrogance; Koch was astonished at Pasteur's casualness towards technical competence; Pasteur lamented Koch's narrow conceptual appreciation. Soft-edged, fluid ecology and Darwinian dynamics were welcome in Paris; precision, differentiation, and reductionism prospered in Berlin.

In 1866 Koch graduated with an M.D. from the University of Göttingen, and later served as a medical officer in the Franco-Prussian War of 1870–1871. His interest in microbiology began when he became the district physician in rural Wollstein. He had much free time to tinker with anthrax bacilli in a small laboratory in his home. Koch was able to solve the mystery of the disappearing bacilli in dead livestock by discovering their ability to form spores. In 1876 this country doctor demonstrated the life cycle of the anthrax bacillus before Ferdinand Cohn, a leading authority on bacteria, who not only published Koch's research, but helped him obtain a position in 1880 with the Imperial Office of Public Health in Berlin. In 1885, after discovering the tubercle bacillus and fully establishing the microbial etiology of cholera (Filippo Facini first described and named the cholera vibrio in 1854), Koch became Professor of Hygiene at the Berlin Hygienic Institute. His laboratory became the mecca of bacteriology for researchers around the world, and his many works received appropriate accolades of the international press, governments, other social institutions, and the common citizen. Apparently the praise was insufficient. Pasteur's famous rabies vaccine led to the creation of the Pasteur Institute, officially dedicated on November 14, 1888. Koch keenly recognized that public esteem and political power can be achieved through a human cure or vaccine.

In 1889 and through most of 1890 Koch was suspicious, secretive, and seclusive. He told his students that no one in the institute except himself was permitted to work on tuberculosis. Finally, at the International Medical Congress of August 1890 in Berlin he offered an explanation of his strange behavior. He calmly told his audience that he had been searching for a remedy against tuberculosis, listing the sundry chemicals which he tested in vitro. He then pronounced the electric words: "I have at last hit upon a substance that has the power of preventing the growth of tubercle bacilli, not only in a test tube, but in the body of an animal." Koch then reported that the substance acts both prophylactically and therapeutically in guinea pigs without harm, and stated that his sole purpose in making the preliminary announcement was to encourage further research.

The response was ambivalence. Rejoicing and cheer rocked the Congress, but the lack of details haunted the gathering, especially when shortly afterwards Kitasato and Behring published in some detail their development of serum therapy (see Part 1). Rumors and later evidence suggested that Koch was under great pressure by the Minister of Education to make the Berlin meeting a historic event, and that the announcement would also exert pressure on the government to build him his own bacteriological institute and research hospital. Indeed, in 1891 he became Director of the new Institute for Infective Diseases.

The public was awed by Koch's announced therapy for tuberculosis. It was the first hope for curing a major infectious disease. Over 1500 physicians, including Joseph Lister, came to Berlin to acquire the remedy. Crowds gathered in the streets in Berlin to chant hymns in Koch's honor and to shout his name. But what exactly was this remedy? Koch's publication of November 1890 added little detail, citing work on human patients. Of especial importance was his observation that the remedy will "in future be an indispensable aid to diagnosis." At last in January 1891, the second installment of the report, which is the following milestone, described the composition of the remedy to a disappointed scientific and medical community.

The simple culture extract soon was referred to as Koch's Lymph and later it became known as tuberculin. Its diagnostic advantage, which was almost immediately confirmed, was furthered by Clemens von Pirquet in 1907 with the development of a skin scratch test and in 1908 by Charles Mantoux's intradermal test.

Large-scale skin testing among cattle helped control bovine tuberculosis, and such tests remain the best indicator of subclinical infection. However, far from being curative, tuberculin was a disaster. Soon reports of overdoses, virulent reactions, and even death appeared. Opposition mounted to the lack of controlled studies, the secrecy, and mismanagement, and the poor results. Koch, nevertheless, continued his work through 1901 creating new tuberculins. His public glory was fleeting, but he went on to further microbiologic fame. He received the Nobel Prize in 1905 in honor of his bacterial discoveries and techniques.

This collection features Koch's major immunological contribution: the discovery of delayed-type hypersensitivity, in this instance a specific and complex cellular reaction to the waxy surface of *Mycobacterium tuberculosis.* The reaction to this substance can enhance immune responses to other antigens; killed tubercle bacilli are a component of Complete Freund's Adjuvant, for example. Thymus-derived lymphocytes and macrophages rather than the antibody-forming B-lymphocytes are primarily associated with the phenomenon, which also occurs with certain fungal and viral infections and in the rejection of transplanted tissue. A related effect, contact dermititis, may develop after repeated skin contact with poison oak, certain drugs, or nickel salts. The characteristic necrosis of delayed hypersensitivity is a result of the interaction of mononuclear cells, which release lymphokines such as lymphotoxin. Killer T-lymphocytes, natural killer cells, and the nonspecific cytotoxic action of activated macrophages also contribute to tissue damage.

For further information:

Brock, T. D. 1988. *Robert Koch: A Life in Medicine and Bacteriology.* Science Tech Publishers, Madison, WI. 348 p.

Brown, L. 1935. Robert Koch (1843–1910). An American tribute. *Annals of Medical History* Series II. 7:99–112; 292–304; 385–401.

Dubovsky, H. 1973. Koch's remedy for tuberculosis. *South African Medical Journal* 47:1609–1614.

Foster, W. D. 1968. Robert Koch and his contribution to bacteriology. *Scientia* 103:53–71.

The Paper*

Since the publication of my experiments with a new remedy for tuberculosis two months ago, many doctors have obtained possession of the remedy, and have thus been able to acquaint themselves with its qualities by their own studies. . . . That the remedy exercises a specific action on tuberculous tissue, and consequently can be employed as a very sensitive and conclusive reagent in searching out hidden, and diagnosing doubtful, tuberculous processes, is agreed on all sides. In regard to the therapeutic effect of the remedy, most accounts also agree that, in spite of the relatively short duration of the treatment, many patients show improvement, varying only in degree. I am informed that cure even has been attained in a few instances. Only in some exceptional cases has it been affirmed that the remedy may not only be dangerous in too far advanced conditions—which is freely admitted—but that it directly speeds the tuberculous process, that it is in fact harmful. . . .

If a healthy guinea pig is inoculated with a pure culture of tubercle bacilli, the inoculation site is sealed with a scab and appears to heal during the next few days. After 10 to 14 days a hard nodule is formed, which soon develops into an open ulcer that persists until the animal dies. However, the case is very different if an already tuberculous animal is inoculated. The most suitable animals for this experiment are those that have already been successfully inoculated 4 to 6 weeks previously. With such an animal, the small inoculation site also is first sealed with a scab,

but no nodule forms, a peculiar change instead taking place at the point of inoculation. Within the first or second day, the spot becomes hard and dark. This is not confined to the point of inoculation, but extends to a diameter of 0.5 to 1 cm. During the next few days it becomes increasingly clear that the epidermis thus altered is necrotic. Finally it sloughs off, leaving a flat, ulcerated surface, which generally heals quickly and completely without infecting the neighboring lymph nodes. Thus the inoculated tubercle bacilli act quite differently on the skin of a healthy guinea pig and that of a tuberculous one. Yet this remarkable effect is not limited to living tubercle bacilli, but also in equal fashion to dead ones, whether killed by long exposure to low temperatures, which I at first tried, or by boiling, or by certain chemicals.

This peculiar fact having been ascertained, . . . it was then further found that pure cultures of tubercle bacilli thus killed, after they have been ground and suspended in water, can be injected under the skin of healthy guinea pigs in large quantities with the production of only local suppuration. Tuberculous guinea pigs, on the other hand, can be killed by an injection of very small quantities of such suspended cultures. According to dose, the time of death varied from 6 to 48 hours. A dose which is just insufficient to kill the animal is sufficient to produce an extensive necrosis of the skin in the inoculation site. If the suspended material is further diluted until it is scarcely turbid to the eye, the animals remain alive. If the injections are then continued at intervals of one or two days, a noticeable improvement in their skin condition soon occurs; the ulcer at the point of inoculation becomes smaller and finally forms a scar. . . .

The remedy is . . . a glycerol extract of pure cultures of tubercle bacilli.

[I]t is possible to separate from the extract a colorless, dry substance that contains greater activity than the original glycerol solution. . . . The quantity of active principle present in the extract is probably very small; I estimate it at a fraction of 1 percent. Therefore if my assumption is correct, we are dealing with a substance whose action on the tuberculous organism far surpasses that of the strongest drugs known. . . .

---

*Koch, R. 1891. Fortsetzung der Mittheilungen über ein Heilmittel gegen Tuberculose. *Deutsche Medizinische Wochenschrift* 9:101–102. [With permission of Georg Thieme Verlag.]

The anaphylactic action of certain venoms

1902 • *Paul Portier and Charles Richet*

Comment

It is not unusual for research begun in one scientific discipline to advance another, even distantly related field. The following milestone is the first of two examples by which invertebrate zoology has by chance contributed to the science of immunity. Both investigations would eventually lead their authors to Stockholm and the Nobel Prize. Our first paper concerns the discovery of the very important phenomenon of anaphylaxis.

Charles Richet (1850–1935), the son of a noted surgeon, began his medical training in 1869, but chose the physiology laboratory over clinical practice after witnessing and then inducing hypnosis in patients. By the time he completed his M.D. in 1877, he had investigated conditioned reflexes in digestion and had discovered that gastric juice contains hydrochloric acid. He became a professor of physiology at the University of Paris ten years afterward. Richet's early interest in immunology is evident from his treatment of human tuberculosis in 1890 by the inoculation of serum from a dog immunized to the avian tubercle bacillus. This was the first attempt at serum therapy in humans. Eleven years later, while on an oceanographic expedition of regions around the Azores and Cape Verde, organized by Prince Albert I of Monaco, he met Paul Portier (1866–1962), a friend of the Prince and an assistant in the physiology laboratory at the Sorbonne. Portier had earned his degrees in science and medicine at the University of Paris in 1891 and 1897, and became in 1906 a professor at the Oceanographic Institute in Paris.

The prince suggested that the two physiologists investigate the immobilizing poison of the Portuguese man-of-war. This colony structure of specialized jellyfish contains tentacles that support adhesive cups and inner venomous pins. By grinding the animals with sand and extracting the toxin (dubbed "hypnotoxin") with glycerol, they were able to study quantitatively its physiological effect on some of the pigeons, ducks, guinea pigs, and frogs carried on board their two-masted, steam-powered yacht.

Richet and Portier decided to continue the research when they returned to Paris. Since the hydrozoan was not indigenous to European waters, they substituted it with the very plentiful sea anemone, which contains a similar toxin. They cut off the tentacles close to the body, and placed them in glycerol. The chemical dissolved and extracted the toxin as before. To bring their study to a modern conclusion, Portier suggested that they attempt to immunize animals against the agent. When heated toxin or low doses of native toxin failed to confer resistance on pigeons and guinea pigs, they switched to dogs.

The following brief milestone seems to describe the surprising discovery of anaphylaxis when a dog, which had previously received a sublethal dose of the toxin, rapidly weakened and died upon a second injection. Although not reported in the paper, the first victim of experimental anaphylaxis was actually a pigeon. This event, coupled with the recognition that the higher sensitivity of animals to secondary injections seemed to be related to the interval between inoculations, led the team to the test described here. In one instance, a dog, named Neptune, which received 0.05 cc/kg and three days later 0.1 cc/kg, became ill within seconds after being given a third injection with 0.1 cc/kg of toxin 26 days after the first inoculation. It gasped for air, dragging itself along the floor until immobilized on its side. Moments later it suffered diarrhea, vomited blood, and died. Only 25 minutes had elapsed since the fatal inoculation. Such a dramatic display was a shock to the investigator as well as the animal. Anaphylaxis bore no resemblance to the death throes that followed a primary toxic injection. The necessity of an incubation period for sensitization to occur was readily verified. In 1907 Richet confirmed the discovery made that year by Richard Otto, an associate of Paul Ehrlich, that the sensitized state could be passively acquired by the injection of serum. Richet continued his studies of anaphylaxis, but Portier was obliged to return to teaching duties. In 1913 the older and more prominent Richet alone was honored with the Nobel Prize. Richet's other contributions were in psychology and parapsychology, statistics, aeronautics, and literature.

Not all animals manifest the same anaphylactic symptoms as dogs. Guinea pigs mainly suffer respiratory constriction, while rabbits have intestinal congestion and heart failure. Anaphylaxis in humans is characterized by laryngeal swelling, rash and itching, and circulatory collapse. The form of symptoms is host-rather than antigen-specific, and the presence of a toxin *per se* is not required. Dosage was important in Portier and Richet's example, since they dealt with a poison. With other antigens, a moderately high dose is necessary to induce anaphylactic shock, and a very low dose can have no effect. Repeated injection of low doses of the antigen can temporarily desensitize an individual by depleting available reactive antibody. The three-week interval necessary for sensitizing the dogs in Portier and Richet's study is not a constant; the period will vary with each test system.

Anaphylaxis can also be demonstrated in vitro. In 1910 William H. Schultz and Sir Henry H. Dale removed strips of small intestine, uterus, and heart from sensitized animals, and after removing all traces of blood, suspended them in physiological saline. When the sensitizing antigen alone was introduced into the solution, the smooth muscles of these organs contracted. The researchers concluded that anaphylaxis is antigen-specific and is initiated by the interaction of antigen and antibody, the latter being tissue bound.

Portier and Richet had pried open a Pandoran box, exposing the detrimental effects of the immune response. Scientists now could study the mechanisms behind the rash that sometimes develops after eating strawberries, the watery eyes and nasal congestion associated with animal hair, and the life-threatening bronchial constriction following a bee sting or an injection of penicillin.

For further information:

Besredka, A. 1919. *Anaphylaxis and Anti-anaphylaxis and their Experimental Foundations* (S. R. Gloyne, translator). William Heinemann Medical Books, London. 143 p.

May, C. D. 1985. The ancestry of allergy: being an account of the original experimental induction of hypersensitivity recognizing the contribution of Paul Portier. *Journal of Allergy and Clinical Immunology* 75:485–495.

Richet, C. 1913. *Anaphylaxis* (J. M. Bligh, translator). The University Press, Liverpool. 266 p.

The Paper*

We call anaphylactic (contrary to protection) the property, with which a venom is endowed, of diminishing rather than reenforcing immunity, when nonlethal doses are injected.

It is probable that many venoms (or toxins) are of this type; but, as one is concerned principally with their prophylactic or vaccinating action, there are yet very few attempts to study them methodically from this point of view.

The poison extracted from the tentacles of Actinia [sea anemones] offers a striking example of the anaphylactic effect.

---

*Portier, P. and C. Richet. 1902. De l'action anaphylactique de certains venins. *Comptes Rendus la Société de Biologie* (Paris) 54:170–172. [With permission of the Society.]

We will not describe here the course of poisoning by this actinotoxin. As a whole, the effects are somewhat close to those of the toxin extracted from the tentacles of Physalia [Portuguese man-of-war], a toxin which we studied during an expedition organized by Prince Albert of Monaco on the [ship] Princesse-Alice. It is sufficient to say that the poison of the tentacles of Actinia, in glycerol solution, is lethal by intravenous injection in the dog, when the injected dose exceeds 0.15 cc per kilogram. When the dose is between 0.15 cc and 0.30 cc/kg, death follows in 4 or 5 days. Above 0.30 cc/kg, it is within a few hours. For doses less than 0.15 cc/kg, the animals, with few exceptions, survive after a period of illness that lasts 4 or 5 days.

But if, instead of injecting normal dogs, one injects dogs that 2 or 3 weeks previously have received nonlethal injections, doses of 0.08 to 0.25 cc/kg bring about death very rapidly. This demonstrates the anaphylactic effect of the first injection. . . .

Our experiments also proved another unexpected fact: the anaphylactic effect is slow to develop. If the second injection is made a few days after the first, the animal behaves as if normal.

We have at this moment several dogs which have received 0.12 cc/kg at first, then 0.12 cc/kg three, four, or five days afterwards, and which are in good health. If this second injection was instead given 15 or 20 or 25 days after the first, these dogs would probably have died as rapidly as the dogs given in the above examples. . . .

Several hypotheses to explain these facts, which are surprising at first glance, will be determined in the course of experiments. We are content merely to call attention to the similarity between this diminished immunity (anaphylaxis) after the injection of actinotoxin and the extremely reduced immunity in tuberculous animals to tuberculin.

Repeated injection of horse serum into rabbits

1903 • Maurice Arthus

Comment

Koch's delayed hypersensitivity was a local manifestation of system sensitization. Cellular infusion of mononuclear cells followed by necrosis was its characteristic. Richet's anaphylaxis, however, was immediate and systemically manifested, although it could also be demonstrated by isolated tissues in vitro. In addition, a transfusion of antibody could passively sensitize a healthy animal. This nice dichotomy of cellular and humoral responses fell apart when Maurice Arthus (1862–1945) introduced a new phenomenon, which seemed to combine features of the previous two. The Arthus reaction had been a thorn in any attempt to develop a uniform model of allergy, and immunologists found it more convenient to simply put the reaction aside in its own category.

Arthus was also a physiology graduate of the University of Paris in 1890. He accepted the professorship of physiology and microbiology (a unique and insightful combination) at Fribourg University in Switzerland in 1896, but four years later he came to the Pasteur Institute at Lille, where he conducted the research described in the following milestone. In 1907 he returned to Switzerland, joining the faculty of the University of Lausanne. Arthus, who had discovered the need for calcium in blood clotting and introduced sodium citrate as an anticoagulant, became involved in immunology, as Henry Sewall, Albert Calmette, and Hideyo Noguchi, through the study of snake and insect venoms.

In the work reported here, Arthus immunized rabbits to horse serum, which itself was an antiserum to an unspecified toxin. Horses were the typical source of diphtheria antitoxin used to treat human patients. Arthus urged caution in repeating such inoculations in humans, but he gave no evidence of the hazard beyond his animal study. The systemic effects were also not described, but apparently resembled those discussed by Portier and Richet. It is the local phenomenon, however, that is known as the Arthus reaction. In addition, Arthus's description of the developing lesion applies only to rabbits. This immune response in dogs, guinea pigs, rats, and humans appears less distinct. Repeated injections, on principle, are not required for its demonstration; a massive injection of antigen can provide sensitization.

Histological examination shows that the Arthus lesion is characterized by an infiltration of polymorphonuclear neutrophils and damage to small blood vessels. The instigator of such inflammation has been shown to be insoluble immune complexes of antigen and antibody, which settle along the wall of small veins. The initial components of complement bind to the complex, activating the complement cascade and attracting the inflammatory leukocytes and platelets. Subsequent release of lysosomal enzymes expose the basement membrane of blood vessels to the immune complexes and their accompanying agents. The floodgates are thereby opened; seeping humoral fluids damage the surrounding tissue resulting in necrosis and retarded healing.

The Arthus reaction is more than a laboratory phenomenon. Pulmonary inflammations have been associated with such an immune response to the repeated exposure of airborne microbial spores. Increasingly more inflammatory and skin-damaging reactions have been observed with repeated injections of toxoids, antitoxins, and bacterial vaccines. Although not exact in its activating components, rheumatoid arthritis is mediated by a similar deposit of immune complexes in the synovial membrane of joints.

For further information:

Cochrane, C. G. and D. Koffler. 1973. Immune complex disease in experimental animals and man. *Advances in Immunology* 16:185–264.

Coombs, R. R. A. and P. G. H. Gell. 1968. Classification of allergic reactions responsible for clinical hypersensitivity and disease. In: *Clinical Aspects of Immunology*, 2nd edition (P. G. H. Gell and R. R. A. Coombs, editors). Blackwell Scientific Publications, Oxford, p. 575.

The Paper*

If one injects rabbits with sterile horse serum (experiments are conducted with anti-toxic sera), fresh or stored, heated to 57°C or unheated, below the skin, into the peritoneal cavity, or into the veins, no early or delayed response is produced. Horse serum injected in this way is not toxic for the rabbit. If this injection of horse serum is repeated after an interval of a few days, one finds that after several injections of the same or weaker dose, injuries are produced, which according to the degree of treatment of the animal, are benign or severe, and which according to the route of introduction, are local or systemic, immediate or delayed. Horse serum is toxic for the rabbit rendered anaphylactic by and for horse serum.

A rabbit received 5 cc of horse serum under the skin every 6 days. After the first three injections, absorption occurs in a few hours; after the fourth injection, at the site of injection a soft infiltration takes place that does not disappear before 2 or 3 days; after the fifth injection, the infiltration which occurs again, is harder, edematous, and does not resorb until at least 5 to 6 days; after the sixth injection, the edematous infiltration is transformed very rapidly into a profound alteration of the subcutaneous cellular tissue, which yields a thick, compact, solid, white mass (absolutely sterile and not with pus), persisting unaltered for weeks; after the seventh injection, the same but enhanced alterations occur: The skin above the induration very rapidly becomes red, more pale and drier; a gangrenous plaque develops, from which tissues are very slowly eliminated (over several weeks) and leave an uneven deep wound that heals with difficulty. The general state of the animal remains good.

This is a typical experiment. However, the stages could be less clearly marked. Necrosis may not occur before the seventh injection; the first signs may not

---

*Arthus, M. 1903. Injections repetée de serum de cheval chez le lapin. *Comptes rendus de la Société de Biologie* (Paris) 55:817–820. [With permission of the Society.]

appear after the fifth, sixth or even seventh injection.

These local phenomena are not simply the consequence of repetitive injections at the same point, because they can occur under the skin after previous injections had been made in the peritoneal cavity. These phenomena likewise are not the consequence of the mere accumulation of serum in the rabbit nor of the presence of a large quantity of the injected serum. . . .

If in a rabbit rendered anaphylactic by subcutaneous or intraperitoneal injections of horse serum, one injects into the vein of the ear 2 cc of horse serum, injuries are produced which, according to the anaphylactic state of the animal, are lethal or nonlethal, and which, in the latter instance, comprise the immediate and delayed responses. . . .

Anaphylactic phenomena have been observed in the guinea pig and in the rat under the influence of repeated injections of horse serum; the observed injuries in these animals will be described later.

Similar results have been observed in rabbits that have received several spaced injections of milk skimmed and sterilized at 110°C. . . . Rabbits rendered anaphylactic for and by horse serum are not so for milk, and vice versa. . . .

Serum sickness

1905 • Clemens von Pirquet and Bela Schick

Comment

It seems to reoccur with each advance in technology: the unexpected side effect. In the first years of this century, diphtheria, a fearful disease of children, was treated with antitoxins produced in horses. Horse antiserum was also being used to cure another common childhood ailment, scarlet fever. In this instance, the horses were inoculated with streptococcal broth cultures; the existence of the scarlet fever toxin was unknown at the time. However, the shield of serum therapy, commercially available since 1893, now bore some rust. By 1895, the reported complications to injections of animal antisera included hives and skin hemorrhages, gastrointestinal disorders, joint pains, paralysis, vomiting, and even death. Two pediatricians in Vienna, having performed numerous such inoculations, recognized for themselves the occasional untoward effect mentioned in the medical literature. They soon realized that this serum sickness had not a toxic, but an acquired immune origin. The following milestone was published as a small book summarizing their clinical investigations on serum sickness. Their interpretation of etiology spurred on research in allergy, which ultimately validated their novel notions.

The senior author was Clemens von Pirquet (1874–1929). He began his college education in theology and philosophy, but turned to medicine, completing his M.D. in 1900 at the University of Graz in Austria. The following year he served as Assistant to Theodor Escherich, a professor of pediatrics at the University of Vienna whose name is immortalized by the common intestinal and laboratory bacterium *Escherichia coli*. Pirquet was soon introduced to immunology in 1902, when he studied with Rudolf Kraus at the Serotherapeutic Institute. Pirquet's first observation of serum sickness following an inoculation of scarlet fever antiserum occurred at this time. In 1903 Pirquet, who was noted for his quick analytical mind, collaborated with Max von Gruber in criticizing Paul Ehrlich's method of quantifying antitoxins. That year he laid out the theory that would carry his research through the next decade. He declared that both the host and the foreign substance contribute to the incubation time of the given disease; that its manifestation was related to the presence of antibody; and that the time required for the formation of such antibodies governs the incubation time. Pirquet was not a microbiologist, and he seemed to ignore the direct tissue damage caused by microbial secretions. However, the concept of an immunological contribution to the disease was a correct and significant step forward. In 1908 he followed through on Koch's tuberculin report, developing an effective skin test for tuberculosis. After serving as Clinical Assistant at the Kinderklinik in Vienna from 1903 to 1909, he declined a clinically restrictive appointment at the Pasteur Institute to become the first professor of pediatrics at The Johns Hopkins University. Despite the pleas and efforts of the Johns Hopkins staff and alumni, he returned to Vienna in 1910 to become a professor at the University there. He had returned due to the incentive of a large salary increase and the opportunity to succeed Escherich. For the rest of his life Pirquet focused his research on nutrition and biostatistics. In 1929 his work at the University of Vienna came to a tragic, unexpected end when he and his wife committed suicide by swallowing cyanide.

Pirquet's associate and good friend, Bela Schick, also became a highly esteemed pediatrician. Born 1877 in Hungary, he also went to the University of Graz for his initial medical training, completed in 1900. Schick joined Pirquet at the University of Vienna, later becoming an adjunct professor and head of the Kinderklinik. In 1923 he emigrated to the United States to chair the Department of Pediatrics at Mount Sinai Hospital in New York City. A mild-mannered, humorous but rigorous teacher, Schick retired in 1942 and died in 1967.

In addition to his work on serum sickness, Schick is noted for the development in 1913 of a skin test (the Schick test) designed to ascertain susceptibility to diphtheria. Active immunization with toxin-antitoxin complexes had been introduced at this time. Schick had compassionately devised his method, using a very low dose of diphtheria toxin, in order to identify those patients who would not need the vaccine and, as later learned, risk the dissociation of the complex to free, active toxin.

In 1907 Schick accurately postulated the immunological origin of the delayed sequelae to streptococcal infections, which include rheumatic fever and glomerulonephritis. Like serum sickness, they are part of a systemic Arthus-type reaction, and hence are diseases caused by circulating immune complexes. The antitoxin-toxin unit *per se* is not involved in serum sickness; horse and other animal serum globulins are antigenic in humans. Experiments in animals have largely reproduced the effect, and acute and chronic forms, based either on single, large, or repetitive, small dose injections, are recognized. Inflammation of the heart arteries and glomerulonephritis are common complications resulting from the deposit of immune complexes and complement cascades along blood vessels.

For further information:

Gronowicz, A. 1954. *Bela Schick and the World of Children*. Abelard-Schuman, New York. 216 p.

Schick, B. 1967. Physiologic and pathologic allergy. In: *Reflection on Biologic Research* (G. Gabbiani, editor). Warren H. Green, St. Louis, pp. 180–190.

Wagner, R. 1968. *Clemens von Pirquet. His Life and Work*. Johns Hopkins Press, Baltimore. 214 p.

Wolf, I. J. 1965. *Aphorisms and Facetiae of Bela Schick*. Knoll Pharmaceutical Company, Orange, NJ. 50 p.

The Paper*

Among all of the symptoms following serum injections, the occurrence of rashes was so prevalent that all symptoms were named serum exanthema. . . .

*von Pirquet, C. and B. Schick. 1950. *Die Serumkrankheit*. Franz Denticke, Leipzig. 144 p. (Translated by B. Schick: Williams & Wilkins, Baltimore, 1951. 130 p., copyright by Williams & Wilkins.)

Besides the possibility of following the fate of the injected serum and the reaction of the organism to it, we have, in the study of this disease, the further advantage that we are able to vary voluntarily the amount of the pathogenic agents. We have abandoned the expression "serum exanthema" because we think that this name could easily lead to the idea that the rash was the most important symptom of the disease; in its place we have proposed the name "serum disease" or "serum sickness. . . . "

[T]he disease proper starts with an eruption of skin manifestations which almost always belong to the urticaria group. Generally they are first seen at the site of the injection and its neighborhood. The rash spreads rapidly over the body and is frequently found at the same time in symmetrical regions. . . . If the eruption of hives is very dense they may become confluent; then the whole environment appears infiltrated by edema. The edema may disfigure the face. The intensive itching makes the patient restless and unhappy.

All eruptions disappear quickly, the single urtica lasting only several hours, the whole eruption of hives rarely longer than 2 or 3 days. . . .

Meanwhile the temperature has risen to a more or less high figure, being a sign of the participation of the rest of the organism. . . . [T]he lymph nodes, regional to the site of the injection, become larger during the period of incubation. This swelling increases rapidly with the onset of the temperature and the rash and may later spread to other lymph glands of the organism. . . .

Whereas the symptoms mentioned are constant, all other symptoms are less frequent. Only the joint pain should be mentioned which due to its injury to the patient's general well-being was noticed from the beginning as one of the most striking symptoms. . . .

The serum sickness shares with many other diseases the peculiarity that the symptoms of the disease do not appear immediately after subcutaneous or intravenous introduction of the pathogenic agent. Between the injection of the agent and the appearance of clinical symptoms, an incubation time exists. . . .

Hartung has already observed that in more than half of his cases the serum symptoms did not appear until 10 days after injection. . . . The incubation period after reinjection is always shorter than after the first injection. . . .

The swelling of the glands [lymph nodes] precedes the onset of the disease and starts to recede before its termination. Herein, in this behavior of the lymph glands, lies its prognostic value. . . .

Those cases, in which any really more significant alteration in the leukocyte count occurred, showed a very uniform behavior. The leukocyte count rises moderately during the incubation period and suddenly falls considerably with the onset of the symptoms of serum sickness. The leukocyte curve reaches a low point from which the curve rises towards the end of the sickness to normal. . . .

[T]he intensive drop in the number of leukocytes is due almost exclusively to the reduction of the number of polynuclear cells. . . . The mononuclear cells seem to be at first sight rather unchanged. But upon closer examination we see that they are altered too. With the onset of the relative lymphocytosis many large mononuclear cells appear with broad protoplasma as well as transition forms, which disappear when the total number of leukocytes again rises. . . .

Those authors, who until now have studied serum sickness, did not pay special attention to the symptoms after reinjection, but dealt with them statistically and clinically in the same way as with the symptoms after the first injection. Likewise it was only in the course of our observations that our attention was drawn to the important difference between first and reinjection, which exist, mainly in connection with the time of onset and intensity of symptoms. . . .

What these cases have in common is that, after an immediate reaction, several days of complete latency follow, which period is concluded by an eruption of new symptoms on the 5th or 6th day. We encounter here again an incubation period which shows a substantial difference from the incubation time after the first injection; it is shortened. Another peculiarity . . . is revealed in the clinical picture: the accelerated reaction sets in with violent, frequently stormy symptoms, and is terminated more rapidly than the normally timed reaction after a first injection. . . .

The double picture of the "immediate" and "accelerated reaction" leads us to a third form of reaction observed in a reinjected person, which consists of the accelerated reaction only. The immediate reaction is left out. This picture is seen after a reinjection following a long interval. . . .

We possess, therefore in the immediate or accelerated reactivity, a new criterium for the diagnosis that a patient has formerly had the same disease. This statement is not only valid for serum sickness, but . . . for many other toxic and infectious diseases. We refer in this respect particularly to the behavior of the human to revaccination. The accelerated and modified reaction to smallpox vaccine proves a previously successfully performed first vaccination.

On the preceding pages we have limited ourselves to clinical observations and have purposely avoided mingling our theories with the facts. The difference in the reactivity between the first injection and the reinjection forced us to the formation of some the-

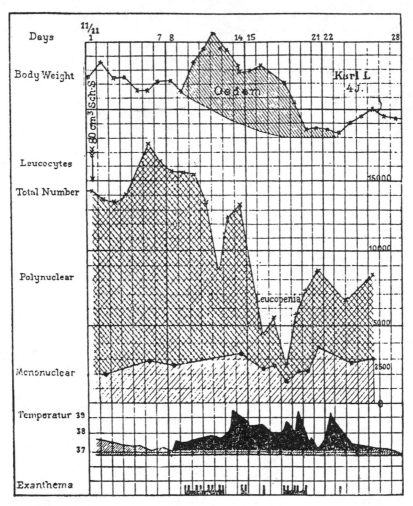

Chart XVIII The leukocyte count rises moderately during the incubation period and suddenly falls considerably with the onset of the symptoms of serum sickness.

oretical explanations of this difference. This difference could not be due to the antigen (injected serum) . . . since the same serum caused different kinds of and differently timed reactions, depending on whether it was injected into the organism for the first time or was reinjected. Thus we came to the conclusion that it was the human organism which has become specifically altered, due to the first injection of a foreign serum, and that it has acquired a new property in consequence of which the second reaction occurs more quickly than the first.

We now ask ourselves what kind of alterations developed in the organism after it was injected with a foreign serum. We know from the results of biological research, that specific substances are formed in the injected organism. When these substances are brought in contact with the antigen in a test tube, they bring about a precipitation. . . .

Hamburger and Moro were the first to prove that humans also form precipitins. . . . However they dropped this idea because Rostoski, Michaelis, and Oppenheimer proved that no precipitation takes place in the blood of living organisms. . . .

As we shall see later it is not simple to show a causal connection between precipitin formation and serum sickness. In most cases precipitin appear much later than the disease and even very intensive serum sickness symptoms run their course without the formation of precipitin. . . .

We therefore state the theory that there exists a causal connection between the formation of antibodies and disease, whereby we stress the point that we do not identify the term antibody with precipitin, on the contrary we give the term antibody a much wider meaning. . . .

The accelerated reaction differs from the normally timed reaction in that the antibodies are reproduced more quickly and therefore the disease starts earlier. The clinical observation of the accelerated reaction shows another analogy between antibody formation and disease. As the curve of precipitin after reinjection not only starts after a short incubation time but also rises more steeply and to a higher point, so the accelerated serum sickness starts not only more quickly but also more stormy.

On this basis a further characteristic sign of the immediate reaction can be understood, i.e., hypersensitiveness. . . .

Studies on supersensitivity

1921 • Carl Prausnitz and Heinz Küstner

Comment

Is food allergy an anaphylactic response, or is it another unique form of hypersensitivity? Carl Prausnitz (1876–1963) pondered this question when confronted with the extraordinary sensitivity to cooked fish of his associate, Heinz Küstner (1897–1963). The general symptoms and speed of inception strongly resembled the classic anaphylactic response, but attempts to find antibodies even by sensitive complement-fixation methods failed. Tests to passively sensitize guinea pigs to fish protein by transfer of Küstner's serum also yielded negative results.

Prausnitz and Küstner were cautious, avoiding any wild speculation. The two physicians recognized that their test system might not have been appropriate. Indeed, we now know that the responsible antibodies, initially called "atopic reagins" by Arthur F. Coca and E. F. Grove and later classified as immunoglobulin class E (IgE), were of insufficient concentration to be detected by the then current in-vitro techniques. In addition, guinea pig tissues will not bind human immunoglobulin; the only suitable animals are primates.

In the delightful milestone that follows, Prausnitz and Küstner describe their clever and elegantly simple approach to the problem. A healthy nonallergic human replaced the guinea pig, and both sensitization and initiation were by intradermal injections in the same area. Serum was thus demonstrated to contain the sensitizing substance, and food allergy, therefore, appeared to be a minor variant of classic anaphylaxis. A key point of differentiation is that anaphylaxis can be experimentally generated in nearly all individuals, while food sensitivity, hay fever, asthma, and allergy to animal dander naturally occur in only some 10 percent of humans. Other individuals can not acquire these disorders, which are categorized under "atopy." The term atopy, referring to strangeness, was first used by Coca upon the suggestion of Edward D. Perry. Atopic individuals generally have elevated levels of serum IgE, and are predisposed to chronic cutaneous fungal infections and other skin diseases.

One anomaly appears in Prausnitz and Küstner's report. They were unable to demonstrate passive cutaneous anaphylaxis to hay fever-inducing pollen. Aware of the inconsistency, they suggested that sera from more sensitive persons may provide positive results. However, Coca and E. F. Grove in 1925, carrying on this research, found another explanation. They determined that about 11 percent of people can not be sensitized by the injection of atopic serum, and another 5 percent are only weakly receptive. Prausnitz and Küstner probably had encountered such an unreceptive subject in their attempts to transfer pollen sensitivity.

Atopy is commonly ascertained by skin tests, performed by patch application, scratching in, or intradermal injections of sets of antigens, also known as allergens. The P-K test, as it became known, is used to screen young children or patients with disseminated skin disease. Monkeys are the preferred passive subjects.

Küstner, who became a professor of obstetrics and gynecology at the University of Leipzig, contributed no other study on immunology. Prausnitz in 1926 rose to the rank of professor at the Hygiene Institute of the University at Breslau, continuing his research in allergy. In 1933 he left Germany for England, where he established a general practice. Prausnitz adopted his mother's maiden name, Giles, in 1939 when he became a British citizen.

For further information:

Coca, A. F. 1951. The development of theories of familial allergies. *CIBA Symposia* 11:1390–1397; 1412.

Middleton, E., Jr., C. E. Reed, and E. F. Ellis (editors). 1983. *Allergy: Principles and Practice*, 2nd edition. C. V. Mosby Company, St. Louis. 1440 p.

The Paper*

Among the idiosyncracies to food stuffs, the supersensitivity to fish has so far received little attention. Since one of us (K.) suffers from this affection, we took this opportunity of investigating the mechanism

----

*Prausnitz, C. and H. Küstner. 1921. Studien über die Ueberempfindlichkeit. *Zentralblat für Bakteriologie, Parasitenkunde, Infektionskrankheiten und Hygiene*. Abteilung 1. 86:160–169. [Translated by C. Prausnitz, in: *Clinical Aspects of Immunology* (P. G. H. Gell and R. R. A. Coombs, editors). Blackwell Scientific Publications, Oxford, 1962. pp. 808–816; with permission of Gustav Fischer Verlag and Blackwell Scientific Publications.]

of the reaction and the serological conditions concerned. In the course of the work, a series of controlled tests were carried out on the other one (P.), who is a hay fever patient; and on several nonsensitive colleagues. . . .

The active substance appears to occur practically only in the muscle flesh of bony fish. It occupies a peculiar position among the agents of supersensitivity, since for our patient fish is completely harmless in the raw state and only becomes poisonous when heated (cooked, baked or fried).

Starting from these observations it was first tried to produce the signs of supersensitivity by parenteral administration of the fish antigen. A standard solution was prepared by mincing fresh marine fish (usually haddock), boiling it in ten times its weight of distilled water, filtering through paper and sterilizing the filtrate for half an hour in the steam sterilizer. The clear, nonopalescent fluid thus obtained proved inactive on the patient's conjunctiva, but highly active on intradermal injection. After intradermal injection of 0.1 cc of the standard solution (the utmost care being taken to avoid subcutaneous injection) there developed at the site of injection within 10 minutes a very itching wheal which rapidly, under our eyes, grew to about 4 cm in diameter. The fully developed wheal was raised high about the surrounding skin, white, with an indented margin; it was surrounded by a deep red flare about 10 cm wide. After 20 minutes there developed the syndrome of severe generalized intoxication . . . (urticaria of the entire body, intense congestion of the conjunctivae and upper air passages, irritating cough, dyspnoea). The generalized signs, which we were able to produce repeatedly in the same form, gradually faded away after several hours. Subcutaneous injection of 1 mg atropine sulphate quickly and completely relieves the respiratory symptoms, 0.1 mg "suprarenin" the urticaria. But even after a day, sometimes even 2 days, edematous infiltration of the injection site persists. . . .

With hay fever similar severe reactions have been described by Dunbar, Prausnitz and others after subcutaneous injection of the active pollen protein. But according to our investigations the same severe syndrome can be produced even by the intradermal injection of pollen protein. . . .

In view of the strictly specific character of the reaction described, the serum of the supersensitive individual was tested for the presence of antibodies. With the most varied testing arrangements it was impossible to demonstrate in vitro precipitins or complement-binding substances in [the subject's] serum or in that of normal persons.

Following the observation of Bauer that in serum sickness the patient's serum agglutinates the corresponding erythrocytes, we tested our patient's serum for activity against fish red blood corpuscles, but with no result. Nor could we discover in a test on the human being any neutralizing substances in the serum. . . .

These results show a close agreement with the similar behavior of pollen protein in the hay fever patient. . . . Both substances are strictly specific for the corresponding supersensitive person, although they show a considerable quantitative difference in their active dose. . . .

The reactions observed show a remarkable resemblance to those of genuine anaphylaxis. True, there is one difference: in fish- and pollen-supersensitive persons, after intradermal injection the reaction sets in almost without any incubation period—within a few minutes—and fades relatively soon; in the person sensitive to serum or tuberculin the intradermal reaction only begins after several hours and remains at its height for days. Still, these differences might only be of a quantitative nature. Whether the forms of supersensitivity discussed here comes under the heading of true anaphylaxis would most readily be decided if they could be passively transferred to nonsusceptible beings. In guinea pigs it was possible to produce passive anaphylaxis by intraperitoneal injection (1 to 2 cc) of the fish-supersensitive patient's serum followed 24 hours later by intravenous injection of 0.5 cc standard fish solution. . . . The attempt was therefore made to transfer the supersensitive state passively to nonsusceptible human beings. The technique used in guinea pigs was out of the question, since corresponding to the weight of the individual to be tested far too much serum would have to be taken from the donor, and above all because of the danger of producing a severe anaphylactic shock. We therefore tried to localize the anaphylactic reaction within the skin by injecting both reactants (serum and antigen) intradermally into the same spot of skin.

1. Mixtures of standard fish solution with the fish-sensitive patient's serum in varying proportions, injected intradermally to normal persons in 0.1 cc amounts, were inactive. . . .

3. A positive result was only achieved when, conforming exactly to the passive anaphylactic experiment in the guinea pig, the serum was first injected intradermally and the standard fish solution was injected the following day into the same spot of skin.

On July 19th, 1920, a person not sensitive to fish solution received into the abdominal skin intradermal injections of 0.1 cc of the following substances:

(1) Serum of the fish-sensitive patient, undiluted;

(2) Serum of the fish-sensitive patient, diluted 1 in 10;

(3) Serum of the fish-sensitive patient, diluted 1 in 100;

(4) Serum of a healthy person, free from any idiosyncrasy;

(5) Normal saline solution.

On July 20th, 1920, 0.1 cc of standard fish solution was injected into each of these spots and (6) into an untreated spot of skin. . . .

After 15 minutes a marked subjective and objective reaction was present only in the spots 1, 2, and 3 pretreated with the specific serum. It was strongest where the undiluted serum had been administered. The control wheals 4, 5, and 6 showed only a trifling traumatic reaction.

After 1 hour the wheal and flare in the skin spots 1, 2, and 3, pretreated with specific serum, were still about the same size as after 15 minutes, but already the border between wheal and flare had become indistinct and the flare was starting to fade. On the next day there was still in these spots the distinct edema which was always seen in the fish-sensitive patient after intradermal injection of the fish antigen. But the spots 4, 5 and 6 remained free from any trace of oedema.

The experiment was repeated in this person, who incidentally is supersensitive to pollen, and in two others, one male and one female, who are free from any idiosyncrasy; the result was the same. . . .

It has thus been proved by this test that, according to the technique which we have elaborated, the state of supersensitivity can be transferred passively to normal persons by the serum of the supersensitive individual.

It had now become obvious to try out the technique in other forms of supersensitivity. For this purpose we chose hay fever and sensitivity to tuberculin and to horse serum. In all of them the result of numerous tests was negative. . . .

Agammaglobulinemia

1952 • Ogden C. Bruton

Comment

A common expression declares that the exception proves the rule, i.e., insight into a complex general mechanism may be attained by ascertaining the reasons why the more accessible exception exists. Typically it is a matter of an aberrant component. Bruton's agammaglobulinemia, the first scientifically established immunodeficiency disease, was the start of a wonderful stream of discoveries that led to the recognition of the two main branches of interacting lymphocytes, the B and T cells.

Ogden C. Bruton (1907–   ) was a senior military physician at Walter Reed Army Medical Center. In the paper that follows, he summarized the case history of a young boy who suffered recurrent bacterial infections. The child's inability to produce antibodies against these infectious agents or upon injections of vaccines was strikingly verified by electrophoretic analysis. The entire gamma fraction of serum was absent. The child apparently could not produce antibodies against any foreign substance. However, in later studies with more sensitive techniques, researchers detected trace amounts of immunoglobulins.

Within four years of this publication, physicians found 40 more children who were suffering this deficiency. Further investigations correlated with absence of antibodies with the lack of plasma cells (fully developed B lymphocytes). Two remarkable anomalies also surfaced: the children seemed to resist viral infections as well as their healthy playmates did, and they demonstrated normal delayed-hypersensitivity responses, including the rejection of allogeneic skin grafts. Immunity, which first was considered a single mechanism, if excluding phagocytes, now appeared to be divided into at least two distinct arms. Bruton's agammaglobulinemia soon was recognized as a congenital disease when all the cases were found to occur in boys. It is a sex-linked recessive characteristic with women as carriers of the trait.

Bruton's successful, athough temporary, treatment of his patient by injections of gamma globulin allowed a quantitative study of the amount of gamma globulin required to resist bacterial infections. Results indicated that the level can drop to about 17 percent of normal before a serious hazard arises.

Now attuned to the possibility of immunological deficiency as the underlying etiology to a variety of disorders, physicians quickly added new types to a still expanding list: Patients with Nezelof syndrome, another congenital disorder, have normal antibody production; it is cell-mediated immunity that they lack. The same conditions occur in the DiGeorge syndrome, which is noted by the congenital absence of the thymus. Other patients were unable to produce a single class of immunoglobulin, and some chronic infections were linked to failures in phagocytic activity. Recently it has been established that in certain hypogammaglobulinemias, B cells are present, but the disorder affects a particular population of T cells that governs the activation of B lymphocytes. Swiss-type Agammaglobulinemia is characterized by combined immune deficiency. Such a lethal condition was also found by Robert A. Good in 1952 in one of his patients, who had a thymus tumor. Normal hypogammaglobulinemia occurs in neonates, whose cellular development remains inadequate for antibody production until about four months of age; the infants are protected by maternally acquired antibodies. Transitory immune deficiency can also occur with certain infections and malignancies, such as Hodgkin's disease. And then there is acquired immune deficiency syndrome (AIDS), a venereal disease whose viral agent attacks, among other targets, a subset of T lymphocytes.

Images of David, "the boy in a bubble," a victim of combined immune deficiency who for years resided in a large, sealed, environmentally controlled chamber in vain attempt to avoid contact with pathogenic microorganisms, and the societal hysteria arising in response to the epidemic of AIDS, whose mortality rate compares to rabies, underscore the protective power of the immune response. We have seen in the previous milestones how enhanced immunological activity can be a seasonal or an avoidable nuisance and only rarely a lethal threat; chronic immunodeficiency, however, is deadly. The loss of immunity is tantamount to a loss of physiological self-nonself differentiation. The physical integrity of the individual is thus not only at risk, open to microorganisms and aberrant constitutive cells, but the pattern of individuality is also gravely challenged. If such a condition prevails, organismal death occurs.

For further information:

Fettner, A. G. and W. A. Check. 1985. *The Truth About AIDS. Evolution of an Epidemic.* 2nd edition. Henry Holt and Company, New York. 306 p.

Gitlin, D. and C. A. Janeway. 1957. Agammaglobulinemia. *Scientific American* 197(1):93–104.

Gold, E. 1974. Infections associated with immunologic deficiency diseases. *Medical Clinics of North America* 58:649–659.

Seligmann, M., H. H. Fudenberg, and R. A. Good. 1968. A proposed classification of primary immunologic deficiencies. *American Journal of Medicine* 45:817–825.

Shilts, R. 1987. *And the Band Played On: Politics, People, and the AIDS Epidemic.* St. Martin's Press, New York. 630 p.

The Paper*

The complete absence of gamma globulin in human serum with a normal total protein as determined by electrophoretic analysis does not appear to have as yet been reported in the literature. Stern mentions two cases of hypoproteinemia in children who had "almost complete absence of gamma globulin and were singularly free from infection." Schick reported a similar congenital case without nephrosis with a review of the literature in which the total protein was low, the gamma globulin fraction low, and edema present. The latter findings in nephrosis are well known. Krebs reported a case in which there was a "depression of gamma globulin in hypoproteinemia due to malnutrition." The present author had the opportunity of following a patient without nephrotic syndrome, with normal nutrition, with complete absence of the gamma globulin fraction and normal total serum protein through several years of many infections, including 19 episodes of clinical sepsis in which some type pneumococcus was recovered by blood culture 10 times. This entity, which, it was found, could be controlled by supplying gamma globulin as contained in concentrated immune human serum globulin, appears to be unique.

The 8-year-old male was first admitted to this hospital at the age of 4½ years. His past history was rather normal. He had varicella 8 months before admission with uneventful recovery and rubeola complicated by pneumonia 6 months previously. His birth and developmental history were entirely normal and a general survey of the major systems revealed nothing of note. The family history revealed no deviation from normal and a 1-year-old sibling was in good health. He was considered a normal and healthy child until 2 nights before admission when he came in from play and had a short shaking chill followed by a rise in temperature to 38.1°C. The next day he vomited. His fever continued and he complained of pain in the left knee. . . .

His hemogram showed RBC count 4.2 million/cmm, Hgb. 12.4/100 cc, WBC count 16.4 thousand/cmm, with 88% neutrophiles (5 stabs), 8% lymphocytes and 4% monocytes. Urine was normal. Blood culture was negative after 10 days' incubation. RGs of both lower extremities including hips were normal. ECG was normal.

The impression was that he had either a septic joint or osteomyelitis. After the initial studies, he was given penicillin. . . .

*Bruton, O. C. 1953. Agammaglobulinemia. *Pediatrics* 9:722–728. [Reproduced by permission of Pediatrics.]

He remained well at home for approximately 2 weeks at which time he developed an upper respiratory infection which is said to have developed into pneumonia. [The account follows with further episodes of infectious disease symptoms, which were treated by antibiotics.]. . . .

During the admission he was thoroughly studied for any possible focus of infection or other pathology by systematically going through each system. These studies included ear, nose, and throat surveys with RGs of sinuses and mastoids, dental examination with RGs, spinal tap, skull RG, EEG, ECG, bronchograms, intravenous pyelograms, repeated urine examinations, urine cultures, stool cultures and examination for ova and parasites, blood chemistry including urea nitrogen, serum protein, chlorides, CO_2 combining power, sugar, bromosulphalein liver function test, sedimentation rate, febrile agglutinations, antistreptolyin titer, Brucellergin and tuberculin skin tests, malaria thick drop preparation, and complete roentgenographic skeletal survey. . . .

The first approach to this problem was by a thorough search for foci of infection. However, with different organisms being isolated, one had to hypothecate the existence of a mutation of organism, and in the absence of demonstrable focus this possibility seemed highly untenable. . . .

When he repeated the same type organism in an illness, it was suggested that he failed to build antibodies for that particular organism and an autogenous vaccine was prepared of pneumococci. This

was given over a planned period of 5 months, but no antibody titer could be demonstrated in his blood serum at the end of this period. . . . It seemed possible that such a prepared vaccine would not contain sufficient immunizing antigen, i.e., the polysaccharides. Consequently the pneumococcal polysaccharide solution of Squibb, containing types I, II, III, V, VII and VIII in one for adults and types I, IV, VI, XIV, XVII and XIX in the other for children, were given at spaced intervals. Again no pneumococcus type antibody could be demonstrated in the patient's serum.

The question naturally arose then as to whether he could build antibodies against any organism. A Schick test was positive at 8 years of age, although the patient had had a diphtheria toxoid series administered in infancy and had booster doses at 3 years of age and again at 6. A third and fourth booster dose failed to produce a negative Schick test. His blood likewise failed to show typhoid antibodies following administration of typhoid vaccine in the usual manner. . . .

With this apparent constant inability to produce antibodies it was suggested that one might expect some derangement in the gamma globulin fraction. By electrophoretic analysis of his blood serum, his blood repeatedly gave completely negative results for gamma globulin. The total serum protein and A–G ratio were entirely normal.

The absence of gamma globulin gave the most hopeful clue to a possible prophylaxis. Accordingly

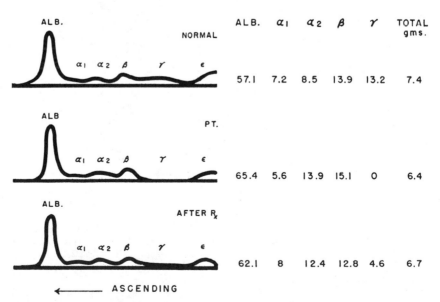

ALB.	α_1	α_2	β	γ	TOTAL gms.
57.1	7.2	8.5	13.9	13.2	7.4
65.4	5.6	13.9	15.1	0	6.4
62.1	8	12.4	12.8	4.6	6.7

Figure 2 Normal electrophoretic pattern compared with that of patient before and after giving gamma globulin.

he was given subcutaneously immune human serum globulin 20 cc containing 3.2 g gamma globulin. Six days later a surprisingly large amount of gamma globulin was demonstrated in his blood serum by electrophoretic analysis. The gamma globulin content of his blood serum was then followed at approximately weekly intervals for the next 6 weeks and . . . there was a gradual loss to negative results. . . .

For the past 14 months the patient has had monthly injections of gamma globulin, without benefit of other prophylactic measures, and has suffered no attack of sepsis.

With the demonstration of the absence of gamma globulin, and the apparent control of infection by furnishing gamma globulin, there seems little doubt of the existence of a direct relationship in this case. It is not possible to present a proved cause for the defective protein fraction. However, two possibilities seem apparent: (1) a congenital dysfunction in the mechanism of gamma globulin production and (2) an acquired dysfunction in this mechanism. The fact that the patient survived 4½ years and without severe infection appears to make the first unlikely. Although no abnormality has been demonstrated in his liver or reticuloendothelial system, we must assume that a functional abnormality exists if we are to accept the present-day thinking as to the production of immune bodies. Felton has postulated such an acquired dysfunction in man, and in mice has produced "immunological paralysis" by an appropriate dose of antigenic polysaccharide. It may then be postulated that this patient's antibody mechanism has by some influence been altered so that it is no longer able to synthesize and/or hold antibody to a specific organism. . . .

On paroxysmal hemoglobinuria

1904 • Julius Donath and Karl Landsteiner

Comment

Oh, what a curious phenomenon! Paroxysmal hemoglobinuria, more common in the nineteenth century than now, is characterized by a series of recurrent attacks whose result is the discharge of massive amounts of hemoglobin, not intact red blood cells, into the urine. The attacks begin when a patient's external tissues are exposed to cold temperatures; drinking cold beverages will not trigger the response, but making a snowman will. Other symptoms include gastrointestinal pain, headache, weakness, fever, and chills. Paroxysmal hemoglobinuria was the first autoimmune disease to be identified and examined in detail.

As for many diseases, recognition of the specific disorder had to emerge from a background of similar blood-related phenomena. By 1866 W. W. Gull established the link with chilling, and in 1880 O. Rosenbach instituted differential diagnosis: He artificially induced an attack by immersing the patient's feet in ice water for 10 minutes. The previous year B. Küssner ascertained that hemolysis took place within the blood vessels rather than in the kidney or urinary tract. The last important fact leading to the following milestone was that most patients also had syphilis. Later, with the development of the Wassermann test, over 90 percent of cases were found to be syphilitic, especially congenitally.

Julius Donath (1870–1950), Assistant at the University of Vienna First Medical Clinic, and Karl Landsteiner (1868–1943), working at the University Institute of Pathological Anatomy, collaborated on this investigation of the mechanism of cold-induced hemolysis. Landsteiner is a giant in the annals of immunology; three other reports of his can be found elsewhere in this book. After earning his doctorate in general medicine in 1891 with emphasis in chemistry, Landsteiner continued his education in organic chemistry under Emil Fischer and Eugen von Bamberger among others. When in 1896 he accepted the appointment of Assistant in Max von Gruber's Institute of Hygiene, he entered the realm of immunology and serology, which remained his life work. Two years afterward, Landsteiner transferred to pathology. Donath, who received his own medical degree in 1896, was a clinical investigator. After two years at the Vienna Poliklinik and nine years at the First Medical Clinic, he continued medical service and teaching at various hospitals in Vienna. Donath and Landsteiner co-authored nine papers.

Their report on paroxysmal hemoglobinuria has the stamp of Landsteiner's caution and typical thoroughness. The experimental design was varied to test the role of each component and each physical condition. Complement was the hemolytic trigger, but what was the primer? Sensitization of erythrocytes seemed to occur only in cold temperatures; hemolysis appeared only after warming. Two years earlier Landsteiner had encountered the quirks of cold agglutinins to erythrocytes: The readily visible clumps that formed in the cold would disperse even at room temperature. The two phenomena seemed to be similar, although the hemolytic reaction was more complex.

We know today that the cold-sensitive antibodies, as well as the antibodies of the Coombs test, a diagnostic test for autoimmune hemolytic anemia, have different low affinities for the erythrocytes. Antibody avidity, or strength of bonding, and distribution and concentration of accessible antigens on the erythrocyte surface differentiate the responses. Thermodynamics is the first factor: complexes of Coombs antibodies and their antigen on or adsorbed onto erythrocytes are unable to form strong bridges, requiring the intervention of rabbit anti-human antibodies to link and agglutinate the red blood cells. Some reactions occur only in the cold because cellular antigens are hidden at higher temperatures. Other cold reactants, whether able to bridge—for agglutination—or not—for sensitization—are insufficiently avid to endure the enhanced molecular agitation resulting from increased heat. Yet it is this heat that is required for complement proteins to effectively penetrate and rupture the erythrocyte membrane.

Subsequent studies of paroxysmal hemoglobinuria determined that erythrocytes of all blood types are susceptible and that natural isohemolysins are not involved. While most cold antibodies are of the IgM class, Donath-Landsteiner antibodies are IgG. As Landsteiner believed, complement (the first components) stabilizes the association of sensitizing antibody and blood cell at cold temperatures; in its absence some dissociation occurs when the temperature is raised. With warmth, the remaining complement cascade is activated.

The relationship with syphilis is the most mysterious aspect of this disease. A higher correlation of the disorder exists with congenital than acquired syphilis. In 1926 M. Namba developed an interesting model by injecting emulsions of guinea pig organs into rabbits, which subsequently produced cold hemolysins and became Wassermann positive. Ten years later, Landsteiner suggested that following infection with syphilis autoimmunization occurs against components of infection-altered tissues. The low affinity of these anti-self antibodies suggests that they are merely cross-reactive to normal cells.

The origin of any autoimmune disease has yet to be satisfactorily explained. The small percentage of cases of paroxysmal hemoglobinuria not associated with syphilis are most likely a result of somatic mutation, perhaps involving T suppressor cells. Current speculation considers low-level autoimmunity as a normal, indeed integral, activity within the immune response.

For further information:

Glynn, L. E. and E. J. Holborow. 1965. *Autoimmunity and Disease*. Blackwell Scientific Publications, Oxford. 420 p.

Heidelberger, M. 1969. Karl Landsteiner. June 14, 1868–June 26, 1943. *National Academy of Sciences Biographical Memoirs* 40:177–210.

Mackenzie, G. M. 1929. Paroxysmal hemoglobinuria. *Medicine* 8:159–191.

Roitt, I. M. 1984. *Essential Immunology,* 5th edition. Blackwell Scientific Publications, Oxford. 369 p.

Silverstein, A. M. 1986. The Donath-Landsteiner autoantibody: the incommensurable languages of early immunologic dispute. *Cellular Immunology* 97:173–188.

The Paper*

Different theories have been proposed to explain the pathogenesis of paroxysmal hemoglobinuria, a peculiar illness whose attack under the influence of cold leads to hemoglobinuria and removal of blood pigment through the urine.

Other, older explanations state that hemoglobinuria is caused by the destruction of blood corpuscles in the kidney. Since the only evidence during an attack consists of hemoglobinemia, the cause of the illness was changed to the blood. Hemolysis itself was declared to depend on different factors. The original assumption that cold destroys the more sensitive blood corpuscles has been contradicted by the fact that the blood of these ill people in vitro is not more sensitive to the influence of cold than normal blood. Therefore, research had to be conducted to find other causes of the blood decomposition. Of course, the extended studies of the last few years on blood toxins supported the assumption that this illness is caused by hemolysin. . . .

Different sides declared that hemolysis could or could not be observed when serum from the hemoglobinuria patients during the attack or from the attack-free interval are mixed and incubated with their own or foreign erythrocytes. . . . Donath examined these contradictory statements in a large experimental series with three cases of hemoglobinuria (the same three on which the following examinations have been carried out), but he was unable to show a lytic influence on their own erythrocytes using either the interval serum or the attack serum. After trying various combinations of hemoglobinuric se-

rum and foreign blood corpuscles, a weak lytic activity of the interval serum for foreign erythrocytes occurred. The so-called isolysis also appeared with normal sera. No increase of this activity occurred during the attack. The erythrocytes of the three cases of hemoglobinuria did not differ from other erythrocytes in their behavior toward foreign human sera. . . .

The only abnormality that could be discovered in the blood of most of these patients is the greater mechanical destruction of their corpuscles. . . .

In the experiments to be described . . . We used a method that allows a quite far-reaching analysis of the event of blood decomposition by hemoglobinuria. This method led to the certain result that this dissolution is caused by hemolysin.

The experiment was a simple initiation in vitro of the conditions occurring during an attack. With blood cells added to a calcium oxalate solution or a mixture of serum and erythrocytes removed from hemoglobinurics during an attack-free period, one can store the blood for a long duration in cold or warm temperature without the appearance of hemolysis. A totally different result was obtained when the oxalated blood or blood with serum was cooled first and then placed into the incubator. In this experiment, which we carried out on the three patients, intensive hemolysis appeared regularly. . . .

As an example, the following experiments are given:

Oxalated blood from Case K—Tube A is placed in ice water for 1/2 hr and then incubated for 2 hr; Tube B is placed in the incubator with Tube A, without being cooled previously. After sedimentation, the liquid in tube A is ruby red and in tube B it is pure yellow.

Serum from Case N—15 drops of serum + 5 drops with 0.85% NaCl solution of washed erythrocytes (dense pellet). Tubes A and B are heated as above. After the sedimentation of the blood cells, the liquid in A is ruby red and in B, pure yellow.

This dissolution is not the consequence of the temperature change because when washed erythrocytes from the same cases were alone subjected to the same temperature changes, not the least dissolution appeared. It is much easier to accept that in this experiment the serum is an important factor. Heating these sera can abolish the hemolysis. . . .

After heating for 1/4 hr, the temperature for total inactivation for the same volume of oxalated solution of diluted plasma lies between 45° and 55°C, but already at 45° a remarkable decrease of activity takes place.

This behavior corresponds totally to the one of the thermosensitive portions of lytic sera, so that hemolysis in our experiments should be regarded as

*Donath, J. and K. Landsteiner. 1904. Ueber paroxysmale Hämoglobinurie. *Muenchener Medizinische Wochenschrift* 51:1590–1593. [With permission.]

a so-called complement activity. The following experiment can be used as proof:

Tube A: 20 drops of oxalated blood placed 1/2 hr in ice water, then 2 hr at 37°C.

Tube B: The same quantity of oxalated blood kept at 37°C for 3 hr.

Tube C: The same volume of oxalated blood placed 1/2 hr in ice water; after centrifugation, plasma is withdrawn and replaced with 1% NaCl solution; tubes are then incubated for 2 hr.

Tube D: As with tube C, but with inactivated serum and NaCl solution.

Tube E: As with tube C, but with oxalated plasma of a normal individual.

Tube F: As with tube E, plasma from normal subject.

Tube G: As with tube E, plasma from another normal person.

Result: Color of liquid—(A) ruby red, (B) pure yellow, (C) colorless, (D) pure yellow, (E, F, G) ruby red.

[The series] shows that cold blood corpuscles mixed with plasma later dissolve when warmed in untreated plasma, but not in NaCl solution, nor in inactivated serum. It also should be stated that it did not occur even when the serum was diluted with NaCl solution 4–8 fold as before. The mutual cooling of erythrocytes and serum (or plasma) of the hemoglobinurics is sufficient to make the erythrocytes susceptible to dissolution through active serum (or plasma) of other individuals. (The cooling of the blood-free plasma from patients has as little hemolytic effect as the cooling of serum-free erythrocytes from these cases.)

The result also is analogous to the phenomenon that can be observed with hemolytic sera. It is now established that the whole hemolytic reaction in this experiment occurs in 2 phases. The second part of the process takes place on heating, and here the serum of the patients can be replaced with any other human serum. The question arises whether the same is true for the first phase, and if here the presence of patient erythrocytes or serum or both are necessary.

This question could easily be answered, when, on one hand, centrifuged washed erythrocytes of hemoglobinurics were brought together with other human sera and, on the other hand, patient sera were brought together with the blood cells of other people, both sets, as described before, first cooled and then heated. The experiment gave an unambiguous result. . . .

It showed that in this experimental design erythrocytes of other individuals are lysed by the serum of hemoglobinurics, even if present in a smaller amount than normal; whereas with foreign serum, the cooled erythrocytes of the patients do not dissolve when heated. Therefore, the peculiar attribute of hemoglobinuric blood that causes the dissolution befits the serum (or plasma), even when the erythrocytes can be lysed easier (as in our Case K). The serum (plasma) of the patients contains a lytic substance that works on their own and foreign blood corpuscles. This lysin cannot be demonstrated by directly mixing together the hemoglobinuric serum with blood cells, but it can be after considering the temperature-dependence of its activity.

For a better clarification of the cold-associated reaction, we carried out the following experiments. We took 2 equal portions of oxalated blood from patient K, cooling one for 1/2 hour in ice water and keeping the other at room temperature; then both tubes were centrifuged, the first being at 0°C. The plasma of both were removed and exchanged, and after mixing, the tubes were placed in the incubator. When observing them after 2 hr, the tube that contained the erythrocytes that were present with the previously cooled plasma showed a very strong hemolysis; the other tube showed none at all. The experiment indicates that the erythrocytes take out an active substance from the plasma in the cold, and shows that neither the red blood cells nor the leukocytes supply a hemolysin to the serum.

The following experimental design led to the same result: Oxalated blood of the patients were cooled in ice water for 1/2 hr, and then under ice water centrifuged. The removed plasma was added to [ambient] blood cells of the same individual. When the mixtures were cooled and then heated, no dissolution took place as would usually occur under the same conditions. . . . The appearance corresponds to the absorption of a hemolysin by the [first] cells. The amount of hemolysin on the cells can, as described above, bring about the effect in the presence of any active human serum.

Analysis of our experiments led us to the following conclusion: During cooling of the serum or plasma of hemoglobinuria patients, the given erythrocytes, be they self or foreign, take up a substance through whose absorption they become capable of lysing in not only the patient serum, but also in other human sera. The act of dissolution occurs with the help of agents in the serum, designated as complement (alexine, cytase, etc.).

To explain this process, one can call up already known phenomena. Through the studies of one of us, it has been established that agglutinations are often dissociated, and that active substances of the serum, namely agglutinin, can be absorbed better by cells when the temperature is decreased. In an examined case of isoagglutination, this behavior appears even more so, since the agglutination is only possible at a low temperature and not observed at body temperature. In this reaction dissociation increases with a rise of temperature. . . .

For lysis of the erythrocytes to be possible, it seems necessary that the substance absorbed during cooling, under natural conditions as well as in our experiments, does not leave the cells upon heating. Since blood dissolution really occurs, it led us to conclude that a reversal of the process on warming does not take place or only to a small extent. In the meantime, the thermolabile substances of the serum, the complement, approach the union of erythrocytes and poison and prevent their separation. . . . It is also possible that the complex of poison and erythrocytes, once built, can not be separated anymore, so that the process of binding is not totally reversible. . . .

An objection to our equivalency of experimental conditions with those of an attack could be stated by the fact that under natural conditions the cooling of a part of the body to 0°C does not happen. In regard to this we tried to determine the temperature limit that needs to be reached to allow dissolution in vitro. . . . Since, when cooling to 10°C . . . a high level of hemolysis could be observed, it is clear that this temperature does not represent the upper border, and that in suitable cases at considerably higher temperatures the described mechanism of hemolysis occurs, too. In one case . . . we also observed a trace of dissociation when erythrocytes, which were mixed with serum for a while at room temperature, were heated to 37°C. . . .

We now come to the question of the source of the lytic substance in the blood of hemoglobinuria patients, but we are not yet able to give an explanation. Obviously, the tissue origin of the patient himself can be taken into consideration as can an exogenous origin, probably in connection with an enduring infection, perhaps syphilis. . . .

Chronic thyroiditis and autoimmunization

1957 • Ernest Witebsky, Noel R. Rose, Kornel Terplan, John R. Paine, and Richard W. Egan

Comment

Within the same year two research groups, representing each side of the Atlantic, independently established Hashimoto's chronic thyroiditis as an autoimmune disease. Their respective reports follow. The first team approached the subject as a scientific study of autoimmunity, selecting thyroglobulin as a unique candidate and developing an animal model. The other team examined patients, utilizing the immunochemical techniques then available to identify the associated antigen, thyroglobulin. Together, these articles pioneered the methodology and strategy for understanding autoimmune processes. They also nicely demonstrate that there is more than one path to the solution of a scientific problem, particularly when serendipity lends a hand.

In 1912 H. Hashimoto, a Japanese surgeon, first described the lymphoid goiter or struma. The disorder is noted by the infiltration of mononuclear cells and the progressive destruction of the follicular cells and germinal centers of the organ. Inflammation and regeneration produce the indurated tissue. Hashimoto's thyroiditis, like similar autoimmune diseases of the thyroid gland, chiefly affects women aged over 30, especially those aged over 50. It has a genetic rather than an infectious origin. Predisposition in certain families was acutely verified by the acquisition of the disease in two sets of uniovular twins.

Ernest Witebsky (1901–1969), Noel R. Rose (1927–   ), and colleagues had come to this study by examining immunological tolerance.

This term refers to the failure of the immune system to recognize a normally foreign antigen. Several experimental ploys can produce this condition. One involves the continuing presence of low levels of the antigen. These researchers considered that tolerance to self antigens might have a similar origin. They thus removed the thyroid from rabbits, and after a suitable cleansing period, injected thyroglobulin, the iodine-containing hormone specific to the thyroid gland, back into the animals. Their working hypothesis collapsed, since tolerance was not broken even after using Freund's adjuvant. However, minor disappointment turned to pleasant surprise when the control rabbits, those with an intact thyroid, developed antibodies and thyroiditis. Their report, which is presented next, concludes with four criteria for establishing an autoimmune etiology of a disease, much like the famous four postulates of Robert Koch, which pertain to infectious diseases.

Witebsky, who attended the University of Frankfurt from 1920 to 1925 and earned his M.D. at the University of Heidelberg in 1926, emigrated to the United States in 1934. He joined the bacteriology faculty at the University of Buffalo in 1936, rising to Professor four years later. He served as Dean of the medical school in 1960. His colleague Rose graduated from Yale University in 1948. Three years later Rose completed his Ph.D. at the University of Pennsylvania, and in 1964 he attained the M.D. at the Buffalo campus of the State University of New York, where he advanced to Professor. In 1973 Rose became the chairman of the Department of Immunology and Microbiology at Wayne State University, and is presently at The Johns Hopkins University School of Medicine. He has maintained his interest in autoimmunity throughout his career.

For further information:

Allison, A. C. 1976. Self-tolerance and autoimmunity in the thyroid. *New England Journal of Medicine* 295:821–827.

Glynn, L. E. and E. J. Hoborow. 1965. *Autoimmunity and Disease.* Blackwell Scientific Publications, Oxford. 420 p.

Rose, N. R. 1981. Autoimmune disease. *Scientific American* 244(2):80–103.

Rose, N. R. and I. R. Mackay (editors). 1985. *The Autoimmune Diseases.* Academic Press, Orlando. 727 p.

The Paper*

For many years only foreign proteins were considered to be true antigens. Horse serum, for instance, proved to be a powerful antigen when injected into human beings, but it did not elicit antibody formation when injected into horses. . . . Landsteiner's discovery of the human blood groups revealed the fact that agglutinins directed against blood group factors within the human race but not within the same individual are present in human serums. Such antibodies have been called isoantibodies. Ehrlich and Morgenroth succeeded in producing isoantibodies in goats by injecting certain goats with red blood cells of other goats, thus producing immune isoantibodies. Attempts to immunize goats against their own red blood cells, however, did not succeed. The inability to produce antibodies against constituents of one's own body was interpreted by Ehrlich as the expression of a biological law referred to by him as "horror autotoxicus. . . ."

In recent years the pathogenesis of several diseases has been ascribed to an interaction between supposed autoantibodies and antigens present in the tissues. Most conspicuous among a number of diseases in this category are certain blood dyscrasias, frequently referred to as "autoimmune blood diseases." Several observations, indeed, seem to support this concept, such as the positive direct Coombs test in acquired hemolytic anemia. The experimental evidence, however, is still incomplete. Yet there are several known instances where autoantibodies have been produced experimentally, such as by the injection of brain tissue. . . .

Because of the unusual immunological position of thyroglobulin, we tried to test the validity of Ehr-

---

*Witebsky, E., R. R. Rose, K. Kerplan, J. R. Paine, and R. W. Egan. 1957. Chronic thyroiditis and autoimmunization. *Journal of the American Medical Association* 164:1439–1447. [Copyright 1957, American Medical Association.]

lich's "horror autotoxicus" law in this case by injecting experimental animals with thyroid extract of their own species. . . .

For the demonstration of circulating antibodies, three major serological procedures were used: (1) precipitation, (2) complement fixation, and (3) tanned-cell hemagglutination. The precipitation test, carried out by mixing undiluted rabbit serum with serial dilutions of thyroid extract, though positive in some instances, proved to be the least sensitive technique. . . . Of 35 serums of rabbits injected with rabbit thyroid extract examined by [tanned-cell hemagglutination], 32 (91%) revealed the presence of thyroid antibodies, in some instances exhibiting titers 10 to 100 times as high as those obtained when tested by complement fixation.

In order to study further the organ specificity of antiserums obtained by injecting rabbits with rabbit thyroid extracts, the rabbit antiserums were tested with thyroid extracts prepared from more than 20 individual rabbits. . . . In some instances, the thyroid gland was removed from the rabbits before immunization with pooled thyroid extract was initiated. Antiserums produced in this way, when examined serologically, gave equally strong reactions with extracts of the thyroid gland from the antibody-forming animal itself. The antigenicity of extracts of the thyroid gland for the same individual rabbit was further investigated by subjecting rabbits to total thyroidectomy and injecting them with an extract of their own thyroid gland. Of 15 rabbits treated in this way, the serums of 4 were positive on complement

fixation tests, and 7 out of 10 gave positive hemagglutination reactions with rabbit thyroid extract, proving the potential antigenicity of the thyroid extract for the same rabbit. . . . [Additional studies with purified thyroglobulin demonstrated this antigen to be responsible for immunization and histopathological effects.]

In addition, four dogs received in all four footpads an initial series of intradermal injections of dog thyroid extract incorporated into Freund adjuvants. One animal developed a strong circulating thyroid antibody that was demonstrable by complement fixation. . . . At the end of nine months . . . the [three remaining] dogs were then killed. On postmortem examination, the thyroid glands of all were found to be hard and small. . . .

Histological changes in the thyroids of guinea pigs, basically similar to those in rabbits and dogs, have also been observed after injections with thyroid extract from guinea pigs. Circulating thyroid antibodies were found in some instances, but none of the guinea pigs produced antibodies as strongly as did the rabbits. . . .

As soon as the first histological section of thyroid glands of animals immunized with extracts of their own thyroid glands were examined in our laboratory in 1954, it became evident that the histological changes resembled in certain respects those seen in chronic thyroiditis in man. During the past two years we have had an opportunity to examine the serums of certain individuals suffering from various kinds of thyroid disease, including several patients in whom

TABLE 2.—*Reaction of Serums of Patients with Thyroiditis to Tanned Human Erythrocytes Coated with Human Thyroid Extract or Human Serum*

Dilutions of Patient's Serum or Rabbit Serum	Erythrocytes Coated with Human Thyroid Extract*					Erythrocytes Coated with Human Serum†
	Serum of Patients with Thyroiditis				Serum of Rabbit 440	Serum of Rabbit 440
	Tre.	Tho.	May.	Bur.		
1:5	++	+++	+++	+++	+++	+++
1:10	+++	+++	+++	+++	+++	++
1:20	+++	+++	+++	+++	+++	++
1:40	+++	+++	++	+	++	++
1:80	++	++	++	−	++	+
1:160	++	++	−	−	++	+
1:320	++	++	−	−	−	+
1:640	++	++	−	−	−	−
1:1,280	−	++	−	−	−	−
1:2,560	−	−	−	−	−	−

* Normal human serums gave negative reaction in all dilutions.
† Serums from all patients and normal human serum gave negative reactions in all dilutions.

a diagnosis of chronic thyroiditis had been made either clinically or histologically. Of this latter group, 12 had circulating antibodies in various titers against human thyroid extract as demonstrated by the tanned-cell hemagglutination test. In none of the patients with other thyroid diseases was a thyroid antibody demonstrable. . . .

The comparison of the histological pictures of experimental thyroiditis in animals with that of thyroiditis in man reveals certain similarities. . . .

The human disease, chronic thyroiditis, might be due, therefore, to a similar mechanism of autoimmunization against constituents of the thyroid gland, specially thyroglobulin, as is thyroiditis in artificially immunized animals. In the case of the animal experimentation, however, the thyroid extracts were incorporated in Freund adjuvants and injected parentally in order to elicit antibody production. . . . One, therefore, might assume that in human chronic thyroiditis a slow but continuous release of thyroglobulin into the circulation acts as a constant antigenic stimulus, resembling the depot effect achieved in animal experiments by means of Freund adju-

vants. Such an assumption is supported by demonstration of a free, thyroglobulin-like protein in the bloodstreams of patients suffering from thyroiditis. . . .

The time seems to have come to establish certain criteria that ideally should be fulfilled in order to prove the role of an autoantibody in the pathogenesis of a particular disease, namely (1) the direct demonstration of free, circulating antibodies that are active at body temperature or of cell-bound antibodies by indirect means; (2) the recognition of the specific antigen against which this antibody is directed; (3) the production of antibodies against the same antigen in experimental animals; (4) the appearance of pathological changes in the corresponding tissues of an actively sensitized experimental animal that are basically similar to those in the human disease. We believe that these requirements have come close to fulfillment in certain cases of human chronic thyroiditis. Nevertheless, what circumstances trigger the release of intact thyroglobulin into the bloodstream remain an unsolved problem.

Auto-immunity in Hashimoto's disease and its implications

1957 • Deborah Doniach and Ivan M. Roitt

Comment

While in their fundamental studies of organ-specific antigens Witebsky and Rose were performing experiments on rabbits, dogs, and guinea pigs, a group of English investigators were trying to determine the cause of thyroiditis in their patients and its correlation with circulating gamma globulins. The clinically directed team included Ivan M. Roitt (1927–   ). A Doctor of Science graduate of Oxford University, Roitt joined Middlesex Hospital Medical School in 1953, where he began his own research on autoimmunity. He later advanced to Professor and Head of a newly created Department of Immunology. The Royal Society elected him to fellowship in 1983. He has writ-

ten a most successful textbook on immunology, which has been translated into 10 languages. In 1950 Deborah Doniach (1912–   ) received her M.D. with specialty in chemical pathology from the University of London. She is presently Professor Emeritus of Clinical Immunology at Middlesex.

Both the English and American research groups found thyroglobulin to be the primary antigen of circulating autoantibodies. Two additional antigens were later detected. One is a minor protein of the gelatinous material within the small ducts of the gland. The second, a microsomal lipoprotein, is a component of the endoplasmic reticulum normally hidden from blood lymphocytes, being located on the apical portion of thyroid cells. It elicits complement-mediated cytotoxic antibodies when exposed as a result of previous tissue damage.

Delayed hypersensitivity is also related to Hashimoto's disease, as determined by the injection of thyroid extracts into the skin of patients. The animal model of thyroiditis, as developed by Witebsky, requires the use of complete Freund's adjuvant, which incorporates killed tubercle bacilli and activates the cellular immune responses. Leaving out these bacteria (incomplete Freund's adjuvant) usually results in experimental failure. Further studies determined that normal humans and animals possess thyroglobulin-binding T cells. The injection of thyroglobulin without adjuvant induces the proliferation of suppressor T lymphocytes, such that the reinjection of the antigen, this time with Freund's adjuvant, will not produce antibodies nor thyroiditis. These specific regulating T cells are the target of the monoclonal antibodies used in experimental immunotherapy of autoimmune disease.

For further information:

Allison, A. C. 1976. Self-tolerance and autoimmunity in the thyroid. *New England Journal of Medicine* 295:821–827.

Glynn, L. E. and E. J. Hoborow. 1965. *Autoimmunity and Disease*. Blackwell Scientific Publications, Oxford. 420 p.

Rose, N. R. 1981. Autoimmune disease. *Scientific American* 244(2):80–103.

Rose, N. R. and I. R. Mackay (editors). 1985. *The Autoimmune Diseases*. Academic Press, Orlando. 727 p.

The Paper*

Recent workers have described abnormalities in the serum proteins of patients with Hashimoto's disease, namely, high values for gamma globulins and for the results of flocculation tests. The highest values were obtained in untreated patients with large goiters. During the months following removal of the goiter, these abnormal levels slowly returned to the normal range.

The known association of gamma globulins with circulating antibodies and the infiltration of the diseased thyroid gland with plasma cells and lymphoid tissue (which are known to produce antibodies) suggested that the disease process and the postoperative finding might be explained if it were postulated that these patients were immunized against an antigen in the thyroid gland. Confirmation of this hypothesis is provided by the results of the present studies, which demonstrate the presence of thyroid-specific precipitating auto-antibodies in the sera of such patients. . . .

In 25 of 30 patients with Hashimoto's disease, the serum contained precipitins against saline-extracted human thyroid gland. The thyroid specificity of the antibody was proved by the negative results obtained when the sera were tested against saline extracts of human liver, kidney, spleen, lymph nodes, parotid gland and brain. Similar precipitin reactions were observed when purified thyroglobulin was substituted for the crude saline extracts of human thyroid. Thyroglobulin was identified as the active antigen. This was shown by the confluence of the precipitin lines when the crude thyroid extract and purified thyroglobulin reacted with Hashimoto serum in the gel diffusion technique of Ouchterlony. Fractionation of Hashimoto serum by zone electrophoresis, followed by precipitin tests on the eluted fractions, showed that the antibody was located exclusively in the gamma globulins. This was confirmed by the technique of immunoelectrophoresis in agar.

In strongly reacting sera examined by the modified Oudin technique, a compact precipitation zone appeared after 16 to 48 hours and remained stationary when antibody and antigen were present in equivalent proportions. In weakly reacting sera the precipitation bands were more diffuse, took up to two weeks to become clearly visible, and gradually moved downwards as the precipitate redissolved in

*Doniach, D. and I. M. Roitt. 1957. Auto-immunity in Hashimoto's disease and its implications. *Journal of Clinical Endocrinology and Metabolism* 17:1293–1304. [With permission, copyright by the Endocrine Society 1957.]

excess antigen. . . . Frequently 2 precipitin lines were observed even when purified thyroglobulin was used, indicating the presence of two distinct antigenic components.

Previous work had shown that anti-human-thyroglobulin sera obtained from rabbits cross-reacted to a small extent with thyroglobulin from a variety of mammalian species. The sera of Hashimoto patients gave no cross-reactions when tested against extracts of thyroid from the rabbit, rat, sheep, hog, cow and horse. . . .

In the 11 untreated patients, values for flocculation tests and gamma globulins were raised above normal, and strong precipitins were found in 7 cases. In 2 untreated patients the precipitins were weak despite a marked elevation of the flocculation values, and in 2 the sera failed to yield any precipitins by the technique used.

Of the 14 patients treated with desiccated thyroid in doses of 120 to 240 mg daily for one to three years, 7 had strong precipitins in spite of the fact that in all but 1 instance the goiters had regressed almost completely as a result of the treatment, and in some instances the results of flocculation tests and the gamma globulin levels had returned to normal from previously elevated values. In 5 of these patients the precipitins were weak, and in 2 no precipitins could be demonstrated.

The sera in 5 cases of Hashimoto's disease were examined within a year of partial thyroidectomy. In 3 instances the precipitin reaction was strong, in 1 it was weak, and in 1 there was no reaction though the test was made only three weeks after incomplete removal of the goiter. . . .

[T]he proportion of cases in which there were no precipitins increased with the amount of thyroid tissue removed at operation and with the length of time that had elapsed since thyroidectomy. . . .

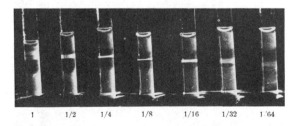

| 1 | 1/2 | 1/4 | 1/8 | 1/16 | 1/32 | 1/64 |

Figure 2 Thyroglobulin precipitin test performed on serial dilutions of serum from a patient with Hashimoto's disease, using a single antigen concentration. Precipitins were visible to 1/64 dilutions of the serum. The compact band seen in 1/8 dilution indicates equivalence of antigen and antibody. The leading edge of the precipitate approaches the serum layer with progressive dilution. Photographed after three weeks at 2°C.

The results of precipitin tests performed on the sera of patients with other thyroid diseases . . . were negative in 105 thyrotoxic patients whether active, postoperative, radioiodine-treated or in a state of prolonged remission after treatment with anti-thyroid drugs. In all of the 103 patients with nontoxic nodular goiter the results were negative.

Precipitins were found in 6 cases of spontaneous myxedema without goiter in which there was no history of previous thyroid disease; but in 27 other cases of myxedema the results were negative.

The present results show that in the majority of cases the serum of patients with Hashimoto's disease gives a precipitin reaction when it is mixed with either crude or refined extracts of the human thyroid gland. This suggests an imunization against human thyroglobulin. . . .

Structural alteration in a body constituent is not a prerequisite for the induction of auto-antibodies. The inability of animals to form antibodies against their own body constituents under normal conditions is considered to be the result of an immunologic tolerance acquired in early life, before the maturation of the faculty of immunologic response. Exposure to antigenic stimuli during this period causes a specific weakening or suppression of the immune reaction to these antigens in later life. The concept of immunologic tolerance provides a rational basis for the phenomenon of auto-antibody formation, since animals may fail to acquire this tolerance of constituents which do not gain access to the sites of antibody formation during their critical developing period, and may therefore produce antibodies in response to any subsequent release of the constituents. The auto-antigenic properties of spermatozoa, lens protein, casein, and brain extracts accord well with this theory. The failure to detect circulating thyroglobulin under normal conditions suggests that human beings may not be immunologically tolerant to this protein and may react to its release from the thyroid by auto-antibody formation.

The present demonstration of circulating antibodies against the patient's own thyroid lymphadenoid goiter and the aforementioned destructive effects of auto-antibodies suggest a new approach to the etiology of this disease. It may be supposed that limited extravasation of thyroglobulin stimulates invasion by lymphoid tissue, with local antibody production. Under certain conditions sufficient antibody may be produced to damage adjacent follicles and release more thyroglobulin. This may in time give rise to a general immune response involving distant parts of the reticulo-endothelial system, with a considerable increase in antibody production, leading to further lymphoid hypertrophy and progressive damage to the thyroid gland. Classic Hashimoto's disease may represent a later stage of such a sequence of events, whereas lymphocyte thyroiditis, an analogous condition described in children and young people, is probably an earlier or milder form of the same pathologic process. . . .

Part 3
Immunochemistry

The great discoveries are due to the eruption of genius into a closely related field, and the transfer of the precious knowledge there found to his own domain. —Theobald Smith

Immunology was one of the first biological disciplines to acquire a formal chemical wing. Chemistry, a most ancient science, began with the alteration of substances and the determination of their interactive mechanisms. The physicochemical laws governing the higher structure of inorganic material, such as compounds, crystals, and alloys, had a distinct, seemingly simple order, but examinations of living matter were more like probes into chaos and darkness. Models of life stuff, the myriad synthetics developed in the familiar aromatic laboratories of organic chemistry, were inadequate to explain biological phenomena and the formation and degradation of the unique biological molecules; 2,4-dimethoxybenzaldehyde is not an amino acid, and its crystals are not enzymes. A new chemical science had to arise to specialize in life—biological chemistry, biochemistry. Similarly, chemistry and the biomedical discipline of immunology begot immunochemistry.

The following series of comments and milestones traces the development of immunochemistry and of its paramount objective of associating specific three-dimensional chemical structures with biological function, most particularly antigenic specificity. The approach of immunochemistry has mainly been physicochemical rather than physiological, and methods to quantify, separate, and identify substances have been its requirements as well as its chief application. Immunology, it should be remembered, was founded by the chemist Louis Pasteur. The father of immunochemistry was Paul Ehrlich, a physician.

The first milestone appropriately belongs to Ehrlich, who demonstrated the need for standard measures of antitoxins. His elaborate model, which included the hypothetical presence of toxoids, was based on his conception of unique functional-structural atomic groups on a molecule of toxin. One such group was toxic; an adjacent group was directed against a complementary configuration on the host cells. The poisonous portion could be denatured to form a harmless toxoid while maintaining the agent's ability to attach to the cell, or to an antibody. Ehrlich, one of the most colorful and enthusiastic characters of science, pictured in his mind—and on whatever surface was available for his pen—all biochemicals acting in this fashion. Variation in antibody-antigen avidity was, therefore, a matter of fitness of shapes. These remarkably accurate ideas were pure conjecture; they conformed to the data, but lacked substantiation.

Svante Arrhenius, who coined the term immunochemistry, could not agree with Ehrlich's emphasis on molecular shape, postulating instead that antibodies and antigens combine by a form of electrostatic colloidal binding. He believed that antibody-antigen binding bore a resemblance to interactions of weak acids and bases. This pioneer physical chemist, whose experiments produced sound data despite mistaken principles, gave immunochemistry its first introduction to thermodynamics, equilibrium constants, viscosity coefficients, and other quantitative parameters. Arrhenius truly merged chemistry and immunology.

The next milestone provided the first evidence of Ehrlich's atomic group model. The work was carried out by Karl Landsteiner, who added and then varied the location of functional groups and short peptides. Landsteiner published numerous papers. The one presented here, on methylation of serum proteins, cut a clear path through the jungle of adsorption chemistry. Landsteiner discovered haptenic and carrier functions. He helped explain in chemical terms antigen specificity. He gave the idea of antigenicity a material counterpart.

Proteins and perhaps glycoproteins were at first assumed to be the only chemical structures to elicit antibodies after immunizations with sugars repeatedly failed. Then Michael Heidelberger and Oswald T. Avery, studying a polysaccharide, the specific soluble substance of pneumococci, found otherwise. Initially, these pneumococcal capsular polysaccharides were recognized as haptens, able to bind antibody but incapable alone to produce it. Later with proper dosage and favorable hosts, the polysaccharide was demonstrated to be fully antigenic, indeed, immunogenic. Heidelberger, who was trained as an organic chemist, employed pneumococcal and other complex carbohydrates as tools in the quantitative microanalysis of immunological specificity.

John Marrack questioned the phenomena of flocculation and precipitation and their inhibition in zones of antibody and antigen excess. How do such phenomena occur? Presupposing multiple valence for both antigen and antibody, he came up with the lattice theory. Bridging of antigen particles with antibodies would form complexes of various size that could overcome the forces of water solubility. His hypothesis, based on the Bohr model of the atom, also introduced the concept of hydrophilic or hydrogen-bonding. This radical notion fought the mortally wounded, but still prevalent, colloid theory and the consensus that antibodies are univalent.

A technological advance commenced the immunochemical campaign to at last ascertain the physical nature of the antibody. Arne Tiselius, a student of the ultracentrifuge creator The Svedberg, developed electrophoresis to characterize and purify macromolecular substances by their net charge. Together with Heidelberger's student Elvin A. Kabat, he subjected antisera to his electrophoretic device, separating the constituent proteins into distinct bands. Antibody activity was found in the third globulin band. Using a Greek nomenclature, antibodies were thus dubbed gamma globulins.

With the improvements in purification techniques, isolated gamma globulins could then be treated with specific chemicals in the hope of splitting the unknown structures into simpler functional units. Rodney R. Porter chose enzymes, the classic cleavers of proteins. The data were a little muddy, but he obtained three fragments, two of which had antigen-binding capacity. Gerald M. Edelman and M. D. Poulik then found that the combination of a reducing agent with a dissociating solvent could gently separate the antibody molecule into four chains, two each of two sizes, later termed heavy and light (H and L chains). Shortly thereafter, Porter published the now familiar model of the bivalent, Y-shaped antibody of gamma globulin. The pentavalent beta macroglobulin was next distinguished. A new nomenclature system soon arose that gave this large antibody the name IgM, for immunoglobulin macro; the antibody of the gamma globulin fraction became IgG. In 1965, David S. Rowe and John L. Fahey discovered a new class of antibodies, IgD, which is mainly restricted to immunoregulation on its B-cell membrane perch.

All antibody classes are functionally distinct, and the last two to be isolated were extraordinarily specialized. The old immunological problem of local immunity to pathogenic microorganisms was finally solved when Thomas B. Tomasi, Jr. and colleagues determined that IgA, which was first found in serum, could take on new protein components and be secreted into the various fluids bathing the boundary zones between host and environment. This immunoglobulin exists in 7S single units, 11S dimers, and 18S secretory forms. The final milestone of this series concerns the discovery of IgE and the recognition of it as reagin, the allergy-related, skin-sensitizing antibody of Prausnitz-Küstner tests (see Part 2/Prausnitz, 1921). IgE proved to be the initiator of the mast cell cascade of inflammation. It takes the simultaneous turning of two IgE locks to activate the cellular response.

The immunochemical quest has virtually been fulfilled. A vast accumulation of data has provided three-dimensional models and computer-analyzed representations of the major immunoglobulins. Domains of each H and L immunoglobulin chain have been associated with biological and chemical functions, such as antigen and complement reception, cellular attachment, and flexibility. Many details remain, but the principles are established and confirmed. Immunochemistry continues to play a dominant role in vaccine design and diagnostic methods. Indeed, since modern reductionist biological science prefers to view phenomena at the molecular level, immunology and immunochemistry sometimes blur into equivalency. The cellular immunologists await in the wings to challenge that tendency.

For further information:

Day, E. D. 1966. *Foundations of Immunochemistry*. Williams & Wilkins Company, Baltimore. 209 p.

Kabat, E. A. 1968. *Structural Concepts in Immunology and Immunochemistry*. Holt, Rinehart and Winston, New York. 310 p.

Roitt, I., J. Brostoff, and D. Male. 1985. *Immunology*. Gower Medical Publishing, London.

Silverstein, A. M. 1982–1983. Development of the concept of immunologic specificity: I–IV. *Cellular Immunology* 67:396–409; 71:183–195; 78:174–190; 80:416–425.

The standardization of diphtheria antitoxins and their theoretical foundation

1897 • Paul Ehrlich

Comment

In life and death, Paul Ehrlich (1854–1915) was a controversial and influential scientist. His novel and elaborate biochemical theories invited severe criticism by his fellow researchers, yet his concepts dominated immunology for decades. He was condemned by clergy for interfering with God's justice against sinners by developing the syphilis-curing arsenical Salvarsan, also known as "606," but he opened the frontier of systemic chemotherapy against infectious disease. He shared the Nobel honors of 1908 with Elie Metchnikoff for his work in immunochemistry and his name was heralded around the world. Thus, the Nazi attempt long after his death to make him an unperson, to use the Orwellian Newspeak, was sheer folly. German bureaucrats changed the name of the street that honored him, they destroyed his biographies, and they expunged his mention in the new textbooks of German science. Ehrlich's great offense to the Third Reich to justify such

actions was that he was a Jew. Nevertheless, while other tombstones in the Jewish Cemetery of Frankfurt were defiled, his grave site with its prominent column-mounted Star of David and medical caduceus was unharmed.

Ehrlich was more than a great chemotherapist and immunologist. A pioneer hematologist, he differentiated the various blood cells and discovered the tissue mast cell; an oncologist, he examined the growth dynamics and transplantation of tumors; a stain technologist, he was able to color nerve cells and to detect the tubercle bacillus in tissues by developing the acid-fast dye technique; a clinical chemist, he discovered the diazo reaction and found a useful test for bilirubin. However, Ehrlich is honored here as a genius of immunochemistry and one of the most colorful characters of the science, literally as well as figuratively.

Ehrlich was a cousin of the pathologist Carl Weigert, who helped introduce him to the newly developed aniline dyes when Ehrlich began his own medical training at the University of Breslau. He later transferred to the University of Strassbourg, and finally received the M.D. at the University of Leipzig in 1878. He next went to Berlin's Charité Hospital. Ehrlich was never offered a professorship, but in 1889 Robert Koch asked him to join his laboratory. He had previously met Koch in 1876, when the bacteriologist came to Ferdinand Cohn's Botanical Department at Breslau to demonstrate the life cycle of the anthrax bacillus. Koch's institute in Berlin was one of the few places where classic Prussian military medical officers and Jewish physicians could work together in friendship without restrictive barriers. In 1896 Ehrlich received from Friedrich Althoff of the Prussian Ministry of Ecclesiastical, Educational and Medical Affairs the appointment as the director of the small, insufficiently funded State Institute for Serum Research and Serum Testing in Steglitz. Althoff soon realized that Ehrlich deserved better, and in 1899 he helped him gain the directorship of the Institute of Experimental Therapy in Frankfurt-am-Main and later the directorship of the adjacent Georg Speyer-haus, where Ehrlich at last received the freedom and funding he needed for his creative work. Later, Ehrlich described success in science as due to "*geduld, geschick, geld, und gluck*"—patience, talent, money, and luck.

Indeed, money was one of the issues that broke up the collaboration between Ehrlich and Emil von Behring. Ehrlich's improved technique for producing highly potent diphtheria antitoxin (see Part 1/Behring, 1890) made possible its commercial manufacture and distribution. A chemical company seemed to be ready to contract with both Behring and Ehrlich for commercial rights in return for a percentage of the profits. However, when Ehrlich arrived at the factory, Behring had already reached a separate accord. He persuaded Ehrlich to forgo his share on the promise that he would use his influence to gain Ehrlich the directorship of a state-sponsored research institute, a position that forbade commercial interests. Behring

failed to help Ehrlich, but prospered in his own right. Indeed, Behring loved to gamble, and with the aid of winnings he established his own factory and laboratory. Ehrlich never forgave his old colleague for the subterfuge and deceit, nor for the audacity of seeking free laboratory services at Ehrlich's own institutes.

In the paper presented here, Ehrlich confronted more than a technical problem of quality control; the very unknown nature of the antibody-antigen union loomed darkly. Max von Gruber, an eminent serologist and hygienist, and many others criticized him for conjuring the various toxoid substances as devices of mere convenience. However, these scientists were just as confused as Ehrlich, following erroneous models of colloid adsorption or electrolytic dissociation. The law of definite proportions was incorrectly assumed to hold. Antibodies were seen as uniform chemical reactants constant in valence and structure; therefore, Ehrlich explained his inconsistent test results by ascribing variation to the antigenic, toxic atomic groups. He proposed a spectrum of weakened toxins, which he termed "toxoids," that differed in their affinity to antibodies. Each experimental preparation had a unique composition of toxin and toxoids, whose behavior under different mixing conditions affected neutralization.

Ehrlich had the idea of affinity reversed. It is the antibody that varies in affinity and also in valence. The notion of toxoids, however, was valid, but not to the extent he thought. Denatured, nontoxic molecules derived from toxins can indeed elicit and couple with toxin-specific antibodies. Equally true was the fundamental approach of all of Ehrlich's research: *corpora non agunt nisi fixata*, substances do not react unless they become fixed. He visualized molecules as having two regions of activity, one of which (the haptophore) attaches to complementary receptors on target cells. The other configuration may be a colored dye (the chromophore) or act as a poison (the toxophore). Ricin, a toxin found in castor beans, and diphtheria toxin, which were the focus of Ehrlich's attention, have recently been shown to consist of two distinct molecular domains, and their respective functions conform to Ehrlich's model. Even certain antibodies display such a dual nature, the variable antibody receptors attaching to the antigen and the constant Fc region (the tail of the Y-shaped structure) coupling somewhat nonspecifically to the surface of macrophages or mast cells. Ehrlich had taken the first bold step to bring an immunobiological phenomenon into the realm of chemistry. Considering that biochemistry was still an ocean of dreams with only few islands of reality, his grasp of stereochemical principles and behavior was amazingly clear.

For further information:

Bäumler, E. 1984. *Paul Ehrlich. Scientist for Life* (G. Edwards, translator). Holmes & Meier, New York. 288 p.

Marquardt, M. 1951. *Paul Ehrlich.* Henry Schuman, New York. 255 p.

Mazumdar, P. M. H. 1974. The antigen-antibody reaction and the physics and chemistry of life. *Bulletin of the History of Medicine* 48:1–21.

Pelner, L. 1972. Corpora non agunt nisi fixata. Maxim behind all of Ehrlich's great discoveries. *New York State Journal of Medicine* 72:620–624.

The Paper*

No one argues that the whole problem of diphtheria antitoxins, not only from the standpoint of practical therapy, but also from the purely scientific view, requires sera whose value is accurately determined. . . .

If the antitoxin or the toxin can be attained in pure form, the preparation of standard test solutions may simply depend on weights, and no precautions whatsoever would be required to preserve a standardized solution. We, however, remain far away from this possibility, since diphtheria toxin that provides the basis for antitoxins is a raw product, containing besides toxic substances, material that blocks anal-

*Ehrlich, P. 1897. Die Wertbemessung des Diphtherieheilserums und deren theoretische Grundlagen. *Klinisches Jahrbuch* 6:299–326.

ysis. At least I have never in my research found a single diphtheria toxin that could be accurately ascertained to be a solution of pure toxin.

In this regard, it appeared impossible to correlate the neutralization of toxins by antitoxin in the proper mathematical fashion that is indispensible for a proper assay. Under these circumstances, the institute standard of immunizing power is, for the present, a purely empirical value, which, should it be lost, never can be recovered and, therefore, we are obliged to preserve it with all means in our power. . . .

It was necessary to develop a new functional assay method and to examine the complicated relations involved in the neutralization of toxins and antitoxin. . . .

If a constant standard must be attained, solutions must be avoided, and conservation procedures should be selected that ensure the best possible stability. From practical chemistry, the agents that especially destroy such instable substances include: (1) water (by hydration), (2) oxygen (by oxidation), (3) light, and (4) heat. . . .

Of the dried diphtheria antisera available, that of Behring, excellently prepared in the Hoechst laboratory, seems to be the best initial material. . . .

A large number of tubes were prepared in this manner, each containing 2 g of dried sera valued at 1700 immunity units per gram. Every 2–3 months one of these tubes is opened with care by drilling, and the dried serum is dissolved in 200 cc of a mixture of 10% salt solution and glycerin, the material containing 50–80% glycerin. By such a manner, a test serum yields a potency of exactly 17-fold. Of this 0.94 cc of a 16-fold dilution or 1 cc of a 17-fold dilution is necessary for analyzing 10-fold the hitherto standard dose of toxin. . . .

It might be assumed a priori . . . that, in a similar way as dried antitoxin, a toxin would serve this purpose. However, in practice there are some reasons [mainly difficulties in manufacturing] that presently support using antitoxin, especially since it is easily acquired by drying it in vacuum over sulphuric acid. . . .

By the present method of the Institute, the measured value of sera is determined by the dose of toxin tested, i.e., the quantity of toxin that is exactly neutralized by 0.1 cc or one unit of serum. . . . In practice, the dose of test toxin is mixed with 4 cc of a suitable dilution of serum and then injected subcutaneously into 250 g guinea pigs. The animal should manifest no signs of illness, and typically there should be no change at the injection site. . . .

To avoid the difficulties of subjective analysis, it appeared necessary to develop a totally objective method. . . .

It appeared simplest to select the occurrence of death as criterion of the measurement, and to determine the test method such that a particular dose of the toxin to be tested, equivalent to ten-fold that employed beforehand, should be neutralized by particular amounts of a serum in such a manner that death of the animal does not take place at all, or least not within a specific period (e.g., 4 days). . . .

During the development of this method, it soon became clear that the processes that take place in the neutralization of diphtheria toxin are exceedingly complicated. Only through a systematic, quantitatively exhaustive study of a series of toxins is it possible to obtain a closer insight into these relationships. . . .

To investigate a certain toxin within a large number of animals by adding increasing doses of toxin to a unit of immune serum, it is almost always possible to find two threshold values (L = limits), which are of the greatest importance for characterizing the toxin. One of these limiting values, L_0, is the dose of toxin that is almost completely neutralized, while the other threshold, L_+, indicates the quantity that, despite antibody, is of such excess toxicity that death of the animal occurs within 4 days. This excess of toxin corresponds to the lethal dose unit, as defined above.

Should the limit values L_0 and L_+ be expressed, not as absolute quantities, but in terms of toxin units contained within, it is a safe assumption, provided the toxin is a pure chemical substance, that $D = L_+ - L_0$ must equal the unit lethal dose. . . .

[Analyses of 11 different toxins are presented.] From these, one may note that toxins yield enormous variation, which apparently cannot be correlated in any way.

I shall only state here that the value L_0, which according to previous assumptions should be 100 lethal doses, in fact equalled a minimum of 27 and a maximum of 108. Similarly, the value of D, which should theoretically correspond to a unit of toxin, showed no less considerable a variation. . . .

Before I can discuss the true significance of these amounts, it is necessary to give a brief outline of the theory of the neutralization of toxin. . . .

In a recent communication I . . . provided preliminary evidence in the case of ricin that a toxin and its antitoxin influence one another by a direct chemical interaction. On continuing this investigation, I have been able to demonstrate by test tube experiments in another case . . . that the interaction of toxin and antibody is much more rapid in concentrated than in dilute solutions, and also that heat accelerates the action and cold retards it. Analogous phenomena are often found in pure chemistry, particularly in the formation of double salts. . . . Especially because it is possible to titrate the antibodies with great accuracy (in favorable circumstances, the

error with the present method is 1%), the reaction between toxin and antitoxin occurs in accordance with the proportions of a simple equivalence. A molecule of toxin combines with a definite and unalterable quantity of antibody.

It must be assumed that this ability to combine with antitoxin is attributable to the presence in the toxin complex of a specific group of atoms with a maximum specific affinity to another group of atoms in the antitoxin complex, the first easily fitting the second like a key in a lock, Emile Fischer's famous analogy. [A preliminary discussion of the side-chain theory is then presented. . . .]

The fact that neutralizing capacity and absolute toxicity are not separably associated has been known to me for many years. Some time ago, I had the opportunity to make observations that indicated an explanation of this phenomenon. My first experiences began in the year 1893, and concerned tetanus toxin.

Following certain theoretical considerations, especially for the substitution of the amino groups of the toxin complex, I treated tetanus broth with carbon sulphide. It was found with this treatment that a relatively rapid and almost complete detoxification of the broth occurred, so that mice could be given 0.5–1.0 cc of the modified toxin without great harm. Mice so treated may acquire relatively quickly, within 8 days, a basic immunity to tetanus toxin, while the same immunity is achieved in mice only with great difficulty and after rather long periods by the use of unaltered toxin. . . . These experiments then suggested to me the notion that the toxin had been changed into a nontoxic form that still had the capacity for specific combination . . . for which I suggest the name toxoid. . . .

As the toxoids arise from the toxins and possess the specific combining capacity, it follows that the characteristic combining group remains wholly intact. Chemical changes must therefore have occurred in the remainder of the atom complex, which cause the more or less complete destruction of the toxicity. Such phenomena are common in toxicology. . . .

From what has been stated, it is self-evident that each toxin may give rise to a great number of toxoids, which must have very different biological properties according to the manner by which they are produced and the consequent alteration of the atom complex. It is certain that some toxoids possess immunizing capacity . . . but it is unlikely that all the possible toxoids have this property. . . .

With respect to the origin of toxoids, . . . they generally occur in relatively large quantities in diphtheria toxins that have been treated with preservatives and stored for a long time. . . . It must be emphasized . . . that even fresh broth (an 8-day culture) is not free from toxoids. . . . Although the mere existence of toxoids explains the fact that the dose of tested toxin, as determined by one immune unit, does not correspond to a constant number of toxin units but to one which varies within wide limits (up to four or five times the number of units of toxin), the explanation adds little to the official technique of testing. . . . I decided that the dose of tested toxin should not rigidly and quantitatively correspond to a single minimal lethal dose. However, it is only during the past year that I have succeeded in finding an explanation for this truly striking finding. . . .

Here one factor is outstanding, namely the varying affinity of the toxoids for the antibody. In this regard, only 3 groups of toxoids can exist: (1) protoxoids, which have a greater affinity for the antibody than the toxin, (2) syntoxoids, with the same affinity as the toxin, and (3) epitoxoids, which show less affinity for the antibody.

Considering protoxoids first . . . serum added gradually to a mixture of protoxoid and toxin will combine first with the protoxoid, and must saturate it completely before the neutralization of the actual toxin can begin. . . .

If to a physiologically neutralized L_0 mixture of toxin and syntoxoid are added further quantities of the original mixture of toxin and syntoxoid, there will be no dissociation, but death will occur if the mixture contains an excess of 1 unit of toxin. . . .

The situation with epitoxoids is very different. Let us consider a physiologically neutralized mixture of toxin and epitoxoid. . . . We see that in this case the added toxin apparently disappears, manifesting itself only when all the epitoxoid that combined with antitoxin has been released. Assuming that a toxic diphtheria solution consists only of toxin and epitoxoid, the differential value, D, after deduction of 1 unit of toxin, is exactly equivalent to the epitoxoid present in the broth. We thus see from this explanation that it is not the presence of protoxoid and syntoxoid, but only the presence of epitoxoid that can raise the value of D. . . .

It is . . . probable that ordinary toxic broths usually contain as components other toxoids, syntoxoids, and protoxoids, in addition to toxin and epitoxoid. The constitution of a diphtheria broth may therefore be expressed in general by the formula x toxoid + y toxin + z epitoxoid. . . .

Immunochemistry. The application of the principles of physical chemistry to the study of the biological antibodies

1907 • Svante Arrhenius

Comment

Before venturing into an unknown corner of biological chemistry, one has to start from someplace. That place of embarkation will always be the familiar and the established. From his training in physiology, Paul Ehrlich was comfortable with Eduard Pflüger's "living" protoplasmic albumin and Emil Fischer's lock-and-key interaction of sugar-splitting enzymes and substrates. On the other hand, inorganic chemistry, so readily accessible, so easily scrutinized in comparison with the mysterious life-stuff, was home for Svante Arrhenius (1859–

1927). Before he examined the antibody question, Arrhenius had helped create physical chemistry, the branch of chemistry that correlates physical properties of materials with their chemical composition and reactions. The Nobel Committee recognized the importance of his chemical work by awarding him the Prize in 1903.

Arrhenius, who even as a youth showed a talent for mathematics, earned the minimal passing marks for his Ph.D. dissertation at the University of Uppsala in 1884, further proving that school grades are not always meaningful. In his graduate thesis, he proposed in rudimentary form his later, more developed theory of electrolytic dissociation, which postulated the existence of free ions in solutions. In 1891 he declined a professorship in Germany to teach at the University of Stockholm. He also served there as rector between 1887 and 1902.

Apparently, Arrhenius first became interested in antibodies (antitoxins and hemolysins) when he met Thorvald Madsen, a Danish bacteriologist. Madsen had studied tetanus antitoxins at Paul Ehrlich's institute in Frankfurt before coming to Stockholm in 1901 to work with Arrhenius. Arrhenius reciprocated the visit later that year by joining Madsen at the State Serum Institute in Copenhagen to conduct collaborative research. When Ehrlich came to the official dedication of the State Serum Institute in 1902, he invited Arrhenius to come to Frankfurt. Thus, in 1903 and early 1904 Arrhenius was able to explore first hand Ehrlich's concepts of the antibody-antigen-complement reaction. Ehrlich, who correctly held that the antibody contained a region that served as a receptor for complement, was countered by Jules Bordet, who also correctly thought that the complex of antibody and antigen must be formed before complement-fixation could occur. Bordet, however, was wrong in assuming that the adherence of complement was merely physical or colloidal, and Ehrlich was mistaken in originally denying the prerequisite of complex formation. Arrhenius participated in some of the research designed to answer Bordet's criticism of the complement receptor concept.

The experimental results did not settle the controversy. Arrhenius could not agree with either Ehrlich's or Bordet's mechanism of hemolysis, the experimental system in which antibody-sensitized red blood cells are dissolved by complement; he preferred his own, which resembles the activity of weak acids and bases. A book of lectures he compiled, excerpts of which follow, discussed these studies. The book and particularly the brief preface laid out the frontiers of immunochemistry, coining the term

itself. Arrhenius observed that antigen-antibody reactions obeyed the law of mass action, being reversible with concentrations proportional to velocity. Ehrlich thought the union to be more durable, like a true chemical bonding. Ehrlich was wrong, although, as was determined some 50 years later with highly sophisticated radioisotope and fluorescent technology, the antibody-antigen equilibrium or affinity constant is extremely high, with range of 10^8 to 10^{12} liters per mole depending on the particular mixture of heterogenous antibody. The strength of this bonding is evident when comparing the constant to that of the weakly soluble salt $BaCO_3$ (10^4) and the insoluble salt PbS (10^{14}). Like a good tactical theoretician, Ehrlich considered the ideas of Arrhenius and modified his stand, permitting reversibility through an intermediate, unstable stage.

Arrhenius and Madsen continued their collaboration on various immunological subjects for several more years. Although they attacked Ehrlich's views, no heated polemic ensued; the investigators respected each other too much. Furthermore, interpretations, not data, were contested. As in the case of many early controversies, the core of both positions was essentially correct as manifested by the actual mechanisms: in this instance, the electrostatics of hydrogen bonding, hydrophobic rejection, and van der Waal forces are all involved in the largely complementary atomic interactions.

After again refusing a professorship and laboratory in Germany, Arrhenius in 1905 accepted the appointment as Director of the Nobel Institute of Physical Chemistry in Stockholm. His scientific interests also extended to cosmology, astronomy, and meteorology, in which he made some important contributions, such as the influence of pressure exerted by solar light on comet tails. Arrhenius's emphasis on quantitation, mathematical and graphic evaluation, and physics is his foremost contribution to immunology. He helped bring the science out of the nineteenth-century age of description and empiricism into the modern period of mechanism and analysis.

For further information:

Kohler, R. E. 1975. The history of biochemistry: a survey. *Journal of the History of Biology* 8:275–318.

Riesenfeld, E. H. 1931. *Svante Arrhenius.* Akademische Verlagsgesellschaft B.M.H., Leipzig. 110 p.

Rubin, L. P. 1980. Styles in scientific explanation: Paul Ehrlich and Svante Arrhenius on immunochemistry. *Journal of the History of Medicine* 35:397–425.

Walker, J. 1928. Arrhenius memorial lecture. *Journal of the Chemical Society* 3:1380–1401.

The Paper*

The following pages contain a summary of six lectures on the Immunity Reactions delivered at the University of California, in Berkeley, California, during the summer session of 1904. The object of the lectures was to illustrate the application of the methods of physical chemistry to the study of the theory of toxins and antitoxins. The idea that the reciprocal action of toxin and antitoxin is of the same nature as a chemical reaction is nearly as old as the study of these phenomena, which was inaugurated by the discovery of the diphtheria antitoxin by Behring and Kitasato in 1890. The German school, led by Ehrlich, the renowned Director of the Prussian Serum Institute in Frankfort-on-the-Main, has in particular done much work in support of the opinion that the interaction of toxin and antitoxin is of the nature of a chemical reaction; whereas the French school, led by Metschnikoff, tried to show that the effect of an antitoxin is chiefly of physiological order, an antitoxin was supposed to stimulate in some way the organic tissues in their struggle against the attack of the poison. . . . . The chemical hypothesis is now generally accepted, and has been adopted recently by Bordet, who originally expressed idea similar to those held by Metchnikoff.

*Arrhenius, S. 1907. *Immunochemistry. The application of the principles of physical chemistry to the study of the biological antibodies.* Macmillan, New York. 309 p.

Nevertheless, many difficulties to the chemical hypothesis remained. Nothing was more natural, therefore, than that the further elucidation of the problem should be sought through the aid of the modern theories of solution. To this end Madsen and Ehrlich invited me to join in their work. . . . [I]t was determined that the laws of equilibrium found their applications. It would seem, therefore, that the adherents of the chemical hypothesis should have felt wholly satisfied with the results. However, one of the strange incidents with which the history of science is replete occurred. In our explanation of the investigated phenomena, especially regarding the diphtheria toxin, Madsen and I, in accordance with the usual rule in the exact sciences, tried to employ as few hypotheses as possible, and in this we followed the example of Bordet. We tried to show that the phenomena observed might be explained on the supposition that diphtheria toxin is a simple substance which slowly decomposes into an innocuous material that still neutralizes antitoxin. In his explanation Ehrlich had previously assumed the presence in the diphtheria poison of a large number of poisonous substances of different strength. Now Ehrlich did not wish to yield this explanation. . . .

I have given to these lectures the title "Immunochemistry," and wish with this word to indicate that the chemical reactions of the substances that are produced by the injection of foreign substances into the blood of animals, i.e., by immunization, are under discussion in these pages. From this it follows also that the substances with which these products react, as proteins and ferments, are to be here considered with respect to their chemical properties. And for the purpose of a clarification of ideas, other substances that behave in an analogous manner will be given a consideration in the discussion.

It is evident that the objection recently raised by Ehrlich and Sachs to this manner of investigation, namely, that it does not enter upon the mode by which the living body produces these so-called antibodies, is quite true. An investigation of the chemical relations of toxin and antitoxin need not carry with it an elucidation of the synthesis of the antitoxin. But I fancy that there are many who are so deeply interested in the chemical behavior of these substances that they will find an investigation of this question well worthy of study. And for myself, furthermore, I believe that the physiological side of the problem, alluded to by Ehrlich, will not find a satisfactory solution until the more simple chemical aspect is elucidated. . . .

The antigenic properties of methylated protein

1917 • Karl Landsteiner

Comment

To read the next milestone is to plunge the mind's eye into the very small and view in awe the then fuzzy new realm of molecules that immunochemistry was beginning to probe. Karl Landsteiner first put flesh on Paul Ehrlich's skeletal conceptions. After Landsteiner, antigens could no longer be considered amorphous globs; they possessed distinct, recognizable atomic groups. In 1914 Landsteiner discovered and soon fashioned an extraordinary tool to explore the mechanisms and characteristics of immunological specificity. He chemically manipulated and modified antigens as a sculptor, testing their aesthetics on an audience of antibody-forming animals. In molecules as in higher organisms, shape relates to function, and with the contribution of Landsteiner's large body of immunochemical research, immunology became a science of shape recognition and response.

At the time of writing the article presented here, Landsteiner was Chief of Pathology at the Wilhelmina Hospital in Vienna and Adjunct (unpaid) Professor in the medical faculty at the University of Vienna. After World War I, the new Republic of Austria was in a state of chaos, with fuel and food shortages and accelerating inflation. Finding the situation hopeless and disruptive, Landsteiner departed to The Hague in 1919 for a position at the Catholic Hospital. Soon, on recommendation by Dutch authorities and with the support of Simon Flexner, its Director, the Rockefeller Institute of Medical Research beckoned Landsteiner. Arriving in New York in 1923, he was presented with full membership and a small laboratory. His research interests in Austria had included microbiology and pathology, especially poliomyelitis; however, the administration insisted that he restrict his investigations to immunochemistry and serology. It was a wise decision.

As the technology and knowledge of organic chemistry expanded, Landsteiner was able to examine in detail the influence of position on attached radicals. Ortho, meta, and para configurations on aromatic rings altered the immunological as well as the physicochemical characteristics of stereoisomers. Changes were especially pronounced with the acidic groups $-COOH$, $-SO_3H$, and $-AsO_3H_2$. For example, an antiserum to m-aminobenzene sulphonate reacted almost as well to the ortho isomer but poorly to the para configuration as the homologous antigen. Substitution of the arsonyl group ($-AsO_3H_2$) in the meta position would still permit coupling with the antibodies, although the reaction would be somewhat weaker.

Landsteiner ascertained that small structures, which were unable to elicit antibodies on their own, were able to combine with antibody receptors made against the entire antigen. He called the combining group a "determinant" (now termed an epitope); its supporting structure was named a "hapten," based on Paul Ehrlich's haptophore and derived from the Greek word meaning "to grasp." A hapten can comprise more than one determinant, although typically the number is one or two. Haptens bound to a "carrier" molecule are antigenic. As his paper indicated, cross-reactivity of antibodies can occur when dissimilar antigens, such as obtained from different animal species, comprise the same or sufficiently alike haptens. He later cleverly exploited this fact to differentiate carrier-specific and hapten-specific antibodies.

By the time Landsteiner wrote his classic and still inspiringly grand summation, the book *The Specificity of Serological Reactions,* he had collected and tested an extensive variety of protein derivatives. He also produced and analyzed sequenced peptides of two to five amino acids for linkage with carrier antigens, as synthetic versions of Ehrlich's side chains. Furthermore, complex proteins were degraded to locate their antigenic and haptenic components. The discovery that haptens can combine with existing antibodies led to experiments in allergic desensitization. Thus, the approach of Landsteiner and his associates was thoroughly modern, except for the absence of rigorous quantitation. Precision rested with his experimental design and with the sharply defined qualitative data. Any quantification was in the form of relative values and first-order approximations. Further precision was not necessary, for the principle and the pattern were far more important.

One of the new approaches to immunotherapy and molecular probes, as mentioned previously, involves the construction of synthetic vaccines. The haptenic spatial structure of known antigens is analyzed in detail with the assistance of computer graphics. Haptenic clefts and protrusions may be formed by a continuous segment of a protein chain or by the juxtaposition of separated segments brought together by chain-folding. Peptides of the continuous variety are easily synthesized for immunization, but different and far more difficult strategies must be used for haptens formed by adjacent domains or chains. In one possible approach, the circumscribed space is mimicked by a specifically designed peptide or glycopeptide, whose component features are chosen from a preanalyzed collection as a crime artist selects noses and beards from a group of standard overlays to match the description of witnesses. The antibodies elicited by this hapten, complexed with a carrier, may then cross-react with the target microbial pathogen or host cellular antigen. Synthetic vaccines, hence,

would be a most fitting application of Landsteiner's research.

For further information:

Kabat, E. A. 1968. *Structural Concepts in Immunology and Immunochemistry.* Holt, Rinehart and Winston, New York. 310 p.

Landsteiner, K. 1945. *The Specificity of Serological Reactions.* Revised edition. Harvard University Press, Cambridge. 310 p.

Lerner, R. A. 1983. Synthetic vaccines. *Scientific American* 248(2):66–74.

Speiser, P. and F. G. Smekal. 1975. *Karl Landsteiner* (R. Rickett, translator). Verlag Brüder Hollinek, Vienna. 198 p.

The Paper*

The following will relate the results of a serological examination of methylated protein, which has been carried out like the earlier study of acetylated protein. . . .

We found that the methylation of protein is easy to achieve at a uniform temperature and under conditions that exclude decomposition. The method consists of reacting diazomethane (CH_2N_2) with protein in an ether solution (containing a little methyl alcohol). In this way, the representative substances of serum protein—casein, edestin, gelatin, silk, and protamine—were examined. . . . We found a considerable amount of methyl groups that were bound to oxygen and nitrogen. For example, protein of horse serum treated twice with diazomethane contained almost 4% OCH_3 and more than 3% nitrogen-bound CH_3. . . .

The methylated product is easy to dissolve in salt solution, easier than the original alcohol-precipitated protein. The suspension is pure white and reacts poorly in base. As with the acetylated serum protein, the Biuret reaction, xanthoprotein reaction, and the reactions with potassium nitric acid, alkaline lead solution, dimethylamidobenzaldehyde, and dia-

---

*Landsteiner, K. 1917. Ueber die Antigeneigenschaften von methyliertem Eiweiss. VII. Mitteilung über Antigene. *Zeitschrift für Immunitätsforschung.* Orig. 26:122–133. [With permission of Springer-Verlag, Wien.]

zobenzolsulfonic acid are positive. As earlier stated, the ninhydrin reaction is weak. . . .

For immunization, 5 rabbits were intraperitoneally injected 4 times with 10 cc of serum and the corresponding amount of the emulsion at intervals of about 10 days. All animals yielded potent immune sera as determined by complement-fixation experiments.

The obtained immune sera showed distinct structure specificity similar to the previously examined antibodies against acetyl protein. The fact that the sera reacted only with the homologous antigen when it was strongly diluted obviously leads, as already mentioned, to the conclusion that the antigen being used was a suspension and not in solution. The same behavior was observed on all antigens of this form. It can be assumed that, besides any possible dissolved portions of the substance (as colloid), a reaction takes place only on the surface of the suspended particles. Large amounts of the substances were still ineffective.

[A table is introduced that shows specificity of antisera to methylated horse serum against homologous antigen in contrast with negative complement-fixation reactions to native protein; proteins treated with alcohol, alcoholic acids, or hydrochloric acid; and acetylated and diazolated proteins.]

The very distinct structural specificity of the methylated protein can also be found with the inverted experimental arrangement, namely, bringing together methylated protein from horse serum with different immune sera, which were produced through injection of differently treated horse serum proteins.

As we can see in these results, the horse methylated protein reacted only with structurally homologous antiserum or immune sera obtained by injections of esterified protein. [A weak reaction was recorded.] This phenomenon is not rare, but has already been observed by others and in our own experiments, namely reciprocal behavior [cross-reactivity] of a pair of antigens and antibodies. While the reaction of the methylated protein with the mentioned immune sera was very pronounced, the inverted reaction—antiserum to methylated protein against protein ester—could not be established, not even with the use of simple hemolysins. From this it may be concluded that the binding and immunogenic functions of an antigen often does not fully manifest parallelism. Since the recognition of such a reaction only becomes possible by knowing its intensity, it surely would not be easy to assert a total failure in detecting it.

A quantitative examination gave the following result. [Progressive dilutions of methylated proteins are reacted respectively with antisera to protein ester, methylated protein, and saline control; a series

of dilutions of ester protein are mixed respectively with antisera to esterified protein, methylated protein, and saline.]

A second analogous experiment had a similar outcome. The effect of the protein ester antisera on the heterologous antigens (at about the same concentrations) appeared noticeably stronger than with the homologous antigen. . . . The fact that the ester antisera can cross-react with methylated protein is presumably explainable through the close chemical relationship of both antigens, since the influence of alcoholic acids on protein causes the formation of alkyl groups. On the other hand, it should be remembered that antisera against acetylated protein mixed with protein ester may not necessarily yield a very intense reaction.

The immune sera were also reacted with a preparation that is produced analogously to methyl derivatives. Horse serum protein was treated with nitrosoethylurethane to create an ethylated protein. The immune sera reacted well with this preparation, but in experiments with decreasing antigenic concentrations, the reaction clearly was weaker than with the methylated product.

The examination of species specificity with methylated protein resulted in a significant change. The antibodies against methylated horse protein reacted not only with this antigen, but also with methylated protein from chickens and even rabbits. The quantitative proportions were similar, as they have been found with acetylated proteins. In a test with decreasing amounts of antigen and a constant and sufficient quantity of immune serum, the differences found between the several species of protein were small and variable; whereas, when a given antigen concentration was used and titration was performed by reducing the serum concentration, the decreasing strength of reactivity resulted in the following ranking: horse, chicken, and rabbit.

Again, as in the previous studies, the effect of immune sera on plant protein, namely methylated edestin, was determined. . . . The experiment showed a weak reaction of the methylated protein antisera on methylated edestin, but considering the control tests with other immune sera, it cannot be ignored. . . . [Assays by flaky precipitation, flocculation, were next examined. Results were similar but less specific.]

The earlier mentioned observations on the antigenic properties of the methylated protein show that certain chemical alterations—even if they do not cause a splitting of the protein molecule and do not disturb the structure of the amino acids—initiate corresponding changes in the antigenic properties, so that specific antibodies correspond to particular protein derivatives. The examination of the serological attributes of the methylated protein go further, since the kind of chemical changes in an antigen can be demonstrated more accurately than in most of the previous instances. . . .

The entry of methyl groups appears most surely with COOH, OH, NH_2, and perhaps NH– groups. Therefore, it can be put forward that the attachment of alkyl groups to the salt-forming groups of the protein greatly changes the antigenic characteristics, abolishing species specificity and producing a new structural specificity. . . . The described extensive changes in antigenic properties presumably can be caused through the substitution of different groups.

The soluble specific substance of pneumococcus

1923 • Michael Heidelberger and Oswald T. Avery

Comment

Oswald T. Avery (1877–1955) knew how to lure talented scientists to assist his investigation of bacterial pneumonia. He would carry in his pocket, or have strategically placed in a desk drawer, a small vial of powdered pneumococcal capsular material. This constituent was designated the soluble specific substance (SSS) because it precipitated in the presence of antipneumococcal antiserum of the same serological type as the cultured bacterium from which the material was derived. Avery had little doubt that SSS, which was so readily and profusely produced by the bacteria and found in the blood and urine of pneumonia patients, was crucial to understanding this infectious disease and its specificity. Preliminary analysis, as presented in the following paper, indicated that SSS was a polysaccharide with possible protein contamination. Approaching his victim, Avery would take out the bottle and gently shake its brownish contents. Urging, charming words, and the magical prop of mysterious, shifting grains enticed, for example, Rene J. Dubos, a young graduate student in soil microbiology at the New Jersey Agricultural Experiment Station to work with him. Dubos' assigned task was to find an enzyme that would split the polysaccharide; the ensuing loss of immunological reactivity would be further evidence that polysaccharide alone was responsible for type specificity, an unorthodox concept. Previously, Avery had worn down the resistance of Michael Heidelberger, who had been trying to crystallize oxyhemoglobin for another team at the Rockefeller Institute and convinced him to change fields. Dubos stated many years afterward that his meeting with Avery was the most important event of his career. Heidelberger regarded his own decision to join Avery's project as similarly fortunate.

Avery, who was born in Nova Scotia, Canada, graduated from Colgate University in 1900 and received his M.D. four years later from Columbia University College of Physicians and Surgeons. While in general medical practice, he began to investigate bacteriological problems, which he found more satisfying than treating patients. This led in 1907 to his appointment as associate director of the bacteriology group at the Hoagland Laboratory in Brooklyn. From here, he moved across the East River, where his career at the Rockefeller Institute, from 1913 to 1948, took him from an assistant in the hospital to an esteemed Emeritus Member. Affectionally nicknamed "Professor" or "Fess" by his colleagues, Avery was a persistent and patient investigator. He intuitively felt that the brown powder would eventually explain bacterial antigenic specificity, and was rewarded at the age of 67 with a discovery of even greater depth: the origin of specificity itself. He found that DNA is the hereditary transforming principle—the stuff of dead, virulent, encapsulated pneumococci that when transferred to living, attenuated, capsule-free strains yielded living, virulent, encapsulated bacteria. DNA thus carried the information for forming particular capsular polysaccharides of unique antigenic specificity.

Avery wanted Heidelberger to join his group because he needed a chemist to analyze the composition of the soluble substance. His hunch that the material was the immunological key to pneumococcal infections was later validated when his team established it to be responsible for virulence as well as antigenic specificity. Heidelberger was a native New Yorker. After earning his Ph.D. in organic chemistry at Columbia University, he traveled to the Federal Polytechnic Institute in Zurich for postdoctoral training. Initially planning to accept an appointment at the University of Illinois, he took instead the unexpected job offer at the Rockefeller. Heidelberger found himself becoming first a biochemist and then, after collaborative research with Karl Landsteiner, an immunochemist. With a long, active life, Heidelberger became the dean of immunochemistry, and could often be found at the laboratory bench at the age of 98!

Analytical technology was crude at the time, and Heidelberger and Avery were duly cautious. Nevertheless, the evidence was clear: the capsular substance was protein-free carbohydrate. This result forced a revision in the concept of immunogenicity. It had been almost an axiom that only proteins are antigenic, the few reports of antigenic glycoproteins being the only exceptions. Heidelberger and Avery's publication is thus lauded as the first to unquestionably overturn that rule. However, this is not quite true. They stated that the soluble substance was not antigenic; its ability to precipitate with existing antibodies indicated that it was a hapten. Perhaps protein was necessary

after all. When they later coupled the polysaccharide with a protein carrier, the rabbits produced antibodies. Years afterwards the problem was resolved: it was a matter of dosage. Presented in small to moderate amounts, the pure carbohydrate is antigenic in humans, the natural host, but haptenic in rabbits. Rabbits require very small doses for immunization, for they are especially prone to immunological paralysis, a form of tolerance. At low doses, mice can also become immunized.

Three other examples of antigenic carbohydrates are microbial teichoic acids, the surface polysaccharides of meningococci, and dextrans. The dextrans, which are repeating units of glucose, were the means by which Elvin A. Kabat, a student of Heidelberger, determined the approximate maximum size of the antibody receptor. He found that he could interfere with the coupling of dextran and its antibodies by first mixing the antibodies in turn with appropriate oligosaccharides of various length, from isomaltose to isomaltoheptaose. The hexasaccharide and heptasaccharide yielded maximal inhibition. It so happens that dextran reacts with horse antibodies to Type II pneumococcal polysaccharide, which is composed of methylpeptose rhamnose, glucose, and glucuronic acid. Cross-reactivity is best inhibited with isomaltopentaose. Any definition of antigenicity, in short, must consider the carbohydrates, but it can exclude pure lipids and nucleic acids, although they may be haptenic when complexed with proteins.

For further information:

Dubos, R. J. 1976. *The Professor, the Institute, and DNA*. The Rockefeller University Press, New York. 238 p.

Gill, T. J., III. 1972. The chemistry of antigens and its influence on immunogenicity. In: *Immunogenicity* (F. Borek, editor). North-Holland Publishing Company, Amsterdam. pp. 5–44.

Goebel, W. F. 1975. The golden era of immunology at the Rockefeller Institute. *Perspectives in Biology and Medicine* 18:419–426.

Heidelberger, M. 1977. A "pure" organic chemist's downward path. *Annual Review of Microbiology* 31:1–12.

***

The Paper*

In 1917 Dochez and Avery showed that whenever pneumococci are grown in fluid media, there is present in the cultural fluid a substance which precipitates specifically in antipneumococcus serum of the homologous type. This soluble substance is demonstrable in culture filtrates during the initial growth phase of the organisms; that is, during the period of their maximum rate of multiplication when little or no cell death or disintegration is occurring. The formation of this soluble material by pneumococci on growth *in vitro* suggested the probability of an analogous substance being formed on growth of the organism in the animal body. Examination of the blood and urine of experimentally infected animals gave proof of the presence of this substance in considerable quantities in the body fluids following intraperitoneal infection with pneumococcus. In other words, this soluble material elaborated at the focus of the disease readily diffuses throughout the body, is taken up in the blood, passes the kidney, and appears in the urine unchanged in specificity. Similarly, a study of the serum of patients suffering from lobar pneumonia has revealed a substance of like nature in the circulating blood during the course of the disease in man. Furthermore, examination of the urine of patients having pneumonia due to pneumococci of Types I, II, and III has shown the presence of this substance in some stage of the disease in approximately two-thirds of the cases. Recently from filtered alkaline extracts of pulverized bacteria of several varieties, including pneumococci, Zinsser and Parker have prepared substances which appear free from coagulable protein. These substances, called "residue antigens," are specifically precipitable by homologous antisera. These observers consider these acid- and heat-resistant antigenic materials analogous to the soluble specific substances of pneumococcus described by Dochez and Avery. In spite of the fact that these "residue antigens" are precipitable by homologous sera produced by immunization with the whole bacteria, Zinsser and Parker have so far failed to produce antibodies in animals by injecting the residues.

In the earlier studies by Dochez and Avery certain facts were ascertained concerning the chemical characteristics of the substance. It was found that the specific substance is not destroyed by boiling; that it is readily soluble in water, and precipitable by acetone, alcohol, and ether; that it is precipitated by colloidal iron, and does not dialyze through parchment; and that the serological reactions of the substance are not affected by proteolytic digestion by trypsin. Since the substance is easily soluble, thermostable, and type-specific in the highest degree, it seemed an ideal basis for the beginning of a study of the relation between bacterial specificity and chemical constitution. The present report deals with the work done in this direction.

The organism used in the present work was Pneumococcus Type II. The most abundant source of the soluble specific substance appeared to be an 8-day autolyzed broth culture; hence this material was used as the principal source of supply. . . .

The process for the isolation of the soluble specific substance consisted in concentration of the broth, precipitation with alcohol, repeated re-solution and reprecipitation, followed by a careful series of fractional precipitations with alcohol or acetone after acidification of the solution with acetic acid, and, finally, repeated fractional precipitation with ammonium sulfate and dialysis of the aqueous solution of the active fractions. . . .

By the method outlined above all substances precipitable with phosphotungstic acid or capable of giving the biuret reaction were eliminated. The residual material for which no claim of purity is made . . . contained, on the ash-free basis, 1.2 per cent of nitrogen. It was essentially a polysaccharide, as shown by the formation of 79 per cent of reducing sugars on hydrolysis, and by the isolation and identification of glucosazone from the products of hydrolysis. . . .

The aqueous solution of the substance gave the Molisch reaction out to the limit of delicacy of the test. Reduction of Fehling's solution occurred only after hydrolysis. Phosphorous was present only in traces; sulfur and pentoses were absent. A 1 per cent solution gave no biuret reaction, no precipitate with phosphotungstic acid, mercuric chloride, or neutral lead acetate, precipitated heavily with basic lead acetate, and gave a faint turbidity with tannic acid. Calcium is very tenaciously retained, but does not appear to be an essential part of the molecule, as the specific reaction was also given by calcium-free preparations. No color is given by iodine solution.

The soluble specific substance is remarkably stable to acids. A solution in 0.5 N hydrochloric acid maintained its activity undiminished and failed to reduce

***

*Heidelberger, M. and O. T. Avery. 1923. The soluble specific substances of pneumococcus. *Journal of Experimental Medicine* 38:73–79. [By copyright permission of The Rockefeller University Press.]

TABLE I.

Summary of the Properties of Various Preparations of the Soluble Specific Substance of Pneumococcus Type II.

Preparation No.	Total N.	Hydrolysis.			S	P	Specific rotation $[\alpha]_D$	Precipitation with immune serum.*	Molisch reaction.†
		NH₂ N	NH₂ N	Reducing sugars.					
	per cent	per cent	per cent	per cent	per cent	per cent			
4‡	6.1	3.5			1.5		Too dark.	1:80,000	
4A§	4.7			63.0		1.0‖	−20.6°	1:640,000	1:320,000
8¶	2.9			++			+19.8°	1:1,250,000	1:640,000
9	6.6				1.8		−8.6°	1:640,000	
11	2.1	0.9	1.3				+31.6°	1:2,500,000	1:1,250,000
15	2.0			49.0		0.9‖	+30.8°	1:2,500,000	1:1,250,000
17	1.2	C = 46.2 per cent.	H = 6.1 per cent.	79.0	None.	Tr.	+55.7°	1:3,000,000	1:1,500,000

* After 2 hours at 37°C. and over night at 4°.

† Unless the α-naphthol solution is fresh, other colors will mask the purple at high dilutions. The figures represent the dilution of the preparation itself; in other words, the highest dilution giving the reaction in the previous column.

‡ From urine.

§ Preparation 4 repurified.

‖ Due to incomplete dialysis.

¶ From dissolved pneumococci.

Fehling's solution after 36 hours at room temperature, but showed reducing sugars and absence of precipitation with immune serum after transfer to the water bath. . . .

Attempts to stimulate antibody production by the immunization of animals with the purified substance yielded negative results.

While it has long been known that the capsular material of many microorganisms consists, at least in part, of carbohydrates, any connection between this carbohydrate material and the specificity relationships of bacteria appears to have remained unsuspected. While it cannot be said that the present work establishes this relationship, it certainly points in this direction. Evidence in favor of the probable carbohydrate nature of this soluble specific substance is the increase in specific activity with reduction of the nitrogen content, the increase in optical rotation with increase in specific activity, the parallelism between the Molisch reaction and specific activity, the high yield of reducing sugars on hydrolysis, and the actual isolation of glucosazone from a small quantity of the material. The small amounts of substance available up to the present have hindered the solution of the problem, and it is hoped that efforts at further purification of the soluble specific substance, now in progress with larger amounts of material, will definitely settle the question.

The chemistry of antigens and antibodies

1934 • John R. Marrack

Comment

Immunology, which long had been regarded primarily as a medical study with therapeutic goals, also became by the late 1920s an exciting field of purely chemical inquiry. In 1925 H. Gideon Wells published *The Chemical Aspects of Immunity* under the aegis of the American Chemical Society. It was translated into German and French, and sold so well that a second and enlarged edition appeared four years later. At this time, the entire scope of physics and chemistry was in flux. A crescendo, which would provide immunochemistry with a new conceptual superstructure, was mounting. Colloidal chemistry was at the peak of its popularity, but already the idea of polar, hydrophilic bonds was taking root.

By the close of the decade, chemists were witnessing some interesting developments: the crystallization of an enzyme and the recognition of proteins as macromolecules. The analytical ultracentrifuge, X-ray crystallography, and simple chromatography also appeared. Progress in the understanding of chemical interactions was now integrally associated with advances in biochemical technology. Thermodynamics and free energy calculations offered quantitative explanations of molecular binding and solubility. Of prime significance to the new science was the initial atomic model of Niels Bohr with its image of shells of electrons. The Bohr atom introduced the idea of electro-valency. Theories of covalent bonding and coordinated or hydrogen bonding were gradually gaining acceptance because of their simplicity and sophistication. Polar forces, usually characterized as hydrogen binding with respect to water, determined solubility of proteins and the formation of surface films by oils and lipids. Thus, new tools, techniques, and theories were

available for the increasing number of chemists who wandered into the field of immunology and for the physician-researchers who were anxious to explore and expand the biochemical foundation of medicine. Although quantum mechanics and its first standard interpretation were also developed during this era, biomedical scientists today are only just beginning to incorporate the paradigm into their disciplines.

John R. Marrack (1886–1976) was, like Karl Landsteiner, a physician with a deep interest in immunochemistry. A medical graduate of Cambridge University, he rose to Professor of Chemical Pathology at London Hospital Medical College. After returning to Cambridge as a University Lecturer, he continued his professorship of chemical pathology in the newly organized London University, where he remained until his death. In 1934 the Bacteriology Committee of the Medical Research Council asked him to write a review of the present state of immunochemistry to provide a more thorough understanding of infectious diseases and host responses. Marrack found the nuclear chemical and physio-chemical conceptions to be powerful tools in formulating his own novel hypotheses.

In his review, which is the following milestone, he proposed hydrophilic forces (hydrogen bonding) as a means of antigen-antibody union. He furthermore discovered that if antigens and particularly antibodies could have a valence greater than one, he could explain a variety of puzzling immunological phenomena, including flocculation, precipitation, and the solubility of antigen-antibody complexes in zones of excess antigen and antibody. Denaturation or significant distortion of antibody protein, which was thought responsible for insolubility and hence flocculation, had no place in his conception. Although he mentioned but did not discuss the Danysz effect, here, too, his model was appropriate. In 1902 Jean Danysz at the Pasteur Institute observed that the amount of antigen bound to antibody differed according to mixing procedure. If, to use his example, diphtheria toxin is added all at once to a like quantity of antitoxin, the poison will be neutralized. If, however, the same amount of toxin is first divided into several fractions and then with 15- to 30-minute intervals each portion is added in turn to antibody, the final solution will be toxic.

Marrack's milestone was the advent of the lattice theory of antibody-antigen coupling. Its fundamental requirement was that antibody must have at least two antigen-combining sites. From our modern perspective, the theory, so simple and understandable, indeed so probable, should have been adopted immediately as the explanation for the various phenomena of antibody-antigen complexes. However, no clear evidence existed that an antibody had two or more receptors that could bridge antigens. Furthermore, no one at the time could even isolate antibodies free of antigen or serum globulins. The antibody molecule was terra incognita: unknown composition, unknown shape, unknown size, unknown electrical charge. The subsequent discovery of van der Waals forces strengthened the lattice concept. Michael Heidelberger, Linus Pauling, and William C. Boyd appreciated Marrack's insight and shortly afterwards developed their own versions: the mutual multivalence, the framework, and the alternation theories. The biomedical community and also a few noted chemists, nevertheless, missed the point of valency, shared electrons, and the concomitant proximity of interacting molecules; they only discussed the possibility of hydrophilic and hydrophobic forces in relation to the archaic notion of colloids. Except for the group of astute young biochemists who were spanning the gap, Marrack's model would have to await another 25 years before it would be accepted in principle.

The antibody itself would have to be isolated and dissected.

For further information:

Fruton, J. S. 1976. The emergence of biochemistry. *Science* 192:327–334.

Kohler, R. E. 1975. The history of biochemistry: a survey. *Journal of the History of Biology* 8:275–318.

Pauling, L. 1946. Molecular structure and intermolecular forces. In: *The Specificity of Serological Reactions.* Revised edition. (K. Landsteiner). Harvard University Press, Cambridge. pp. 275–293.

The Paper*

Since the antibody globulin coats sensitized particulate antigens and forms the greater part of antigen-antibody precipitates, these new properties of the antigen-antibody complex may be ascribed to changes in the antibody globulin. It appears that these properties are very similar to those of proteins denatured, for example, by heat. . . .

When we consider the close packing of antibody molecules round the antigen, it does not appear necessary to invoke any special process of denaturation. When the antibody molecules are attacked to antigen (Figure XXII A), the polar groups, on which the solubility of the antibody globulin normally depends, are brought into apposition with each other, and attract each other instead of water molecules. The effect of such close packing on the accessibility of polar groups to water is well illustrated in the case of the fibrous proteins. Only the polar groups on the free surface are left available for binding water. If these are insufficient to keep the complex in solution, the complexes will aggregate if the surface potential is below a critical level. If the antibody molecule has more than one adsorbing site, it is possible that the complexes may be bound together in a coarse lattice such as is shown diagrammatically in two dimensions in Fig. XXII B. This view differs from the hypothesis that the antibody globulin is denatured in that the hydrophobe character of the particles of antibody combined with antigen is ascribed not only to a loss of attraction for water, but

*Marrack, J. R. 1934. *The Chemistry of Antigens and Antibodies.* Special Report Series no. 194. Medical Research Council, London. 135 p.

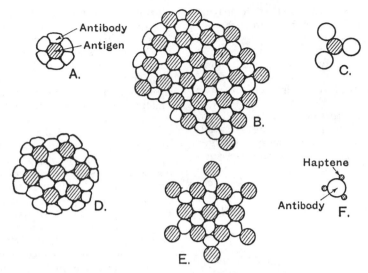

Figure XXII Diagrams of possible arrangements of antigen and antibody molecules in the complex. (A) simple unit; (B) complex structure at optimum proportions; (C) antigen excess; (D) antibody excess; (E) antigen excess; (F) antibody and haptene.

also to a specific attraction between the particles. This mutual attraction is due to the link provided by further antigen molecules. Differences in the structures thus formed would account for the macroscopic differences between the precipitates formed in different reactions. Polysaccharide antigens, for example, which probably form long chain molecules, can bind together a large structure, forming disklike coherent precipitates, unlike the granular precipitates formed by most protein antigens. . . .

Simple haptens do not, as a rule, form a precipitate when mixed with the corresponding antibodies; presumably because they have only one or two active groups per molecule and therefore do not cause the close packing of antibody molecules (Fig. XXII F). . . .

When antigen is in excess, complexes such as C or E in Fig. XXII will appear. Complexes such as C will remain soluble, as the polar groups of the antibody molecules are not brought together, and will therefore not aggregate; complexes such as E surrounded by antigen groups will be soluble and cannot be bound together by specific bonds, as none of the aggregates have any free antibody molecules on the surface. When antibody is in excess complexes such as D will be formed which likewise cannot be bound together by specific bonds. Consequently aggregation will be hindered when either antibody or antigen is in excess, giving rise to the so-called zone phenomenon. . . .

The remarkable point about the zone phenomenon is the difference between the results of antigen and antibody excess. Excess of antigen produces in-

hibition whichever procedure is used. . . . If it is supposed that antibody is denatured on combination with antigen, this difference between the effect of excess antibody and excess antigen would be accounted for on the supposition that antibody was denatured while antigen was not. With antigen in excess the complex formed would be coated and protected by undenatured antigen. . . .

On the supposition illustrated in Fig. XXII this difference between the effects of excess of antigen and antibody would be attributed primarily to the presence of more combining sites on antigen than on antibody. As a result the antigen-antibody precipitate would be mainly composed of antibody. This would mean that in the diagram of Fig. XXII antibody molecules pack tightly round antigen molecules and their polar groups neutralize each other, even when antibody is in excess. They will therefore be aggregated as relatively hydrophobe suspensions even when not bound by specific bonds. On the other hand, with antigen excess, as in C or E in Fig. XXII, no packing of the molecules on the surface occurs as there are not receptor sites on the antibody molecules to hold more antigen; the polar groups are available to attract water and flocculation does not occur.

. . .[N]o precipitation will occur in the post-zone (antigen excess) owing to the formation of small aggregates, such as E in Fig. XXII, protected by the excess of antigen. With smaller quantities of antigen continuously larger aggregates will be formed possibly arranged as a lattice with incomplete packing of the antibody molecules. These may settle, leaving the supernatant fluid cloudy, owing to the presence in it of large aggregates. At optimum proportions a continuous lattice will be formed. When the antigen concentration falls below this level, aggregation will be slower, mainly owing to the reduction in the number of antigen molecules which serve as centres of aggregation, also to some degree because the formation of a continuous lattice fails progressively more and more as no further antigen molecules are available to provide links for the formation of larger structures when aggregates of moderate size, such as D, are formed. Also some polar groups on the surface of particles such as D may not be blocked, and therefore retain their attraction for water, and to some extent inhibit the clumping of the particles as a hydrophobe suspension. . . .

[T]he optimum proportion is considered to be that ratio of antibody to antigen which is capable of forming a stable lattice. This will be determined partly by a question of size. In the instance in which the antigen, serum globulin, is of approximately the same size as the antibody, the ratio is 1 to 4. This would be given by a lattice such as shown in Fig. XXII (but in three dimensions), with each antigen molecule surrounded by 16 antibody molecules, and each antibody molecule by 4 antigen molecules (not three as in the flat figure). It is not necessary that at the proportion that forms a stable lattice all the "receptor sites" on the antibody should be satisfied by "determinant" antigen groups; that is, the most rapid flocculation need not occur in a neutral mixture of antigen and antibody.

In the agglutination of bacteria the formation of a lattice would be of considerably less importance, and therefore the increased rapidity of agglutination at optimum proportions considerably less marked. . . .

Owing to the fewness of their combining groups and to spatial considerations, simple haptene molecules, which are not themselves aggregated, cannot take the place of antigen molecules in the antibody-antigen lattice. Their inhibiting action on flocculation can therefore be compared to the inhibition of crystallization, from supersaturated solutions, by dyes which are adsorbed on the crystal surface. Such adsorbed molecules do not take the place of the essential constituents of the crystal in the crystal lattice, but inhibit crystallization. This affords an explanation of an unpublished observation of the reviewer that "simple haptenes," in amounts insufficient wholly to prevent flocculation, do not alter the "optimum proportions" of antigen to antibody. That is, on the present theory, they do not alter the proportions of antigen and antibody required for building a continuous lattice, although they slow the reaction by forming surface films.

Possible explanations of various other points suggest themselves.

The decreased reversibility on standing may be due to increased building up into a uniform structure, together with the replacement of intermolecular attraction by actual chemical bonds.

Temperature can affect immunity reactions in two ways, apart from actual damage to antigen or antibody at temperatures above 55°C. In the first place, a rise of temperature will increase the number of effective collisions between antigen and antibody, and will therefore accelerate the reaction. In the second place, increased heat vibration will tend to break down the compound of antigen and antibody and complexes built up by them. Hence immunity reactions take place more rapidly at higher temperatures up to a certain limit, but combination becomes firm and may break down at the higher levels.

An electrophoretic study of immune sera and purified antibody preparations

1939 • Arne Tiselius and Elvin A. Kabat

Comment

Of interest to our survey of immunochemistry is the Scandinavian center of physical chemistry. The Golden Age of most continuing scientific or medical disciplines has had a time-space focus. Typically, schools developed around pioneer standard-bearers, a situation also found in the history of art and design. For medical microbiology, it was Louis Pasteur in Paris and Robert Koch in Berlin roughly between 1870 and 1915, the Great War bringing the epoch to a premature close. For psychoanalysis, it was Sigmund Freud, Alfred Adler, and Carl Jung in Austria and Switzerland approximately between 1895 and 1940. The Great War, Part II, along with the deaths of the founders of the field closed that introductory chapter. The Scandinavian chemistry nucleus, arising under the influence of Svante Arrhenius, was especially active between 1900 and (again) 1940, resurging in the mid-1960s.

War, as indicated, has a nasty habit of disrupting orderly scholarship and experimental pursuits while furnishing, in compensation, the impetus for creativity and novel technology. Furthermore, the survival imperative often forces the emigration of many leading scientists to distant havens, shifting and diffusing the congregation of investigators and geographic focus of some research fields. Today with instantaneous communication, rapid transportation, and frequent international assemblies and collaboration, research hubs are scattered or short-lived and extremely local. More than ever, science is a coordinated global effort.

Between the wars, Theodor (The) Svedberg firmly planted the flag of creative chemical technology in Sweden. He was a professor of physical chemistry at the University of Uppsala, where he examined colloids. A winner of the 1926 Nobel Prize, he is best remembered for inventing the ultracentrifuge. Indeed, sedimentation coefficients are named in his honor. Between 1925 and 1932 Svedberg was assisted by Arne Tiselius (1902–1971), who received his own Nobel award in 1948 for another analytical method, electrophoresis.

Tiselius earned his doctorate in 1930. While serving as a lecturer between 1930 and 1938 at the Institute of Physical Chemistry of the University of Uppsala, he resided for one year (1934) at the Institute for Advanced Studies at Princeton University. In 1939 he was appointed Professor of Biochemistry at the University of Uppsala and given an institute newly created for this field. Tiselius was selected in 1947 to be the new vice president of the Nobel Foundation.

His dissertation concerned electrophoresis and the separate, differential migration of molecules within an electric field, but his system was crude and soon put aside. His American visit caused him to reevaluate the concept. In 1937 Tiselius developed an improved apparatus and began to examine serum. He invited Michael Heidelberger to send someone from his laboratory to study the physical chemistry of purified antibodies by the advanced techniques of ultracentrifugation and electrophoresis. Heidelberger did not hesitate to choose Elvin A. Kabat (1914–   ).

Kabat in 1932 had graduated from City College of New York with a major in chemistry, but was unable to find work because of the depression. By chance, Heidelberger's wife Nina bought some clothing from Kabat's mother, and suggested that young Kabat should see her husband. Although Michael Heidelberger considered Kabat to be "over-qualified" for the vacant position of laboratory aide, he accepted him. While still assisting in research, Kabat entered the graduate program in biochemistry at Columbia University College of Physicians and Surgeons. In 1937 he received his doctorate, and went to Sweden. On his return from Uppsala and after visiting other European research laboratories, he accepted the post of Instructor in Pathology at Cornell University Medical College. Three years later, Kabat was back at Columbia University, this time a member of the faculty in the Department of Bacteriology. He was promoted to the rank of Professor of Microbiology in 1952.

The collaboration of Tiselius and Kabat yielded an outstanding, entirely novel means for separating and physically characterizing antibodies from other serum proteins. Its principle has become the basis of a large variety of modifications, including isoelectric focusing and two-dimensional immunoelectrophoresis. As stated in the following milestone, they found antibodies in the third or gamma peak; hence, antibodies were soon termed gamma globulins. When it became known that some globulins of the gamma peak were not antibodies, the term immunoglobulins was introduced, begetting IgG (immunoglobulin gamma). Analysis by ultracentrifugation would establish gamma globulins to have a sedimentation coefficient of 7S, corresponding to a molecular weight of about 150,000 daltons. However, not all antibodies are of this category. Within the faster migrating beta peak are such immunoglobulins, first termed β_2-macroglobulins of γM and now called IgM (immunoglobulin macro). They have a sedimentation coefficient of 19S with molecular weight around 900,000 daltons. Changes in the electrophoretic pattern of serum occur over an immunization period. The first exposure to an antigen initiates IgM formation, which subsides after a delay as IgG increases. Subsequent contact with the antigen will typically produce a similar IgM response but an immediate and much higher IgG level, hence the term "booster shot." A significant finding of the research of Tiselius and Kabat was that antibodies are not uniform in electrical charge or sedimentation characteristics. This was the first indication that antibodies were physically heterogeneous. Correlations of physical properties with antibody specificity and avidity would soon be determined.

For further information:

Kabat, E. A. 1983. Getting started 50 years ago—experiences, perspectives, and problems of the first 21 years. *Annual Review of Immunology* 1:1–32.

Kekwick, R. A. and K. O. Pedersen. 1974. Arne Tiselius 1902–1971. *Biographical Memoirs of Fellows of the Royal Society* 20:401–428.

Tiselius, A. 1967. Introduction at the visit to the Institute of Biochemistry in Uppsala. In: *Gamma Globulins. Structure and Control of Biosynthesis.* Nobel Symposium 3 (J. Killander, editor). Interscience Publishers, New York. pp. 283–286.

Work, T. S. and E. Work (editors). 1970. *Laboratory Techniques in Biochemistry and Molecular Biology.* Vol-

ume I. North-Holland Publishing Company, Amsterdam. 572 p.

The Paper*

Studies on the electrophoresis of serum have shown that besides the albumin normal sera possess three separate globulin components differing in mobility and designated as α, β, and γ. The relationship of antibodies to these components is of considerable importance. Differences in the antibody globulin formed in various animal species have already been found by ultracentrifugal studies and in electrophoresis as well as by immunological means. It has also been shown that in an antiserum to crystalline egg albumin, the antibody migrated with the slowest (γ) component and could be isolated in one of the cells of the apparatus and analyzed for antibody content. The work reported in this communication is an attempt to study and compare the electrochemical properties of the antibody in the original sera with . . . purified antibody preparations . . . and to measure the isoelectric points of these purified preparations. It is also of importance to make use of and correlate the results obtained using both the mutually independent electrophoretic and ultracentrifugal methods since molecular weight homogeneity does not necessarily mean electrochemical homogeneity and *vice versa*. . . .

The new Tiselius electrophoretic apparatus, in which sections of the U tube may be moved with respect to one another and cut off the column of solution into four parts to permit isolation of various components, was used. . . . Two methods of observation of the migrating boundaries were applied, Toepler's *Schlieren* method and the Lamm scale method, both depending on refractive index changes in the solution due to the migrating boundary. The former of these in which each component appears as a black band in the U tube image in the focus of the camera, provides a convenient way of following the experiment by direct visual observation. In the latter method an equidistant scale placed behind the U tube is photographed at intervals through the solution. These photographs are compared microscopically with those from a reference scale photo-

---

*Tiselius, A. and E. A. Kabat. 1939. An electrophoretic study of immune sera and purified antibody preparations. *Journal of Experimental Medicine* 69:119–131. [By copyright permission of The Rockefeller University Press.]

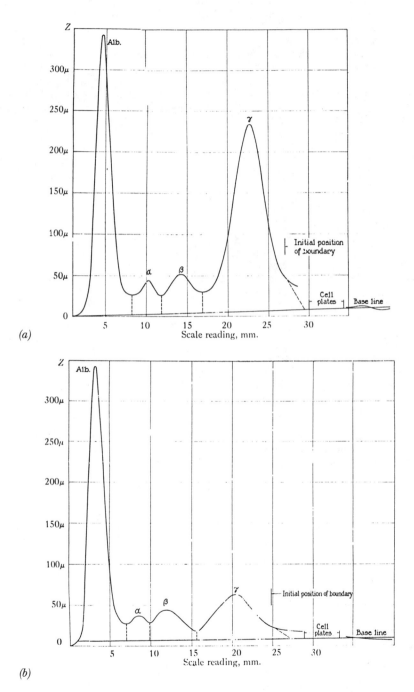

Figure 1 Electrophoresis scale diagram of anti-egg albumin rabbit serum 431–5 1:4 before (a) and after (b) absorption of the antibody.

graphed before the current is started. The displacement of the scale lines, Z, from their positions on the reference scale are plotted as ordinates against the corresponding positions in the U tube cell as abscissae yielding a curve in which each electrochemically distinct component in the solution will have its own peak. . . .

It can be . . . noted that in the horse antipneumococcus sera a new component migrating between β and γ was present. That this component disappeared on removal of the antibody (20.7 percent of the total protein) can be seen from the *Schlieren* photograph . . . before and after absorption of the antibody. No new component was observed in the other sera at the same pH. . . .

[R]esults [were] obtained by electrophoresis of rabbit and monkey antipneumococcus and anti-egg albumin sera before and after removal of the antibody. The type of curves obtained in the case of anti-egg albumin serum 431–5 is shown in Fig. 1 and the marked decrease in the γ component in the absorbed serum is evident. The absence of antibody in the α and β components was also directly established in the case of a rabbit antiserum to crystalline horse serum albumin by isolating the albumin and α and β components and demonstrating the absence of antibody with crystalline serum albumin. . . .

The mobility values obtained for the purified horse, pig, and rabbit antibodies were the same as that observed in serum at the same pH within experimental error. . . .

The results now obtainable with the new electrophoresis technique make it possible to obtain a more quantitative picture of the relationships of immune substances to the serum globulin and more detailed information about the electrochemical properties of immune sera and purified antibodies. [It was indicated] that the mobilities of the various normal components in sera from several animal species are approximately the same. . . .

In those antisera in which the antibody occurs in the slowest migrating fraction, the electrophoresis method could be used to isolate fairly pure antibody. It is of great importance to select antisera in which a very high percentage of the γ component is antibody. On immunization there occurs an increase in total serum protein, as well as in total globulin and antibody; therefore determination of the amount of antibody nitrogen would not be a sufficient guide to purification by the electrophoresis method. . . . The method should be most useful for obtaining purified antibodies to protein antigens since the salt dissociation methods are not applicable. In those cases in which the antibody is not in the slowest component the method is too laborious (such as horse antibody). The purified γ component is usually isolated in lower concentration than in the original serum due to the lack of absolute homogeneity of the globulin components. The advantage of the electrophoretic method is that it is a very mild method and permits isolation of proteins which retain their native state.

The data concerning the degradation of horse antibody in the animal on continued immunization indicate that it is also accompanied by a definite change in mobility as noted by the presence of two antibody components in a later bleeding from an animal which had previously shown one component. Thus 9093 B showed two components in electrophoresis, both in appreciable concentration and a comparison of the original serum absorbed and unabsorbed showed that some of the slower γ component was removed on absorption of the antibody. Similarly in horse antibody 902 E prepared from an earlier bleeding, only one component was observed in electrophoresis and in the centrifuge, while in 902 K prepared in the same way from a bleeding taken after another year of immunization, degraded material was present in the centrifuge and a new component of lower mobility was present in electrophoresis. This is probably a manifestation of a process of degradation and removal of antibody protein in the horse after prolonged immunization.

The hydrolysis of rabbit γ-globulin and antibodies with crystalline papain

1959 • Rodney R. Porter

Comment

When Rodney R. Porter (1917–1985) performed molecular surgery on the antibody, he lit the match to the immunological firecracker. Today the explosive renaissance of the science shows no signs of waning. Indeed, it has touched off secondary bursts in every field that it has entered. In 1972 the Nobel Committee awarded Porter their prestigious prize for his contributions in solving the puzzle of the immunoglobulin, which began with the following milestone.

Porter trained at the University of Liverpool and Cambridge University. Between 1949 and 1960 he worked at the National Institute for Medical Research, Mill Hill. Before taking his final post as Professor of Biochemistry at Trinity College at Oxford in 1967, he was Professor of Immunology at St. Mary's Hospital Medical School of London University.

His report itself is somewhat complicated and enigmatic. What is it about? Within the twenty years since the previous milestone, biochemistry had blossomed with development of knowledge of molecular structure, biosynthetic pathways, enzymic activity, and improved methodology. Such technological advances included radioisotopic tagging, two-dimensional paper chromatography, and column liquid chromatography, which were of two forms. One comprised ion exchange resins that, when followed by a wash of an increasing ionic gradient (pH also may be raised), separate molecules by their differing net electrical charge; the second was in essence a sieve of microbeads that separate a mixture of globular molecules based on their size, a correlate of molecular weight. Proteolytic enzymes were found to split proteins by hydrolyzing peptide bonds at locations unique for each agent. Since proteins are linear arrangements of different amino acids, however folded they may be, they have distinct polar ends of amino (nitrogen) and carboxyl groups. Chemical modification of the N terminal provided a marker for the product of hydrolysis, and was used in sequential analysis of proteins. Porter utilized these new methods in an attempt to pinpoint on antibodies the region or regions of antigen binding.

Porter used the enzyme papain, which required an activating reducing agent, to digest the structure and isolate two apparently similar fractions and one entirely distinct fragment. The dual peaks obtained upon chromatography, which contained the antigen receptors, were an artifact of methodology. The digestion of antibodies under acid conditions was later demonstrated to give fraction I; antibodies under basic conditions yielded fraction II. Thus, the two peaks were due to charge heterogeneity. If only one peak of twice the concentration had been obtained, Porter still would have reached the same conclusions.

The evidence strongly indicated bivalence—the first two fragments each being able to bind antigen without forming a precipitate, as predicted for univalent structures—and Porter noted the possibility that fraction I and II could lie on either side of fraction III, as suggested by Linus Pauling's model. The proportion of 2:1, if the artifact was eliminated, would be even more supportive of a duplicated receptor. Porter did not even consider the possibility of two distinct, covalently linked chains, since at the time all known protein structures were composed of a single polypeptide chain. Today Porter's fractions I and II are termed "Fab" for "fragment antigen-binding." Because the third fragment could be crystallized, it is known as "Fc" or "fragment crystalline." Crystals indicated that Fc fragments derived from antibodies of diverse specificity were virtually homogeneous. Conversely, the inability of fractions I and II to form crystals correlated antigen specificity with structural heterogeneity, i.e., differences in amino acid sequence. If Porter had instead used pepsin without a reducing agent, he would have found only one large peak and a range of small peptides. The substances in this major fraction would be able to precipitate antigens. With the addition of the reducing agent, the peak would be split in two as with papain. The results differ because the susceptible peptide bonds for pepsin are beyond the joint of disulfide bonds in the Fc region, while those for papain are above the disulfide linkage. The larger pepsin fragments are designated Fab', while the unreduced fragment containing dual antibody receptors is called F(ab')$_2$.

Since the primary goal of the research was to reduce the antibody to smaller yet still active structures, Porter succeeded. Beyond this, the complexities of the immunoglobulin remained hidden. Sausage-shaped clay models were built based on Porter's report and the photographs of inadequately prepared specimens of fragments taken by electron microscopy, a field then fresh and naive. Nevertheless, Porter took the first step, encouraging his colleagues on the immunochemical path. He also provided some significant clues and testable hypotheses. Buried within his technique was a chemical tool, the reducing agent, that was being used concurrently in another immunology laboratory. The reduction of disulfide bonds within and between immunoglobulin chains would later literally shake things apart.

For further information:

Kabat, E. A. and M. M. Mayer. 1961. *Experimental Immunochemistry*. 2nd edition. Charles C Thomas, Springfield, IL. 905 p.

Pasternak, C. A. 1985. Rodney Robert Porter. *BioscienceReports* 5:809–813.

Porter, R.R. 1967. The structure of antibodies. *Scientific American* 117(4):81–90.

Porter, R. R. 1973. Structural studies of immunoglobulins. *Science* 180:713–716.

The Paper*

The molecular size of rabbit γ-globulin is such that any direct attempt to relate structure to biological activity is not feasible at present. An alternative approach is to degrade antibody molecules in such a way that activity will persist in smaller fragments and so to reduce the structural problems involved. . . .

It has been found that γ-globulin is split by papain into three large pieces with very little release of amino acids or small peptides. If the γ-globulin contains antibody against any of the several antigens investigated, then two of these pieces retain combining though not precipitating power. The third piece, which may be readily crystallized, has no antibody activity but it has most of the antigenic sites of the original molecule. The isolation and properties of these three fractions will be described. . . .

[T]he recovery of γ-globulin protein taken has fallen in the range 85–95%. In view of the probable handling losses in dialysis and freeze-drying, it is considered that the higher figure is the most accurate. When such a digest examined in the ultracentrifuge in 0.1 M phosphate, pH 6–7, some crystals again formed on dialysis but the supernatant showed only one peak ($S_{20,w}$3.5). As γ-globulin has $S_{20,w}$6.5, it was clear that the protein had been split into large fragments of similar size with very little production of diffusible peptides. Attempts to fractionate this mixture by zone electrophoresis were not successful, the resolution could be achieved by chromatography on carboxylmethylcellulose. Acetate buffer, pH 5.5, was chosen because under these conditions most of the carboxyl groups of the ion-exchanger are dissociated. . . . To help to keep all the material in solution chromatography was carried out at room temperature (20–23°). With a gradient of increasing salt concentration at this pH, three components could be resolved which have been named fractions I, II and III in order of elution from the column.

---

*Porter, R. R. 1959. The hydrolysis of rabbit γ-globulin and antibodies with crystalline papain. *Biochemical Journal* 73:119–126. [Reprinted by permission.]

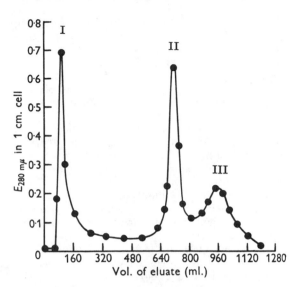

Figure 1   Chromatography of papain-digest of rabbit γ-globulin on carboxymethylcellulose. Weight of digest 150 mg. Column 30 cm × 2.4 cm diameter. Volume of mixing chamber 1200 ml. Gradient from 0.1 M-sodium acetate, pH 5.5, to 0.9 M-sodium acetate, pH 5.5, commencing at 200 ml eluate volume.

If the gradient on the column was reduced, fractions II and III were more spread and III "tailed" badly, but there was no suggestion of any further resolution. Fraction I appeared very close to the solvent front and this was re-run on a diethylaminoethylcellulose column at pH 6.4. No fractionation was obtained but again with a slow gradient there was considerable tailing. By these limited criteria the three fractions appeared to be single components and to be the only significant products of the digestion of γ-globulin by papain. . . .

Yields of the three fractions were measured by summing the absorption at 280 mμ in each peak. The ratios of yield varied somewhat from experiment to experiment but averaged (I:II:III) 1:0.8:0.9, and total recovery from the column was 85–90%. When re-run, fractions I and III were recovered in about 95% yield and fraction II in about 85% yield. The absorptions of peaks I, II and III at 280 mμ at a concentration of 1 mg/ml in water or 0.02 N acetic acid were 1.4, 1.4 and 1.0 respectively. If the relative yields are corrected for the lower recovery of fraction II, and the lower specific absorption at 280 mμ of fraction III, then the corrected relative yields (I:II:III) are 1:0.9:1.25 by weight. . . .

Fraction III is readily identifiable as the material with a low solubility near neutrality. It may be crystallized and recrystallized by dialyzing a solution in 0.02 N acetic acid against sodium phosphate buffer, pH 6.0–7.0, at 2°. The crystals are diamond-shaped plates, often of considerable size but thin and easily broken.

The three fractions were studied in the ultracentrifuge and the results for normal γ-globulin are summarized in Table 1 [γ-globulin, 188,000; I, 50,000; II, 53,000; III, 80,000]. . . . The relative sizes of the three fragments were (I:II:III) 1:1.05;1.6, which is in approximate though not exact agreement with the calculated relative yields of the fragments. . . .

The most striking feature of the analysis is the great similarity of the amino acid content of fraction I and II. With the exception of cystine, differences rarely exceed 10% and . . . this is close to the experimental error. In contrast, fraction III shows considerable differences, most marked in the contents of threonine, proline, glycine, alanine, methionine, isoleucine, tyrosine, cystine, and the three basic amino acids, the differences in several cases being more than 100%. . . .

About two-thirds of the carbohydrate of the original molecule is found with fraction III, one-third with fraction I and a small amount, which may not be significant, is with fraction II. . . . If the total recovery of carbohydrate in the the three fractions is compared with that present in the original, the yields are approximately 110 and 120% for hexose and hexosamine respectively. . . .

The three fractions were prepared from digests of γ-globulin which had been obtained from rabbit antisera against ovalbumin, bovine serum albumin, human serum albumin and antipneumococci polysaccharide type 3. None would precipitate with the corresponding antigen but fractions I and II prepared from γ-globulin containing antiprotein antibodies inhibited the precipitation of the antigen by the homologous antiserum. This effect is specific; for example, I and II from antihuman serum albumin γ-globulin had no effect when added to bovine serum albumin and its antiserum; fraction III, on the contrary, had no effect whatever its source or whatever the test system. . . .

In contrast with these results none of the fractions from antipolysaccharide γ-globulin appeared to have any power to inhibit the combination of polysaccharide with its antiserum. However, when much higher ratios of inhibitor to antibody were used, inhibition of precipitation occurred with fraction I or II. The differences between the antiprotein and antipolysaccharide fractions appears to be quantitative rather than qualitative. . . . Fraction III again appeared to be completely inactive in qualitative tests, but in this case the solubility limitation is greater and it could only be concluded that III has certainly less than half the activity of I or II.

The power of the fractions to precipitate with goat antirabbit γ-globulin serum was now tested and I and II showed neither precipitation nor inhibitory activity. Fraction III precipitated 70% of the antibody precipitated by γ-globulin.

Rat antiserum was prepared against rabbit γ-globulin and fractions I, II and III. Groups of three rats were used for each antigen and, after the immunization course . . . the serum of each group was pooled, and gave antibody contents of 4.2, 7.8, 8.1 and 4.0 mg of antibody/ml for γ-globulin, I, II and III respectively. All the fractions were at least as effective antigens as the original molecule, and I and II were the most effective, but as only three animals were used per group the difference may not be significant.

When rat anti-γ-globulin was tested with the fractions, rather different results from those with goat antiserum were obtained. Fraction III precipitated 50% of the antibody, and I and II 15% each. The antigenic specificities of the fractions were compared by measuring the precipitates from I, II and III with rat anti-II serum. . . . [T]he curves for I and II are almost identical, but III gives almost no precipitate. This again emphasizes the great similarity of I and II and their sharp distinction from III. . . .

The results show that papain-digestion of rabbit γ-globulin causes limited and highly selective splitting to give three large fragments and very few small peptides. As papain shows rather a wide specificity in the digestion of the chain of insulin, it is apparent that the structure of the native molecule must be such that many potentially hydrolyzable bonds are protected by steric and other factors. Ultracentrifuge studies of the splitting of γ-globulins from different species, by a variety of enzymes, have all shown that a small number of fragments are the main products in each. It is possible that in γ-globulins only small parts of the peptide chain are accessible to proteolytic enzymes, so that even though different enzymes break different bonds in these vulnerable sections the principal large digestion products are similar.

Our results with the papain-digestion of rabbit γ-globulin suggest that the single polypeptide chain has been split into three distinct sections, which together comprise some 90% of the original molecule. However, fractions I and II are so similar that the question arises whether they could be derived very largely from the same section of the chain. They are almost indistinguishable in N-terminal amino acid, amino acid analysis, molecular weight, antigenic specificity and, if derived from antibody, in their antigen-binding capacity. They differ in chromatographic behavior and carbohydrate and cystine content.

There are at least three possible ways of splitting a single chain to give results such as this, and they are illustrated in Fig. 6: A shows the obvious split into three distinct sections, B the production of two fractions from the same section of chain and C the result if γ-globulin consists of two types of molecule, such as euglobulin and pseudoglobulin, one of which gives rise to I + III and the other to II + III. If either B or C were correct then the yield of III should exceed the sum of the yield of I and II. In fact the yield of each of the three fractions is very similar, as would be expected in A. In B and C the overall recovery in view of the molecular weights found, would be 130,000/188,000, i.e. 70%, considerably lower than the experimental figure of about 90%, which again is that which would be expected if A were correct. . . .

It follows that two large sections of γ-globulin (each about 30% of the whole) are extremely similar in chemical, physical and biological properties. The finding of such close agreement between the amino acid analysis of these two fragments and also an almost identical antigenic specificity suggests that there may be almost a repeat of the amino acid sequence and configuration. This is in contrast with the properties of fraction III, which differs in every respect, so that there appears to be a large repeating Unit (I or II) joined to a larger section (III) of entirely different character. This unusual make-up of the γ-globulin molecule is presumably related to its antibody activity. . . .

The finding that γ-globulin appears to be built of three sections, one of exceptional stability and the other two containing the antibody-combining sites, is reminiscent of Pauling's theory of antibody formation, in which it is suggested that antibody molecules consist of a rigid centerpiece and two flexible

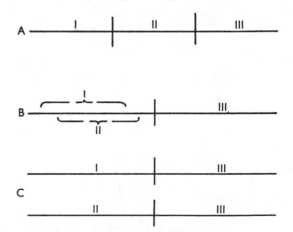

Figure 6 Different ways of splitting rabbit γ-globulin to give three fractions of approximately equal size.

ends capable of taking up configurations complementary to the antigen and hence forming antibody-combining sites on these flexible parts. . . . There is no evidence on the relative positions of fractions I, II and III in the whole molecule, except that II may be from the N-terminal end. Nor is there any evidence on the essential feature of Pauling's theory, that the amino acid sequence of all antibodies is identical and that the different atibody-combining sites are formed only by refolding of the same polypeptide chain. . . .

Studies on structural units of the γ-globulins

1961 • Gerald M. Edelman and M. D. Poulik

Comment

Rodney Porter shared the Nobel Prize in 1972 with Gerald M. Edelman (1929–   ), who used a similar strategy but different tactics in engaging the problem of antibody structure. Edelman's first report on this investigation appeared in 1959, but it is his more developed report of 1961 that follows. A biochemist may find the article a delight, and aficionados of gadgets and technology will also enjoy the work; others, particularly those who are more at home at the cellular and organismal level, may become a little dazzled and uncomfortable, despite the abridgment. Today increasingly technical, ultraspecialized papers have largely replaced the more readable articles of the generalist found in journals of earlier decades. Such is the price of advancement in science as complex concepts and nomenclature are developed to describe ever more complex phenomena.

Edelman came to immunology with an extensive medical background. After earning his M.D. from the University of Pennsylvania in 1954, he trained at Massachusetts General Hospital, served two years in the Army Medical Corps, and then in 1960 obtained the Ph.D. from the Rockefeller Institute, now Rockefeller University. He has remained at the Rockefeller as Professor of Biochemistry.

The second author of this milestone is M. D. (Miroslav Dave) Poulik (1923–   ). Born in Brno, Czechoslovakia, he emigrated to Canada, where he received his M.D. in 1960 from the University of Toronto. In 1961, after assisting Edelman on this research, he was appointed Assistant Director of Research at the American Red Cross facility in Washington, D.C., and then accepted a professorship in pediatrics at Wayne State University. In 1972 he also became Professor of Immunology and Microbiology at that university.

Edelman and Poulik suspected that the antibody was composed of more than one protein chain. If this were true, then the chains would likely be joined by way of disulfide bridges, such as found in the amino acid cystine. Porter used cysteine, itself a mild reducing agent, to activate papain. Edelman and Poulik chose the more potent sulfhydryl reagent, mercaptoethanol, to split the expected disulfide bonds, and added urea as a dissociating solvent for the fractions. Another problem confronted the team: antibody heterogeneity. In order to determine whether antibody specificity is a result of unique foldings of protein chains or whether it is due to the underlying amino acid sequence, a sufficient quantity of a homogeneous antibody was required. Normally large amounts of antibody with single specificity are unobtainable in serum; however, the epitome of cellular abnormality, the tumor cell, provided a solution. Lymphoid tumors, called myelomas, produce massive amounts of a single antibody. Each myeloma is a natural monoclonal antibody factory. Indeed, artificially produced monoclonal antibodies are derived from a fusion of myeloma and normal B cells called a hybridoma (see Part 8/Köhler 1975). However, in 1961, when the present work was done, myeloma proteins were recognized only as being antibody-like. The following year, Edelman and his student Joseph A. Gally established that urinary Bence-Jones proteins were the low molecular weight chains of myeloma proteins, solving a mystery begun in 1847 with their discovery by Henry Bence-Jones.

Edelman and Poulik ascertained through ultracentrifugation, liquid chromatography, and electrophoresis that 3 to 5 protein chains exist in each antibody. Within the next several years, Porter, Edelman, and others clarified the basic structure of IgG. In the currently accepted model, these antibodies consist of four chains: a pair each of heavy and light (H and L) chains. A "Y" configuration was surmised—and eventually proven by electron microscopy and X-ray diffraction data—the Fc being the tail and composed of a section of joined H chains. Each antigen receptor consists of a set of H and L chains, and the Fab was the set minus the tail segment of the H chain. To complete the nomenclature, that portion of the H chain that was included in the Fab was termed the Fd. Still later, two antigenic types of light chains, designated κ and λ, would be found among antibodies but never within the same unit. The macroglobulin, IgM, would be found to consist of five IgG-like structures arranged like a star with tail sections joined at the center by another small polypeptide chain, the J chain. As the report suggested, some of the disulfide bonds were not directly involved in interchain linkage; located in each chain, they served to fold the linear protein into a strong tertiary structure, each globular domain with its own function.

Antibodies are extraordinary structures, far more complicated, diverse, and interesting than

was imagined in 1960. These pioneering contributions of Porter and Edelman concerned merely the gross anatomy of these biological units. Their fine structure, the origins of variation and receptor specificity, the relation of amino acid sequence to function, the method of assembly and related problems would occupy investigators for many years. Like the Herculean Hydra, the immune system answers each research question with the creation of two more.

For further information:

Edelman, G. M. 1973. Antibody structure and molecular immunology. *Science* 180:830–840.

Killander, J. (editor). 1967. *Gamma Globulins. Structure and Control of Biosynthesis.* Proceedings of the Third Nobel Symposium. Interscience Publishers, New York. 643 p.

The Paper*

In studying the molecular structure of the γ-globulins, one is confronted at the outset with the problem of whether these proteins consist of one or of several polypeptide chains. The solution of this problem has significance in determining the chemical basis of antibody specificity, and in formulating a detailed theory of antibody production. In addition, it bears upon the relation between normal γ-globulins and those of disease.

A previous report showed that normal human 7S γ-globulin and a pathological macroglobulin dissociated to components of lower molecular weight when treated with reagents that cleave disulfide bonds. The present study is concerned with an extension of this approach to a variety of normal and abnormal γ-globulins. Partial separation of the dissociation products of γ-globulin has been achieved by means of column chromatography and starch gel electrophoresis. The results suggest that γ-globulin molecules are composed of several discrete subunits or polypeptide chains linked by disulfide bonds. . . .

---

*Edelman, G. M. and M. D. Poulik. 1961. Studies on structural units of the γ-globulins. *Journal of Experimental Medicine* 113:861–884. [By copyright permission of The Rockefeller University Press.]

Reduced alkylated γ-globulin was found to be very insoluble in aqueous solvents except at extremes of the pH scale. Ultracentrifugal patterns of the material that did dissolve usually showed extensive aggregations. . . . A search for effect solvents revealed that the reduced alkylated γ-globulin was soluble in strong urea solutions (6 M or greater), in guanidine-HCl solutions (3 M or greater), in 0.5 to 1 per cent sodium dodecyl sulfate solutions, and in 50 per cent acetic acid. Urea solutions appeared to promote disaggregation effectively and for this reason they were chosen for most of the experiments. . . .

An analysis of the apparent molecular weights of the starting material and of variously treated human γ-globulins was performed. . . . Corresponding to each value of $M_{app}(1 - V)$ is an approximate value of M_{app} calculated on the assumption that $V = 0.74$ and using measured values for the solvent densities. . . . A striking difference was found for γ-globulin reduced in urea. . . . In this case, the apparent molecular weight dropped to about 1/3 of the control value for untreated γ-globulin in urea. . . .

Reduced carboxamidomethylated fraction II human γ-globulin was chromatographed on carboxymethyl cellulose ion exchanger in buffer prepared with 6 M urea. . . . The weight average molecular weight in urea of the products isolated from the first peak was approximately 17,000. Ultracentrifugal analysis in urea of the material from the second peak yielded a weight average molecular weight of 103,000, and indicated the presence of aggregates.

In an attempt to achieve greater resolution, starch gel electrophoresis in urea at acid pH values was employed. . . . Unreduced γ-globulin and unreduced γ-globulin treated with iodoacetamide showed a diffuse slow band with a suggestion of an additional minor band. After reduction and carboxamidomethylation, the pattern was entirely altered. At least 4 bands appeared, and a different feature was the presence of 2 main bands of slightly different mobility. . . .

Partial reduction of γ-globulin with mercaptoethanol in the absence of urea followed by carboxamidomethylation resulted in a product that was soluble in aqueous solutions. Although the molecular weight of this material in aqueous solution was similar to that of untreated γ-globulin, the weight average molecular weight in 6 M urea was approximately 135,000, suggesting partial dissociation in this solvent. After chromatography on carboxymethyl cellulose in 6M urea, a pattern similar to that of more completely reduced γ-globulin emerged. On the starch gel in urea, however, the pattern was somewhat different than that obtained for the more completely reduced γ-globulin. There were fewer components and the mobilities of the bands appeared to be greater. . . .

In view of the relative homogeneity of the myeloma globulins, a comparison was made of their behavior after reduction, using starch gel electrophoresis in urea. . . . A striking difference in the number and position of the bands is apparent, although before reduction the broad diffuse patterns of these proteins were quite similar. Both reduced myeloma proteins had at least one band of mobility similar to one of the bands of reduced normal γ-globulin, yet each reduced myeloma protein had one or more bands different from those of reduced normal γ-globulin. It is notable that the patterns obtained for the myeloma proteins differed from each other. . . . Notwithstanding the differences in their overall patterns, the reduced myeloma proteins appeared to possess certain bands with mobilities in common.

Two methods were used to demonstrate that reduction of γ-globulin by thiol compounds was taking place. Free sulfhydryl groups were titrated amperometrically at a rotating platinum electrode after removal of reducing agent (MEA) on a Dowex 50 ion exchange resin under anaerobic conditions. In some samples, the extent of reduction was determined by estimating the conversion of cystinyl and cysteinyl groups of S-carboxymethylcysteinyl groups using ion exchange chromatography. . . .

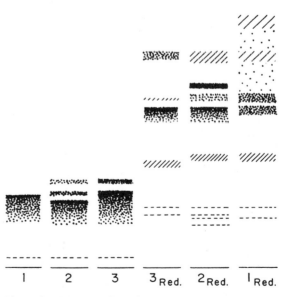

Figure 6a Diagram of starch gel, comparing human fraction II γ-globulin and two myeloma globulins before and after reduction. 1, human fraction II γ-globulin; 2, myeloma globulin; 3, myeloma globulin; $3_{Red.}$, reduced and alkylated myeloma globulin 3; $2_{Red.}$, reduced and alkylated myeloma globulin 2; $1_{Red.}$, reduced and alkylated human fraction II γ-globulin.

Estimation of the number of disulfide bonds cleaved by reduction in urea of 7S γ-globulin for short periods of time yielded values ranging from 7 to 9 disulfide bonds per mole. That not all bonds were cleaved in these instances was shown by the determination of the S-carboxymethylcysteine content of γ-globulin reduced by the bulk dialysis procedure. This appeared to be the most efficient of all procedures employed, yielding a total of 12 bonds cleaved per mole of protein. . . . [IgM was then similarly examined after its reduction and dissociation to 7S units.]

Amino acid analyses were done on fraction II γ-globulin and on the reduction products obtained by the bulk dialysis procedure. . . . No striking differences were found in the amino acid composition of native and reduced protein. The S-carboxymethyl-cysteine content of the reduced alkylated human γ-globulin was 2.86 gm/100 gm of protein corresponding to 24 half-cystine residues per mole of protein. Half-cystine was not detected, suggesting either that both reduction and coverage of free SH groups were complete, or that any residual half-cystine was destroyed in the hydrolysis. . . .

A comparison of the amino acid content of materials from the first and second peaks of chromatographically separated reduced and alkylated γ-globulin [was given]. Material from the first peak which behaved as a single broad band on starch gel electrophoresis had an amino acid composition that was markedly different from both that of the starting material and material from the second peak.

Reduction of γ-globulin conceivably might remove part or all of the carbohydrate portion of the molecule. To test this possibility, the fraction II human γ-globulin and the material recovered from the solutions inside and outside the dialysis sac in the bulk dialysis procedure were examined for carbohydrate.

Unreduced γ-globulin contained 1.4 per cent hexose, 0.8 per cent hexosamine, 0.17 per cent fucose, and 0.2 per cent sialic acid. The reduced γ-globulin from the inside of the dialysis sac showed hexosamine, fucose, and sialic acid contents similar to those of unreduced γ-globulin. . . .

Although the decrease in apparent molecular weight of 7S γ-globulin and macroglobulin was accompanied by an increase in titratable SH groups, it was not definitely established that disulfide bonds linked the frangments together. Other linkages that might be involved include thioester bonds, sugar-protein linkages of various types, and peptide bonds. A number of chemical procedures were used to survey these possibilities . . . [and all] failed to bring about any change in the sedimentation coefficient. . . .

The evidence suggests that the average molecular weight of reduced γ-globulin is 1/3 to 1/4 that of the unreduced protein. In the case of the pathological macroglobulin, the molecular weight of the derivative resulting from reduction in urea was about 1/20 that of the 19S protein. It is notable that the size of these derivatives is in the same range as that of Bence-Jones proteins. . . .

An exact determination of the types and number of bonds holding the various subunits together will require more extensive chemical studies. From the data presented here, the disulfide bond emerges as the most likely possibility. . . . In most cases, reduction of the disulfide bonds was incomplete. Dissociation occurred, despite this fact, suggesting that only certain disulfide bonds serve to link the subunits. . . . Weak forces may also help to link the subunits. . . .

The exact number of polypeptide chains possessed by each type of γ-globulin cannot be determined from the present evidence, although an estimate of 3 to 5 chains per 7S γ-globulin is consistent with the data. . . .

A unifying hypothesis may be formulated for the structure of proteins in the γ-globulin family based on the findings presented above as well as on findings of other investigators. 7S γ-globulin molecules appear to consist of several polypeptide chains linked by disulfide bonds. Bivalent antibodies may contain two chains that are similar or identical in structure. The 19S γ-globulins would be composed of 5 or 6 multichain units [each] of the size of 7S γ-globulin. A provisional explanation for the wide molecular weight range of antigenically related globulins from Bence-Jones proteins to macroglobulins is suggested by this model. Heterogeneity and differences in iso-antigenicity may arise from various combinations of difference chains as well as from differences in the sequence of amino acids within each type of chain. . . .

Characteristics of an immune system common to certain external secretions

1965 • Thomas B. Tomasi, Jr., Eng M. Tan, Alan Solomon, and Robert A. Prendergast

Comment

Perhaps the oldest and certainly the most common metaphor used in describing the immune system is combat: the invading parasite versus the defending phagocyte aided by the magic bullets of antibodies. We can likewise consider the various immunoglobulins as having military functions. IgG is the principal infantry soldier. IgM is the shock trooper, first on the scene with high firepower, low precision, and no reserves. IgE is the engineer, initiating the release of inflammatory agents to slow the progress of pathogens and to attract and aid the access of phagocytic cells, the tanks. IgD seems to be an adjutant or training liaison, located on the surface of unprimed B-cells to assist in activating antibody production. Remarkably, the immune system also includes a specialized perimeter defender or sentry, IgA, that, when fully equipped, patrols the zone between flesh and external environment from outpost garrisons.

IgA is secretory antibody. It is the major immunoglobulin of tears, colostrum, saliva, intestinal fluids, and nasal and genitourinary mucus, and thus it protects the local associated tissues. IgA may also be found in blood, cerebrospinal fluid, and pleural and amniotic secretions in small proportions. The phenomenon of local immunity, wherein serum antibodies are not involved, has been long known; Alexander Besredka, a student of Elie Metchnikoff, was among the first to examine its characteristics beginning in 1919. The discovery of so-called coproantibodies (fecal antibodies) that were said to ward off intestinal bacteria and of antibodies in respiratory mucus directed against influenza virus occurred around 1950, but evidence for their local production was circumstantial. Furthermore, all antibodies were lumped under the banner of gamma globulins, although the macroglobulin IgM was differentiated. When Joseph F. Heremans first described IgA in serum in 1959, he provided another candidate for these secretion-associated antibodies.

The foremost investigator of IgA has been Thomas B. Tomasi, Jr. (1927–   ). He commenced his medical and scientific career at Dartmouth College and the University of Vermont, where he attained his M.D. in 1954. Completing his medical training at Columbia Presbyterian Hospital in New York in 1958, he next joined the Rockefeller Institute. Tomasi went back to Vermont in 1960 to chair the division of experimental medicine. In 1965, after receiving his Ph.D. at the Rockefeller Institute, he became a professor of medicine at the State University of New York at Buffalo. He is now Professor of Immunology at the Mayo Medical and Graduate School in Rochester, Minnesota.

Tomasi and his collaborators, in investigating how these special secretory antibodies migrated from their tissue site of origin to the exterior fluids, noted a profound change in the antibodies' structural characteristics. Indeed, they found IgA to be a most peculiar antibody, varying in Svedberg units—7S, 11S, and 18S—and in antibody valence—2 and 4. The proportion of each form varied with the site of recovery; for example, serum IgA is mainly 7S. Polymerization, the joining of two 7S units, seemed clear, but something else was added.

It was a special J (for joining) chain, similar to that of IgM. The 18S structure, found only in secretions, had a further constituent. This was later known as the SC (secretory component), thought to be necessary for passing the immunoglobulin safely through the cytoplasm of mucosal cells and into the duct of an associated gland. A peptide synthesized by local epithelial cells, the SC covalently combines with IgA dimers, seemingly to render them more resistant to proteolytic enzymes.

Besides the now familiar ultracentrifugation and electrophoresis techniques, Tomasi made his discoveries with the Ouchterlony double-diffusion gel immunoprecipitation technique (see Part 8/Ouchterlony, 1948). The research team was able to recognize antigenic identity, by the observation of smooth-contoured merging of adjacent precipitin bands, and antigenic differences, by discerning separate bands or spurring of an overlapping band. The use in histological studies of fluorescein-labeled antibodies against the immunoglobulin was also instrumental in determining the sequence of events from IgA synthesis to secretion. Radioisotope tags in tissue photomicroscopy (autoradiography) and metabolic and circulatory probes further contributed to this knowledge.

A scientific paper contains more than just facts in its words. The following milestone describes how Tomasi's team identified the three antibody forms as IgA, why they ruled out a serum source of secretory IgA, and what technological evidence assured them that the immunoglobulin acquired unique components. Although moderately technical in style, the report is exciting. It has the quality of a detective story, with each experimental probe revealing a new clue. It also has a flavor of Alice in Wonderland as the immunoglobulin confronts the researchers, teasing them in its various guises. Anyone who has made an unanticipated discovery while researching, or has been in contact with such an individual at the time, will appreciate the spark beneath the objectivity of the written paper.

For further information:

Besredka, A. 1927. *Local Immunization. Specific Dressings* (H. Plotz, editor and translator). Williams & Wilkins Company, Baltimore, 181 p.

Tomasi, T. B., Jr. 1976. *The Immune System of Secretions.* Prentice-Hall, Englewood Cliffs, NJ. 161 p.

The Paper*

It has been demonstrated that γ_1A-globulin is the predominant type of γ-globulin found in human parotid saliva, colostrum, lacrimal secretions and recent evidence suggests nasal and bronchial fluids as well. The γ_2/γ_1A ratio in this group of fluids is less than 1 whereas in normal human serum this ratio is approximately 6, suggesting that there is preferential secretion of γ_1A-globulin into these body fluids. In an attempt to elucidate the mechanisms involved in the secretion of γ_1A-globulin this protein was isolated from two of these fluids (saliva and colostrum) and some of its properties were compared with those of serum γ_1A. Previous work in this laboratory had suggested that salivary and colostral γ_1A may have a higher sedimentation coefficient than that of the majority of serum γ_1A. The current report contains further chemical and immunological studies on purified preparations which indicate that while salivary and colostral γ_1A are similar to each other, certain of their chemical and immunological properties differ significantly from those of serum γ_1A. Using fluorescent antibody and autoradiographic techniques local synthesis of γ_1A has been shown in the parotid gland. In addition, antibody activity (isohemagglutinins) have been demonstrated in purified preparations of γ_1A derived from these fluids. . . . The local production of a unique type of antibody suggests the existence of an immune system characteristic of certain external secretions whose properties differ, at least in part, from those of the immunological system responsible for the production of classical circulating antibody. . . .

There is evidence which suggests that some of the γ_1A-globulin in normal human serum is present in the form of polymers. However, density gradient

*Tomasi, B. T., Jr., E. M. Tan, A. Solomon, and R. A. Prendergast. 1965. Characteristics of an immune system common to certain external secretions. *Journal of Experimental Medicine* 121:101–124. [By copyright permission of the Rockefeller University Press.]

ultracentrifugation followed by quantitative determination of γ_1A on the fractions of three normal sera and the sera from three patients with Laennec's cirrhosis revealed that over 90 per cent of the γ_1A was present in 7S form.

Analysis of ascitic fluid of patients with Laennec's cirrhosis were found to contain γ_2- and γ_1A-globulins in approximately the same ratios as they are present in the patient's serum. . . . [A]scitic fluid was used as a ready source of large quantities of γ_1A- and the γ_1A-globulins derived from it were considered representative of the major type (7S) of γ_1A present in serum.

In the final step in the fractionation of colostrum on sephadex G-200 the γ_1A-containing eluate was divided into three fractions in order to demonstrate any heterogeneity in the size of the colostral γ_1A. Density gradient ultracentrifugation was performed on each of the three fractions and the concentration of γ_1A in the various portions of the gradient determined. . . . From these figures and the protein contents of the fractions it can be estimated that approximately 60 per cent of the γ_1A in the original sample is 11S, 20 per cent 18S, and 20 per cent 7S. . . .

The ultracentrifuge pattern obtained on parotid saliva contained two peaks, a major component having an $S^0_{20,w}$ of 11.4S and a minor component usually consisting of from 5 to 10 per cent of the protein

with a sedimentation coefficient of approximately 18S. The following evidence was obtained indicating that both the 11S and the 18S components were γ_1A: (a) By careful quantitation of the γ_1A it could be demonstrated that the areas under the ultracentrifugal peaks could be explained quantitatively only if both the 11S and 18S components were γ_1A. (b) Density gradient ultracentrifugation using markers of known molecular size shows that the major peak of γ_1A is in a position in the gradient consistent with a molecule having a sedimentation coefficient of 11S. . . . (c) Samples of saliva were obtained from two normal individuals whose sera completely lacked γ_1A. The ultracentrifuge patterns . . . lack both the 11S and 18S components, which are normally present in concentrated saliva. . . .

The electrophoretic mobility of salivary and colostral γ_1A is slightly slower than that of serum γ_1A. This finding is consistent with the lower sialic acid content of the 11S γ_1A. . . .

The 11S components in saliva and colostrum behaved identically in all of the studies to be described. The 11S γ_1A, like the 7S γ_1A derived from ascitic fluid [but unlike the IgA polymers in serum], did not dissociate in disulfide-reducing agents. . . . However, following treatment of the reduced protein with 2 M urea partial dissociation and with 4 M urea complete dissociation occurred to 3.5S units. . . . Treatment of 7S and 11S γ_1A with papain in the

Methods

Collection of Samples.—Parotid fluid was obtained with a Curby parotid cap. Samples of 100 to 200 ml were collected from normal humans and patients with multiple myeloma and concentrated approximately 50-fold by negative pressure dialysis.

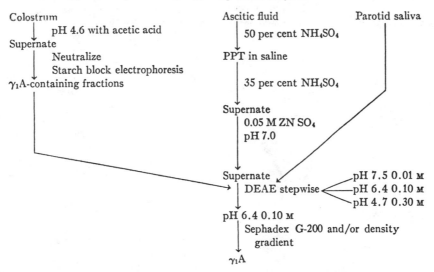

Figure 1 Experimental procedures.

presence of 0.01 M cysteine resulted in units of 3.7S. . . .

Using an antiserum made against serum, (ascitic fluid) $\gamma_1 A$, and four different antisera against isolated $\gamma_1 A$-myeloma proteins, no immunological difference could be detected between serum, saliva, and colostrum. However, using an antiserum made against 11S $\gamma_1 A$ derived from saliva or colostrum, immunological differences could be detected. As shown in Text-Fig. 6 spurring of the colostral and salivary $\gamma_1 A$ over serum indicates the presence in the 11S $\gamma_1 A$ of antigenic determinants not present in serum. Following absorption of [the] antiserum with normal serum, activity remains against saliva and colostrum. The absorbed antiserum failed to react with six normal sera, five $\gamma_1 A$-myeloma sera and the sera from two patients with Sjogrens syndrome, having large amounts of $\gamma_1 A$ with a broad range of electrophoretic mobilities. Antigenic specificity could also be demonstrated in the reduced and alkylated 11S. . . .

Evidence that the specificity of the salivary and colostral $\gamma_1 A$ is associated only with the higher polymers present in saliva and colostrum is suggested by the immunological studies on the $\gamma_1 A$ fraction derived from colostrum. [Ouchterlony plates] show that while the 11S and 18S $\gamma_1 A$-polymers are immunologically identical both have been shown to spur over the 7S colostral $\gamma_1 A$. . . . No immunological differences have as yet been detected between 7S colostral and 7S serum $\gamma_1 A$. . . .

When fluorescein-conjugated anti-11S $\gamma_1 A$ was applied to parotid tissue sections, two types of staining were seen. Cells showing striking cytoplasmic fluorescence were seen in the interstitial tissue between the acini. Some of these cells contained large amounts of cytoplasm and had eccentric nuclei and were probably plasma cells. . . . The second type of tissue staining present in the cytoplasm of the epithelial cells was scattered randomly and was not uniform except in the acini adjacent to the ductules. In this region, there was uniform fluorescence of almost all glandular cytoplasm.

When [11S] antiserum was absorbed with normal human serum, staining of the interstitial cells was entirely removed, leaving only the glandular cytoplasmic staining. Further evidence that the glandular cytoplasmic stain was specific for salivary 11S $\gamma_1 A$ was provided by the conjugate of antiserum against serum 7S $\gamma_1 A$. With the latter conjugate, there was staining of the interstitial cell cytoplasm but no staining of glandular acinar cells. The fluorescein-conjugated 7S $\gamma_2 A$-antiserum showed no staining of parotid tissue.

Radioactivity appeared in the saliva in significant amounts beginning about 15 minutes following the injection of the $I^{131} \gamma_1 A$. The counts per ml of saliva increased rapidly to a maximum at 3 days and then slowly decreased, becoming negligible after 2 weeks. . . . [E]vidence was obtained indicating that the radioactivity in saliva was not bound to protein. . . .

These studies suggest that the radioactivity present in the saliva was associated with free iodine or with small dialyzable molecules or fragments of molecules. Thus no evidence of transport of intact $\gamma_1 A$ from serum to saliva was obtained. Similar studies performed in four subjects using I^{125}-labeled 7S γ_2 likewise showed no evidence of transport of the γ_2-molecule.

Anti-A and Anti-B antibodies were demonstrable in the saliva of individuals of appropriate blood groups. Colostrum also contained isohemagglutinins sometimes in very high titers, often exceeding markedly the serum titers. . . .

The occurrence of myeloma proteins in the salivas of eight patients with $\gamma_1 A$-myeloma were studied. In two patients the predominant serum protein was 11S and in six patients it was 7S, although polymers of other sizes were often present in smaller amounts. In none of the cases was the salivary $\gamma_1 A$-content markedly elevated despite high serum concentrations (30 to 80 per cent of total protein as determined by paper electrophoresis). . . .

There are several possible explanations for the selective occurrence of $\gamma_1 A$ in body fluids: (a) Simple filtration of serum proteins with subsequent reabsorption of γ_2 and most of the other proteins with the exception of $\gamma_1 A$. This mechanism although unlikely cannot be excluded with presently available information. Such a mechanism would be analogous to the filtration which occurs at the renal glomerulus with subsequent reabsorption of much of the filtrate by the renal tubules. . . . (b) Transduction or secre-

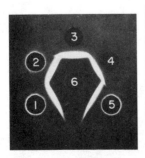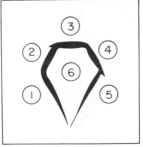

Figure 6 Ouchterlony plate illustrating the immunological specificity of salivary and colostral 11S $\gamma_1 A$. Well 1, normal human serum; 2, ascitic fluid 7S $\gamma_1 A$; 3, salivary 11S $\gamma_1 A$; 4, colostral 11S $\gamma_1 A$; 5, normal human serum; 6, anticolostral 11S$\gamma_1 A$.

tion of serum proteins with selective degradation by proteolytic enzymes present in the fluids, the $\gamma_1 A$ being more resistant to proteolysis than the other proteins. This mechanism can be excluded only in the case of parotid saliva. Previous work indicates that the parotid fluid lacks proteolytic activity. . . . (c) Active transport of $\gamma_1 A$ from serum to fluid. (d) Local synthesis of $\gamma_1 A$ by the corresponding gland. The latter two mechanisms are the most likely. . . .

There are three possible mechanisms of secretion which are consistent with our experimental findings. It is known that there are small amounts of polymeric $\gamma_1 A$ present in normal serum. . . . It is possible therefore that there is selective transport of this minor polymeric form of serum $\gamma_1 A$ by the glandular epithelium. Contrary to this, however, is the finding that the 11S salivary and colostral $\gamma_1 A$ are immunologically specific and did not show identity with any of three $\gamma_1 A$-myeloma polymers (also approximately 11S) or with an intermediate sedimentary $\gamma_1 A$-isohemagglutinin from serum. The serum $\gamma_1 A$-polymers unlike the salivary and colostral 11S $\gamma_1 A$ dissociate on treatment with reducing agents. . . . The second possibility is that the glandular epithelium alters serum 7S $\gamma_1 A$, perhaps by a piece which results in its polymerization and/or transport. This piece presumably would be the immunologically specific

determinant which was detected in the salivary and colostral $\gamma_1 A$ in these studies. This mechanism seems unlikely in view of the lack of evidence of transport of labeled $\gamma_1 A$. . . . The third possibility is the local synthesis of a specific $\gamma_1 A$ by cells present in the interstitium of the gland. The autoradiographic studies demonstrate the local synthesis of $\gamma_1 A$ by normal parotid tissue. . . . The presence of striking fluorescence in the interstitial cells of the salivary gland in our studies is also consistent with the local synthesis hypothesis although the amounts of protein produced and the cell types involved have not been definitely identified. . . . In spite of the demonstration of local synthesis the question still remains however whether the glands synthesize an immunologically specific polymer or a serum type of $\gamma_1 A$ which is subsequently modified by the glandular epithelial cells. This latter mechanism is suggested by the finding of fluorescent staining restricted to acinar and ductule epithelial cells using the anti-11S $\gamma_1 A$-antiserum which had been absorbed with normal human serum. . . .

In view of the relatively high concentrations of $\gamma_1 A$ in certain external secretions and its known antibody activity against microorganisms and allergens it is possible that the $\gamma_1 A$ in these fluids serves a defense function. . . .

Identification of γE antibodies as a carrier of reaginic activity

1967 • Kimishige Ishizaka and Teruko Ishizaka.

Comment

As Thomas Tomasi, Jr. is forever associated with IgA, the research team, indeed, research organization of Kimishige and Teruko Ishizaka are thoroughly and inseparably linked with the antibody of allergy, IgE. IgE has been the bane and source of livelihood of generations of allergists, and it is an immunological trigger of inflammation. Its discovery, chemical characterization, and the determination of its biological function have been a long struggle complicated by a red herring.

Prior to 1962, all attempts to isolate the serum substance, reagin, in atopic individuals (those with a predisposition to hypersensitivity reactions) that could sensitize the skin of normal recipients in the Prausnitz-Küstner test (see Part 2/Prausnitz, 1921) failed utterly. Purified IgG and IgM had no such sensitizing activity. After IgA was discovered, however, many research papers indicated that the immunoglobin possessed reaginic attributes. Seemingly pure preparations derived from atopics were re-

peatedly found active, and the removal of the
IgA fraction of serum also eliminated the reagins. IgA reportedly blocked passive sensitization of normal tissues. In what appeared to
be the key observation, ragweed allergen was
found to couple with IgA by sensitive radioimmunoelectrophoresis. Just when textbooks were
declaring with little reservation that IgA was
indeed the reagin, the Ishizakas observed an
anomaly.

Kimishige Ishizaka (1925–   ) was born in
Japan, earning first his M.D. in 1945 and then
his Dr.Med.Sc. in 1954 from the University of
Tokyo. In 1949 he married Teruko Matsura
(1926–   ), who received her own M.D. that
year. She completed her academic doctorate
along with her husband, and together they have
remained a research unit reminiscent of other
famous husband-wife pairs, Pierre and Marie
Curie, Jacques and Therese Trefouet, and Elie
and Eugene Wollman. The Ishizakas did their
postdoctoral work in 1957 under Dan H.
Campbell at the California Institute of Technology, who steered them into the problem of
antigen-antibody complexes. The necessity of
having two antibodies within complexes to induce skin reactions and also to fix complement
was a valuable lesson, suggesting the concept
of antigen bridging of cell-bound antibody. In
1959 the Ishizakas returned to Japan to work
at the National Institute of Health, and three
years later they moved to Denver at the Children's Asthma Research Institute and Hospital, where Kimishige became research director.
Since 1970, they have worked at the Johns
Hopkins University School of Medicine, where
each has focused on separate but related IgE
projects. Although the Ishizakas remain citizens of Japan, Kimishige was elected President
of the American Association of Immunologists
in 1985.

What the Ishizakas noted back in 1964 was
that IgA against blood group A antigen obtained from hay fever patients had no reaginic
activity. Because by now particular biological
functions were associated with specific immunoglobulin classes, they concluded that the dis-

crenpacy was a result of a minor contaminant
in IgA preparations. They used a subtractive
approach to prove their hypothesis. After immunizing rabbits with a reagin-rich serum fraction of hay fever patients, they absorbed the
harvested antisera with purified IgG, IgM, IgA,
and IgD derived from human myelomas. When
they reacted the antisera, now depleted of all
these immunoglobulins, against the patient sera
by immunoelectrophoresis (see Part 8/Grabar,
1958), a faint precipitin line was detected. They
then succeeded to demonstrate that the antigen in the precipitin line could couple with
radioisotope-labeled ragweed antigen. By 1966,
the Ishizakas were confident that they had discovered a new immunoglobulin class, which they
designated γE (E for erythema-producing), later
changed to IgE. The next year their hypothesis
was substantiated by the demonstration that the
new class of immunoglobins contain κ and λ
chain antigens in addition to unique H chain
determinants.

But was this immunoglobulin a reagin? They
had eliminated all previously known immunoglobulin classes as candidates; they now needed
positive data. What was necessary was the isolation of IgE directed against a specific antigen
and its successful use in P-K testing. Unfortunately, obtaining such purified IgE was not
feasible at the time. They temporarily settled
on removing the reagins to various allergens in
sera from allergy patients with anti-IgE antibodies, establishing that the association of reagin and IgE was not merely limited to ragweed.

The following milestone of 1967 picks up the
story. It provides the final piece of evidence
linking the new immunoblogulin class to reaginic activity. The Ishizakas' characteristic me-
ticulousness and stepwise variations of experimental design are cautions based on the earlier
and erroneous acceptance of IgA as the sensitizing antibody of allergy. Immunologists
won't be fooled again, if they can help it! They
demonstrated that highly purified fractions of
IgE can indeed passively sensitize tissue.

Unfortunately, this research could not be confirmed at first by others. However, when IgE-producing myelomas were finally isolated and when IgE (the Fc portion, to be specific) was found to attach to basophils and mast cells, sensitizing the cells, opposition subsided. Later Teruko Ishizaka discovered that bridging of the cell-bound antibodies by antigen, or bringing them together by whatever method, was the trigger for releasing histamine. As in immune-complex pathology, the association of at least two antibodies were required for skin reactions and allergic responses.

What does IgE do besides mischief? Recent evidence indicates that this system is actually a means of defense against protozoan and metazoan parasites. Mast cell and basophil mediators, released through IgE-antigen activation, alter the otherwise favorable environment, open the vascular system for an influx of IgG and complement, and recruit eosinophils and neutrophils to the area.

For further information:

Ishizaka, K. 1974. Historical aspects of immunoglobulin E. In: *The Biological Role of the Immunoglobulin E System* (K. Ishizaka and D. H. Dayton, Jr., editors). National Institute of Child Health and Human Development. DHEW Publication no. (NIH) 73–502, Washington, D.C. pp. 3–16.

Ishizaka, K. 1985. Twenty years with IgE: from the identification of IgE to regulatory factors for the IgE response. *Journal of Immunology* 135:i–x.

The Paper*

From our previous studies in this series, accumulated evidence has indicated that human reaginic antibodies are associated with γE-globulin. When serum from a ragweed-sensitive individual was fractionated by chromatography on a diethylamino-

---

*Ishizaka, K. and T. Ishizaka. 1967. Identification of γE-antibodies as a carrier of reaginic activity. *Journal of Immunology* 99:1187–1198. [Copyright by William & Wilkins.]

ethyl (DEAE)-cellulose column and examined by gel filtration, sucrose density gradient ultracentrifugation, and zone electrophoresis, the distribution of reaginic activity correlated with that of γE-antibody, which was determined by radioimmunodiffusion. It was also found that reaginic activity in the sera of ragweed-sensitive patients paralleled the concentration of γE-antibody to purified ragweed allergen as measured by antigen-binding activity. No correlation was observed between the reaginic activity and the concentration of either γG-or γA-immunoglobulins. Essentially all the reaginic activity in the sera of ten patients was lost upon absorption of the sera with an anti-γE serum which did not contain any antibody against γG-, γA-, γM- or γD-globulins. Subsequent studies on the antigenic structure of γE-globulin have shown that γE-globulin possesses the antigenic determinants of both κ and λ light polypeptide chains and in addition has characteristic antigenic determinants not shared by any of the other immunoglobulins of known classes and subclasses. These findings indicated that γE-globulin represents a distinct class of immunoglobulins.

Since the major protein components in reagin-rich fractions so far studied were γG- and/or γA-globulin, further purification of γE-globulin in the fractions was attempted to study the relationship between it and reaginic activity, with use of purified ragweed allergen. Although the protein has not been isolated, reagin-rich preparations were obtained in which the antibody against the allergen was associated with γE-globulin alone.

Three serum samples from ragweed-sensitive individuals were employed in the present experiment [serum A, U, and P]. . . .

The globulin fraction was obtained from . . . serum by precipitation with 1/2 saturated ammonium sulfate at pH 7.0. The precipitation was repeated twice and the final precipitates were dissolved in 0.15 M saline. The fraction was dialyzed against 0.005 M phosphate buffer, pH 8.0, and aliquots of the fraction were then applied to a DEAD-cellulose column equilibrated with the same buffer. Proteins were eluted stepwise with phosphate buffers of increasing molarity. . . .

[R]eaginic activity was concentrated in Frs. II and III which were eluted with 0.025 M and 0.035 M buffers respectively, and Fr. II was most active on a weight basis. The distribution of γE-antibody in the chromatographic fractions was tested by radioimmunodiffusion using radioactive antigen E. The γE-antibody was detected in Frs. II and III but not in the other fractions.

Further purification of reaginic antibody was undertaken by gel filtration through Sephadex G 200 columns. About 50 to 60 mg N of Fr. II was applied to the columns. . . . [T]hree protein peaks were obtained. The distribution of γG- and γA-globulins in the fractions was tested by immunodiffusion and the reaginic activity was tested by P-K [Prausnitz-Küstner] reactions. The major protein component in the first and second peaks was γA-globulin but contained some γG-globulin, whereas the third peak was composed of γG-globulin alone. The reaginic activity was detected in Frs. II$_1$ and II$_2$ but not in II$_3$. . . .

Our previous experiments on reaginic antibody indicated that the antibody was not associated with γA-globulin. . . . Therefore, DEAE-Sephadex column chromatography was used for further purification of reaginic antibody. . . . The fractions were concentrated . . . and tested for the presence of γE-antibody by radioimmunodiffusion. Only the fractions containing high skin-sensitizing activity gave the radioactive γE band and the intensity of radioactivity in the γE band formed by the fractions paralleled their skin-sensitizing activity. . . .

In both sera U and A, the highest skin-sensitizing activity was observed in Fr. B, which was about 150 times more active than the original serum on a weight basis. . . .

In order to remove γA- and γG-globulins from the active fractions, Fr. B from serum U and Frs. A and B from serum A were absorbed with rabbit-anti-γA- and anti-γG-antibodies which had been precipitated with goat anti-RGG. . . . The final supernatants, which did not give a precipitin ring in immunoplates containing anti-γA or anti-γG, were concentrated by negative pressure dialysis and tested for skin-sensitizing activity by P-K reactions, using antigen E as a challenging allergen. It [was] evident . . . that the skin-sensitizing activity of the final preparations was 500 to 1000 times more active than the original serum. The most active preparation gave positive P-K reactions with a 1:80,000 dilution. However, the protein concentration[s] . . . did not parallel their reaginic activity. The possibility was therefore considered that the preparations may contain rabbit and/or goat γ-globulin (antibodies), which were used for purification. The preparations were tested for the presence of the proteins by immunodiffusion. All of the preparations contained goat-γ-globulin but not rabbit-γ-globulin. . . .

The presence of human immunoglobulins and of antibodies associated with each immunoglobulin in the preparations was tested by radioimmunodiffusion using radioactive antigen E. One of the three preparations was placed in a center well of an Ouchterlony plate while antibodies specific either for each immunoglobulin or for F$_{ab}$ were placed in peripheral well. After incubation and washing the plates, radioactively-labeled antigen E was added to the antibody well and radioautographs were taken. . . . Fr.

A$_{abs}$ from serum A contained γE-globulin but no detectable amount of other immunoglobulins. In addition to γE-globulin, γD- and a trace amount of γG-globulin were detected in Fr. B$_{abs}$ of both sera. Radioautographs of the Ouchterlony plates showed that the γE precipitin band which formed with all of the three preparations indeed bound radioactive antigen E and that none of the anti-γG, anti-γA, anti-γM or anti-γD preparations gave a radioactive band. It was also found that all the preparations gave a radioactive band with anti-F$_{ab}$ antibody. In order to confirm that γE-antibody has light polypeptide chains of immunoglobulins, radioimmunodiffusion was set up between the two preparations from serum and anti-light chains, i.e., anti-κ- and anti-λ-chains. . . . [A]nti-κ-chain antibody gave an intense radioactive band but anti-λ-chain antibody did not. Lack of antibody activity in immunoglobulins other than γE-globulin indicated that γE-antibody was responsible for the radioactive bands formed with anti-κ-antibody and with anti-F$_{ab}$-antibodies.

The final preparations from serum A were analyzed by radioimmunoelectrophoresis using anti-γE, anti-γD and anti-human serum. It was found that Fr. B$_{abs}$ gave a definite precipitin band and Fr. A$_{abs}$ showed a faint band against anti-γE-serum in stained slides and that the γE-band formed with both prep-

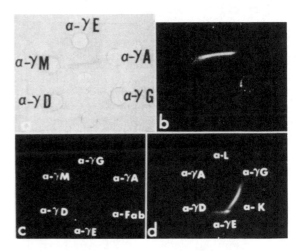

Figure 5 Radioimmunodiffusion analysis of purified reagin-rich preparations. Both the stained slide (a) and corresponding radioautographs (b) are shown for Fr. A$_{abs}$ from serum A, which was placed in center well. Peripheral wells were filled with antibodies specific for each immunoglobulin. Only anti-γE serum (a-γE) gave a visible precipitin band (a), which combined with radioactive antigen E (b). (c) and (d) are radioautographs of the analysis of Fr. B$_{abs}$. Center wells of the plates were filled with Fr. B$_{abs}$ from serum A against anti-immunoglobulin, anti-F$_{ab}$ (a–F$_{ab}$), anti-κ (a-κ) and anti-λ (a-λ) chain antisera in peripheral wells.

TABLE III

Effect of absorption with anti-γE and anti-γA on skin-sensitizing activity of reagin-rich fractions[a]

Fraction	Absorbed with	P-K[b] Reactions with Dilutions of:			
		1000×	2000×	4000×	8000×
A_{abs}	Unabsorbed	ND[b]	45 × 48 (11)	43 × 34 (9.5)	25 × 36 (7)
	Anti-γE[c]	–	–	–	–
		7000×	14000×	28000×	56000×
B_{abs}	Unabsorbed	ND	37 × 34 (10.5)	33 × 36 (8)	22 × 30 (7)
	Anti-γE[c]	–	–	–	–
		500×	1000×	2000×	4000×
D	Unabsorbed	ND	35 × 41 (10)	29 × 36 (8.5)	22 × 32 (7)
	Anti-γA	ND	32 × 37 (10)	28 × 34 (8)	25 × 28 (7)
	Anti-γE[c]	–	–	–	–

[a] Numerals in this table represent diameters of erythema and those in parenthesis represent diameters of wheal in millimeters.

[b] P-K, Prausnitz-Küstner; ND = not done.

[c] Twofold dilutions of Fr. A_{abs} and Fr. D and 1:7 dilution of Fr. B_{abs} were absorbed with an equal volume of anti-γE.

arations bound radioactive antigen E. . . . Anti-human serum gave a diffuse γ_1-band with Frs. A_{abs} and B_{abs}, which combined radioactive antigen E. The position of the band corresponded to the γE-band. When the fractions were analyzed with anti-γD-serum, Fr. B_{abs} but not Fr. A_{abs} showed a visible γD-band but the γD precipitin band did not combine radioactive antigen E. These findings indicate that the antibody against antigen E in the preparations is associated with γE-globulin alone.

In order to confirm that reaginic activity in the preparations is actually associated with γE-globulin, Frs. A_{abs} and B_{abs} from sera A were absorbed with anti-γE serum and the skin sensitizing activity of the supernatants was tested. The preparations diluted in normal human serum albumin were injected into the same individuals as controls. . . . [T]he supernatant failed to induce a P-K reaction in both samples. As Fr. D of serum A contained a high concentration of γA-globulin, it was absorbed with anti-γA-antibody. The supernatant contained no detectable γA-globulin, however, the P-K titer of the fraction did not decrease following the absorption. When the same fraction was absorbed with anti-γE, skin-sensitizing activity was no longer detectable in the supernatants. It was found in radioimmunodiffusion that the supernatants obtained after precipitation of γE-globulin did not show the radioactive γE-band, whereas unabsorbed fractions diluted in saline did. . . .

Part 4
Cells and Interactions

I have yet to see any problem, however complicated, which, when you looked at it in the right way, did not become still more complicated. —Poul Anderson

All existence is a relationship. —Alan Watts

Immersed in the fascinating intricacies of immunochemistry, it is easy to forget that the fundamental unit of life is the cell. For the reductionist, DNA is apt to come first to mind. However important the role of chromosomes of the cell may be in comprehending deep order, however convenient the use of disrupted cell solutions may be for isolating and analyzing fundamental components, cells are the most stable organizations, the bricks of organic structure and process in an unstable, fluctuating cosmos. The principle is also apparent at a lower level of form when considering the relationship of atoms to the diverse nuclear entities found after collisions of elemental matter in particle accelerators. As cellular molecules are ever exchanged with the environment, and are metabolically synthesized and transformed or degraded—and are sometimes short-lived even if isolated in vitro—the function and form of the cell itself endures; as diverse hadrons and leptons of the atom are ever interacting with the surrounding cloud of evanescent "virtual" pi-mesons and with more distant wave-particles, thus arising, transforming, or decaying—and are characteristically transitory when separated—the chemical pattern of the atom itself persists.

The present section, therefore, introduces the cellular managers of immunity. In contrast to the sedentary tissue sheets of epithelial, muscle, and connective cells, the immunological cells are generally independent, actively or passively mobile blood cells. They have the flavor of organisms in their own right, interacting with themselves and their environment in an ecology of immunity. The Russian zoologist Elie Metchnikoff, whose milestone leads the series, was the first to sense the evolutionary significance of this quasi autonomy. He described the roles of the macrophage and the polymorphonuclear neutrophil, the phagocytes, in combating invading microorganisms and in ridding the body of aberrant host tissues, picturing these cells as altruistic protozoans. The macrophage, phylogenetically the premier cell of immunity, has had many ups-and-downs in relative importance. Continually surprising immunologists with its affector and effector activities and secretions, the macrophage is the chief antigen processor. The nonmotile and nonphagocytic dendritic cell of blood and lymphatic tissues has the similar function of antigen presentation.

The discovery of antibodies pushed phagocytes out of the limelight. The cellular origin of humoral agents, not readily identified, was simply ignored for some 60 years. In 1948 Astrid E. Fagraeus finally demonstrated the maturation of lymphocytes into antibody-secreting plasma cells. Six years earlier, when these cell types were only candidates for the source of antibody, cellular immunology was resurrected by Karl Landsteiner and Merrill W. Chase. In two papers presented in this part, they demonstrated that white blood cells in peritoneal exudates from allergic or hypersensitive animals, but not immune sera from such animals, could transfer the immediate and delayed forms of cutaneous sensitivity to normal animals. Antibodies now had to share the stage with activated cells.

Through the 1950s the lymphocyte was considered a single entity having multiple functional attributes. However, in a quiet report in an obscure journal, Bruce Glick and Timothy S. Chang related their discovery that the then mysterious bursa of Fabricius of birds was the site in which developing antibody-synthesizing cells developed. Other investigators soon observed that removal of the bursa did not prevent delayed hypersensitivity reactions nor the rejection of transplanted tissues. Thus, a wedge was driven into the physical order of immunity. Immunology hesitated at the brink: mammals do not have a bursa. The organ associated with the cells responsible for delayed hypersensitivity reactions was also unknown.

The paper of Jacques F. A. P. Miller provided part of the answer: the thymus processes the bursa-equivalent lymphocytes into the mobilizers of phagocytes and the destroyers of transplants. Eventually, bone marrow was established to be the mammalian source of bursa-equivalent cells. Lymphocytes hence no longer would be considered as composed of a single type of cell. Furthermore, the two unique lympocyte populations, thymus- and bursa- or blood marrow-derived cells—T and B cells, respectively—were regarded to have independent functions.

In 1966 Henry N. Claman and his colleagues by their seminal report united the two immunological camps. Seemingly, thymus and bone marrow cells could act synergistically in the production of antibody. The nature of cooperation or communication between these cell types was well beyond conjecture at that time, but the researchers were confident that antibody formation actually *required* the interaction of the two cell types, with the thymus cell being the helper. Immunologists, like Alice, were following a white rabbit into a land of surprising phenomena.

Four years later Richard K. Gershon and K. Kondo observed that such cellular interactions can suppress as well as activate antibody synthesis. The T cells were therefore split into helper, suppressor, and later cytotoxic subtypes. These cells were not only functionally specialized, they also carried unique antigens. Despite the increasing divisions, no hierarchies were created, and all the immune cells, directly or through their secreted mediators, were interactive, forming a regulatory network. The rapid advances in immunological thought were echoed in changes of its philosophically rooted mechanisms: lymphocytes were first monistic, then dualistic, and now holistic. Macrophages, which had been stranded on the sidelines, again became essential.

The next paper presents the peculiar phenomenon of the graft-versus-host reaction. Harvey Cantor and Richard Asofsky found that a graft of large numbers of lymphoid cells into an immunologically compromised or deficient host of sufficiently distant histocompatibility type will cause system disorders, runting, or even death of the host. It was a matter of two selves contesting the same territory. Cantor and Asofsky determined that T cells from thymus and spleen or lymph node were interacting synergistically. T-T activity joined T-B, T-macrophage and dendritic cells, and B-macrophage associations, expanding the network dynamics.

N. Avrion Mitchison and his colleagues kept one foot anchored at the cellular level while stepping down into the molecular realm. They focused on the hapten and carrier portions of the antigen and their respective receptors on cells. In attempting to explain the mechanism of antibody production by interactive cells, they observed distinct differences in cellular sensitivities. T cells seemed to be carrier specific; the immunoglobulin receptors of B cells coupled with haptens. The research team proposed a model of interaction whereby the antigen served as a cellular bridge or preliminary link for cell-to-cell contact. The interaction later was found to be more sophisticated, but immunochemistry and cellular immunology had fused at a common point of mechanism and understanding.

The last milestone of this section describes an additional cellular member of the immune system that was acknowledged around 1975. Called a natural killer cell, or NK for short, it appears morphologically, functionally, and antigenically to be an intermediate form between T lymphocytes and macrophages. The NK cell is not antibody-mediated (although a subtype might act this way), and does not require prior sensitization to destroy tumor and virus-infected cells. Relatively nonspecific in its action, the NK cell is stimulated by interferon. The place of the natural killer cell in the immunological network and its regulatory system are yet to be satisfactorily determined.

For further information:

Cantor, H. 1979. Control of the immune system by inhibitor and inducer T lymphocytes. *Annual Review of Medicine* 30:269–277.

Katz, D. H. 1977. *Lymphocyte Differentiation, Recognition, and Regulation.* Academic Press, New York. 749 p.

Nelson, D. S. 1969. *Macrophages and Immunity.* North-Holland Publishing Company, Amsterdam. 335 p.

Ruben, L. N. and M. E. Gershwin (editors). 1982. *Immune Regulation. Evolutionary and Biological Significance.* Marcel Dekker, New York. 331 p.

A disease of Daphnia caused by a yeast. A contribution to the theory of phagocytes as agents for attack on disease-causing organisms

1884 • Elie Metchnikoff

Comment

Alexandre Kovalevsky welcomed to his laboratory his old friend and colleague in comparative embryology and invertebrate zoology, Elie Metchnikoff (1845–1916). While on holiday in Messina, Italy, after having resigned his professorship at the University of Odessa in protest of the administration's deceit in enlisting his aid to mediate a student strike, the visitor had made a wonderful insightful discovery from a simple test: the insertion of a rose thorn into a transparent starfish larva. As he predicted, amoeboid cells had gathered to remove the offender of self-integrity. However, Metchnikoff felt that these cells and their human equivalent were not mere supernumeraries of the pathological drama, nor were they only transports of damaged tissue. They were active providers of immunity to foreign matter, be it a splinter in the thumb or a microbe. How could this conception be convincingly demonstrated? In the course of happy conversation, the budding immunologist caught sight of his host's aquarium in which Daphnia (water fleas) were behaving strangely. He removed a few affected specimens for microscopic examination and saw large masses of amoeboid cells engulfing the fungal pathogen of the Daphnia. Suddenly the entire spectrum of host-parasite interactions

crystallized. Metchnikoff had his first model for resistance to infectious disease.

Metchnikoff is among the giants of immunology, a winner of the Nobel Prize in 1908, which he shared with Paul Ehrlich, but the scope of his research included physical anthropology, zoology, embryology, pathology, microbiology, microbial pesticides, epidemiology, chemotherapy, and gerontology. His research and writings also helped create the yogurt industry. Indeed, Metchnikoff was, in many ways like Linus Pauling, a media personality of his day, with journalists, including those of the *New York Times,* covering his every move and pronouncements on health and intestinal hygiene. It would be a nice scientific myth to ascribe his popularity simply to the merits of his exciting and diverse research, but discoveries alone, unless they are like rabies vaccine or penicillin, can not provide this. Metchnikoff was more than a creative scientist; he was a phenomenon.

The youngest son of a Russian officer of the Imperial Guard, Metchnikoff even as a child was fascinated with science. At age 15 he translated a German textbook of physics, at age 17 he submitted his first zoological research paper, and his second report, published a year later, appeared in translation in a British microscopy journal. In 1862 he entered Kharkov University, already a *gymnasium* gold medal recipient, and earned his bachelor's degree in two years. During his travels while a graduate student, Metchnikoff studied under leading German zoologists and anatomists, and in 1867 received his master's degree at the University of St. Petersburg. He obtained his doctoral degree the following year. In 1870 he was appointed a professor at the University of Odessa, where his social views were popular with students and liberal faculty members.

A visitor to Metchnikoff's laboratory in 1912 at the Pasteur Institute would often find artists, musicians, scholars, statesmen, actors, philosophers, and a horde of students from seemingly every nation. Whereas Robert Koch was severe and stuffy and Louis Pasteur was aristocratic and awesome, Metchnikoff was accessible to all, even taking time to instruct a peasant woman on the merits and methods of sterilizing salad. His younger associates called him Papa Metch. Friendly and jocular, generous and emotional, this free-spirited romantic Russian contrasted sharply with western European conventions. Metchnikoff's support of student rebels, particularly Poles and Jews, had filled a dossier in the Kremlin, and his advocacy of equal educational rights for women raised concern among administrators. His infectious and exuberant optimism about science would be shattered only by the trenches of World War I.

The paper that follows contains his first full account of his observations of fungus-infected Daphnia. A keen observer and microscopist, Metchnikoff had stared at thousands of slide preparations, and was no stranger to the wandering amoeboid cells that were involved in digestion, in metamorphosis, and in tissue regeneration. He also proposed that they might be the evolutionary source of the mesoderm. Now these cells were given a name, phagocytes, and the further role of defense against pathogenic microorganisms. Rudolf Virchow, a Professor of Pathologic Anatomy at the University of Berlin, was so impressed with the re-

port, it fitting into his scheme of cellular pathology, that he published the article in his famous medical journal. However, the paper was not an instantaneous success. A subsequent issue contained Metchnikoff's report of anthrax bacilli versus phagocytes of frogs, reptiles, and, more importantly, rabbits. The work was closer to human diseases, but it faired no better. That white cells could seek out and actually kill microorganisms was a most radical notion at the time. White cells were thought to favor the growth of microorganisms, and the influential bacteriologist Robert Koch proposed that wandering phagocytes could further harm the host by spreading the pathogen through the tissues. Thus, the noted zoologist-cum-microbiologist found himself largely ignored or derided by the medical establishment.

In 1884 the only proposed mechanism for immunity was Pasteur's crude and unsubstantiated nutrient depletion theory. Antitoxins were unknown, and no one had yet observed any bactericidal activity of whole blood or serum. The germ theory itself was not quite solidified. Metchnikoff, therefore, like all pioneers and theoreticians, suffered from the skepticism of conservers of the status quo. His report on phagocytes, nevertheless, gave vivid proof of microbial destruction. Host cells did resist infections. In another article that year, he suggested that spleen, lymphatic glands, and bone marrow had a role in immunity. Thus Metchnikoff planted the flag of cellular immunology.

Circumstances in 1887 dictated that Metchnikoff leave Russia, despite enticements to remain. Since 1886 he had served as scientific director of the Odessa Bacteriology Station, where he was responsible for the production of vaccines against rabies, fowl cholera, and other diseases. However, the combination of his lack of a medical degree, conflicts with some of his clinical staff, the constant disputes with the local medical society and the conservative press, and the unfounded blame for the deaths of recently vaccinated animals during an epidemic of anthrax, made conditions untolerable for research. Metchnikoff found the offer of a similar post in St. Petersburg fraught with the same problems. He sought a new appointment in western Europe, including at Robert Koch's hygiene institute. Koch was not at all interested, but a courtesy visit to Louis Pasteur produced an unexpected invitation to join the new Institute then under construction. Pasteur's own experience in silkworm diseases and microbial interactions, including antibiosis, probably influenced that decision. Metchnikoff thus emigrated to Paris the next year with his wife Olga, who assisted him in the laboratory and rendered many of his illustrations. Metchnikoff at first had a small laboratory and several Russian students, including Waldemar Haffkine, who later developed the first effective plague and cholera vaccines. Eventually Metchnikoff became the beloved subdirector and Chief of Service of the Institute. His more developed phagocyte theory will be discussed in detail later. It is sufficient to state that Metchnikoff, who never surrendered his Russian citizenship, died a hero of France, a hero of immunology.

For further information:

Hirsch, J. G. 1959. Immunity to infectious diseases: review of some concepts of Metchnikoff. *Bacteriological Reviews* 23:48–60.

Metchnikoff, O. 1921. *Life of Elie Metchnikoff 1845–1916.* Houghton Mifflin, Boston. 297 p.

Silverstein, A. M. 1979. Cellular versus humoral immunity; determinants and consequences of an epic 19th century battle. *Cellular Immunology* 48:208–221.

Zalkind, S. 1959. *Ilya Mechnikov. His Life and Work* (X. Danko, translator). Foreign Languages Publishing House, Moscow. 206 p.

The Paper*

The common water flea or Daphnia seems quite suitable for studies on pathological processes and may be able to throw some light on many general questions in medicine. Although these crustaceans, because of their small body size and delicate nature, have proven to be very unsuitable for the production of all kinds of artificial diseases, they offer many advantages for the study of those disease phenomena with which they become afflicted artificially. Because they are relatively small and fairly transparent animals, they can be observed for many hours at a time without damaging them, and also repeatedly from day to day. . . .

The disease which I wish to describe in the following lines is a disease due to a budding fungus, or loosely, a yeast. So far as I know, this disease has not been described earlier and was even unknown to me two years ago when I described another disease of Daphnia. I first found it last fall in an aquarium in which Vallisneria and Daphnia were almost the only flora and fauna. I noticed many Daphnia that seemed to be ill, and under the microscope I could see that this was a different disease than I had seen earlier. The whole body cavity up to the last antenna was filled with a massive accumulation of fungus cells, which I demonstrated to be different stages of a single species of fungus. I have named this fungus *Monospora bicuspidata.* . . .

From the characteristics of this parasite, it seems to be very similar to the ordinary yeasts, although it is not possible to ascertain its definitive place in the system of fungi, since we know from the recent work of Brefeld that yeast-like stages occur in many different fungi (Ustilago, Tremella, etc.). . . .

I have observed all of the stages of the Monospora in the abdominal cavity of sick Daphnia. In the early period of the disease, one sees predominantly the budding conidia, while in the later stages the ascospores prevail. In spite of many experiments, I have not yet been able to cultivate this fungus on artificial media. I have tried various nutrient media, such as acidified meat extract, orange juice, and soon.

In the individuals dying of the disease, a large number of spores in asci are produced, which are consumed by healthy individuals. Although the asci do not rupture in water, the spores which occur in

*Metchnikoff, E. 1884. Ueber eine Sprosspilzkrankheit der Daphnien. Beitrag zur Lehre über den Kampf der Phagocyten gegan Krankheitserreger. *Archiv für pathologische Anatomie und Physiologie und für klinische Medicin* 96:177–195. [With copyright permission of Springer-Verlag.]

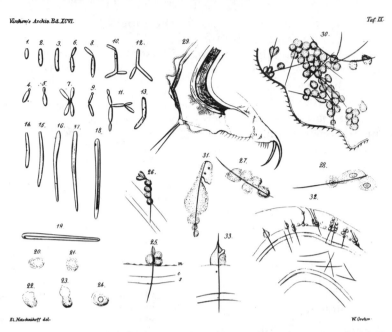

Virchow's Archiv. Bd. XCVI.   Taf. IX.

El. Metschnikoff del.   W. Grehm.

Plate IX   *Figs. 1–14.* Conidia of Monospora in various configurations. *Figs. 15, 16.* Elongated conidia, just before spore formation. *Figs. 17–19.* Formation of the ascospore. *Figs. 20–23.* Blood cells of Daphnia magna, drawn from life. *Fig. 24.* A blood cell treated with acetic acid. *Fig. 25.* A spore that has penetrated the intestinal wall, surrounded by four blood cells. (*m*) Muscle layer of the intestine, (*e*) Epithelial layer, (*s*) Layer of rods. *Fig. 26.* Another spore, as in Fig. 25. *Fig. 27.* A spore surrounded by blood cells from the body cavity of a Daphnia. *Fig. 28.* Another spore after treatment with acetic acid. *Fig. 29.* The abdomen of an infected Daphnia, with many spores in the body cavity surrounded by blood cells. Many spores are also seen in the intestinal wall and in the intestinal cavity. *Fig. 30.* Area of the abdomen of another Daphnia with intense accumulation of phagocytes around the spores. *Fig. 31.* Blood cells that have coalesced around a spore. *Fig. 32* An area from the anterior portion of the body, with many free spores and engulfed spores. *Fig. 33.* A germinating spore and an adherent blood cell.

the intestinal canal are mostly free of the asci, which I believe is due to the action of the digestive juices of the Daphnia on the asci. As a result of peristalsis, the spores penetrate the intestinal wall, so that they are partly in the intestine and partly in the body cavity. The most favorable spores for observation are those that are partly in the body cavity, but with most of the spore in the intestinal wall and intestinal cavity. Hardly has a piece of the spore penetrated into the body cavity, than one or more blood corpuscles attach to it, in order to begin the battle against the intruder. [Footnote: The blood corpuscles of Daphnia, like most vertebrates, are colorless, amoeboid cells which are adapted to the uptake of solid particles. They circulate in a system of cavities and are kept in circulation by a tubelike heart. Daphnia are completely lacking in blood vessels, except for a short outlet tube which several authors have called the aorta.] The blood cells fasten so tightly to the spore that they are seldom broken free by the blood stream.

In this case, they are replaced by new blood cells, so that in most instances the spore is more or less entirely surrounded by them. Often the spores penetrate completely into the body cavity, in which case they are even more likely to fall prey to the blood corpuscles. The number of blood cells that collect around one spore varies considerably. When many spores are in the body cavity at the same time, such a large number of blood cells surround them that the whole area appears highly inflamed, so far as one can speak of inflammation in a vessel-less animal. The blood cells collected around the spore do not always maintain their individuality, and may unite occasionally into a more or less extensive plasmodium (a so-called giant cell). . . .

In the intestinal contents or excrement, one finds that the majority of the spores are intact, which indicates that they are unaffected by the digestive juices. Those that are surrounded by blood cells behave completely otherwise. After a spore has lain for a

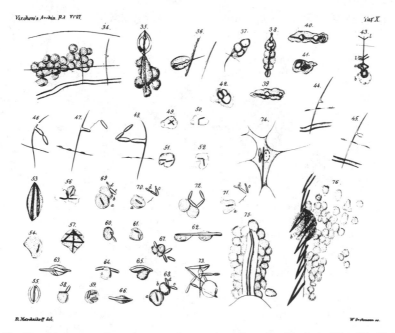

Plate X *Fig. 34.* An area from the posterior portion of another Daphnia. *Figs. 35–42.* Spores in various stages of alteration due to the action of blood cells. *Fig. 43.* A spore partially penetrating the wall: (*a*) small wall opening; (*b*) the lower portion of the spore, engulfed by a blood cell and markedly altered; (*l*) young Leptothrix, which has settled on the free portion of the spore. *Figs. 44–48.* Various stages of spore germination and conidia formation. *Figs. 49–52.* A single blood cell in four different configurations. *Figs. 53–57.* Various blood cells and conidia. *Fig. 58.* A blood cell adjacent to two conidia. *Fig. 59.* The same cell as in Fig. 58, one-half hour later. *Figs. 60–66.* Various blood cells and conidia. *Fig. 67.* A ruptured blood cell, from which the conidia have escaped. *Fig. 68.* Two blood cells, in one of which (*a*) a germinating conidium rests, while in the other (*b*) two conidia (*c, d*) remain in contact outside. *Fig. 69.* The same picture as Fig. 68, one-half hour later. The conidium (*d*) has begun to form a bud. *Fig. 70.* The same as Fig. 69, without blood cell (*b*), which has in the meantime moved away, two hours later than Fig. 69. Conidium (*c*) is beginning to bud. *Fig. 71.* The same picture, one and one-half hours after Fig. 70. *Fig. 72.* Two blood cells adjacent to four conidia. *Fig. 73.* A group of conidia which have brought about the dissolution of a blood cell that had engulfed a spore. All that remains is an empty shell and fine debris. *Fig. 74.* A fibrous phagocyte containing three fungus cells. *Fig. 75.* An injured layer of tissue with many blood cells attached. *Fig. 76.* A disrupted area of another Daphnia, also with many blood cells.

time in the middle of a number of these cells, it begins to undergo regular changes. First it thickens, turns light yellow in color, and its contours become jagged. Then it swells in several places to various sizes, assuming round or irregular shaped balls, which become brownish yellow. Meanwhile the rest of the spore, which is still rod-shaped, seems lighter and yellower. Still later the whole spore comes apart into irregular brownish yellow, dark brown and almost black grains, some large and some small. The connection of these particles to the earlier delicate spore can only be determined through knowledge of the whole process of transformation of one into the other. In the meantime the blood corpuscles have united into a fine-grained, pale plasmodium, which

still has the ability to move by amoeboid motion. Occasionally one can find in certain places in the Daphnia body, whole heaps of these plasmodia, which are especially striking because of the grains which they contain. . . .

I believe that the changes that take place in the spore are the results of the action of the blood cells. This belief is based on the following observations. When a spore remains for a long time with half of it in the intestinal wall and only half ingested by the blood cell, only this latter part undergoes the regressive changes and becomes definitely decomposed, while the portion lying in the wall maintains wholly its normal appearance. Such examples are too frequent to make one doubt of their generality. . . .

From what has been said above, it is evident that spores which reach the body cavity are attacked by blood cells, and—probably through some sort of secretion—are killed and destroyed. In other words, the blood corpuscles have the role of protecting the organism from infectious materials. This does not always occur. In cases in which a large number of spores reach the body cavity, or for some other reason one or more spores remain unaffected by the blood cells, the disease may break out. . . .

Because the process described here can be observed much more favorably than the battle of phagocytes against bacteria, I will make a few additional comments on the observations. In order to obtain certain results, one must observe one organism for many hours. Then one can see that the blood cells really ingest the spores. Sometimes this process occurs very quickly, but other times it is a very slow process. . . . The number of spores that one blood cell can ingest varies; ordinarily one finds only two spores in each cell, but occasionally one can find three, four, or more spores.

The blood cell that ingests a parasitic spore still retains its ability to move. . . . Occasionally spore-containing cells unite together into a small plasmodium, which then harbors more parasites than usual. . . .

The blood cells are able to attack living fungus cells as well as the spores. . . .

Although it is true that the fungus cells are destroyed by the blood cells, it can not be denied, on the other hand, that the blood cells can also be affected by the parasites. Several times I observed a blood cell full of parasites rupture before my eyes, setting the fungus cells free again. Also I could see a number of times that blood cells in the neighborhood of a large number of fungus cells would gradually dissolve and completely disappear. This indicates that the fungus cells produce a substance that is deleterious to blood cells. . . .

The farther along the disease has progressed, the more blood cells that are dissolved, so that at the time when the Daphnia contains a significant number of ripe spores, it reveals only a few or no blood cells.

Aside from the blood cells, only the isolated connective tissue cells play a similar role as phagocytes (eating cells). They behave in the same way as the blood cells in the ingestion of fungus cells. In the same way, they are dissolved by the fungus cells, so that in the later stages of the disease, all of the phagocytes of the animal body disappear. Other tissue elements do not suffer such a remarkable change. One may see a large number of fungus cells develop

on the heart muscle, but the heart continues to contract regularly. . . .

Once the Daphnia has become sick and contains fungus cells, it generally dies without a chance of recovery. In the last period of the disease, so many spores have been formed that the body takes on a diffuse milk-white color. . . . The whole disease takes two weeks to proceed. A young, isolated Daphnia that had just begun to form fungus cells from spores died 16 days later. . . .

From the above it can be seen that the infection and illness of our Daphnias is a battle between two living beings—the fungus and the phagocyte. The first consist of one-celled lower plants, while the latter represent the lowest tissue element and have a great similarity with the simple organisms (Amoeba, Rhizopodium, and so on). Because the phagocytes have retained the primitive property of taking up solid food, they can act as destroyers of parasites. They seem therefore, as the bearers of nature's healing power, which has been known to exist for a long time, and which Virchow first placed in the tissue elements. The whole course of the Daphnia disease fits in with the basic thoughts of this master of cellular pathology, all the more so since the main role has here been found to be an independent cellular element. . . .

As I remarked at the beginning, the yeast disease of Daphnia is of special interest in so far as it helps us to understand the pathological processes of the higher animals. It strengthens the statement that the white blood corpuscles and other phagocytes of vertebrates eat disease producers, and particularly the schizomycetes, and in this way are of considerable service to the organism. Although this conclusion had been drawn from the sum total of our knowledge of this subject, there has not been one conclusive example of the whole process of ingestion and digestion of fungus cells by phagocytes. Therefore we can criticize the conclusions that have been drawn concerning the presence of bacteria in whole blood cells. For example, R. Koch concluded, from his observations of various quantities of septicemia bacteria in the white cells of mice, that the bacteria could "penetrate the white blood cells and reproduce there." The process of penetration and reproduction could not be directly observed by him. . . . It seems to be more probable, that in this case also, the parasites were eaten by the blood cells. . . .

Because of the paucity of knowledge of this subject, it can be concluded that the pathological results obtained through studies on lower animals can be viewed as a new support for certain basic ideas of cellular pathology.

Experiments on transfer of cutaneous sensitivity to simple compounds

1942 • Karl Landsteiner and Merrill W. Chase

Comment

Metchnikoff's cellular approach to immunology began its slide from favor, but not from honor, by the first years of this century. Without the strength of his personality to maintain the defense, research quickly and almost exclusively came to focus on antibodies and their activities. Everyone conceded that these humoral agents, as every other substance of the body, are synthesized by cells, in this case probably mononuclear white cells. However, the cellular contribution to nearly all immunological responses, especially in acquired immunity, seemed only indirect. Furthermore, cell biology was little advanced over the image of organelles within a membrane-surrounded sea of nondescript cytoplasm. Immunologists, and to some extent their administrators and patrons, deemed further research efforts on phagocytes and other blood cells unproductive, relegating them to pathologists and histologists. More promising, rewarding avenues were serology, allergy, and immunochemistry. However, pots put on the back burner and left unattended will eventually boil over.

In 1942 a brief paper from the laboratory of Karl Landsteiner reminded immunologists that there is more to their field than immune sera and nonspecific phagocytes. Stimulated cells from peritoneal exudates could accomplish what had been established for serum: the passive antigenic sensitization of skin. The responsible type of cell was not determined nor was the mixture analyzed for antibody producers. The phenomenon required a large quantity of cells, and even then sensitization was short-lived. Nevertheless, allergy could now be studied at the cellular level.

Three years later, a second similar report by Landsteiner and Merrill W. Chase (1905–) offered evidence that cells alone could transfer sensitivity to tuberculin. This was less surprising, since local cellular migration and changes are symptomatic of this delayed hypersensitivity reaction and serum from sensitive donors can not be used to transfer the reaction. While serum therapy could immediately provide immunity, a lag period was observed with the cellular inoculum. The experiment was a natural extension of the earlier study, which made use of killed tubercle bacilli with the consequent induction of skin sensitivity. It was not the first such report on passive transfer of tuberculin sensitivity; that had appeared in less convincing fashion in 1909. Anaphylactic and delayed hypersensitivity were thus traceable to some constituent of peritoneal exudates, which was now described as comprised of polymorphonuclear neutrophils, lymphocytes, and macrophages. Spleen and lymph node cells from allergic or tuberculin-sensitive animals also could provide the temporary state of immunity. An immunological Sherlock Holmes had not yet appeared to disclose the cellular perpetrator; however, an increasing mass of circumstantial evidence pointed to the lymphocyte.

The first report was among the last written by Landsteiner. He died the following year in 1943. His interest in allergy began when he was in Vienna, and between research on artificial antigens and on blood groups (see Part 3/Landsteiner, 1917, and Part 7/Landsteiner, 1901), he occasionally turned an experiment toward that problem. The leading question was how local contact could sensitize the entire skin. One notion was that the antigen itself spread through the tissues. Landsteiner entered this study convinced that contact sensitivity was a result of tissue-bound antibodies, and vigorously sought their presence in extracts of sensitive skin. In preliminary experiments he tried to loosen the antibodies of peritoneally inserted tissue by irritating the peritoneum with a shock of injected mycobacteria. Clarified exudates failed to transfer sensitivity to normal guinea pigs. A partially clarified exudate, however, had the ability to do so. The microscopic observation of lymphocytes in the exudate abruptly changed Landsteiner's opinion on the allergic mechanism. The publication concerned allergy to picryl chloride (2-chloro-1,3,5-trinitrobenzene), a hapten whose antigenicity is dependent on its combination and concomitant alteration of tissue proteins. Earlier studies had involved the first chemical allergen, 2,4-dinitrochlorobenzene. Assuming now that cells of animals treated with picryl chloride would possess the apparatus of allergy, he hypothesized that a transfer of these cells would render the recipient similarly allergic, much like the transfer of antitoxins could provide passive protection in normal subjects. The use of inbred guinea pigs was an important factor, since some strains were not especially susceptible to sensitization.

For further information:

Chase, M. W. 1985. Immunology and experimental dermatology. *Annual Review of Immunology* 3:1–29.

Corner, G. W. 1964. *A History of the Rockefeller Institute 1901–1953. Origins and Growth.* Rockefeller Institute Press, New York. 635 p.

Heidelberger, M. 1969. Landsteiner June 14, 1868–June 26, 1943. *National Academy of Sciences. Biographical Memoirs.* 40:177–210.

Turk, J. L. 1967. *Delayed Hypersensitivity.* North-Holland Publishing Company, Amsterdam. 252 p.

The Paper*

In the course of experiments to passively transfer skin sensitiveness to simple compounds an attempt was made to induce sensitivity by injecting peritoneal exudates from sensitized animals. Guinea pigs were rendered sensitive to picryl chloride . . . using conjugates (guinea pig stromata treated with picryl chloride) in conjunction with intraperitoneal injections of killed tubercle bacilli. To produce exudates, killed tubercle bacilli (or tuberculin) were injected intraperitoneally about 3 weeks from the beginning of the treatment, when substantial tuberculin hypersensitivity was established.

On injecting such exudates intraperitoneally into normal animals, the recipients in most of the experiments were seen to develop sensitivity to picryl chloride; when then a drop of an oil solution of the substance was put on the skin, erythematous reactions, mostly of high color, were apparent on the next day. The phenomenon was found to be due not to the clarified fluid but to the sediment obtained upon centrifugation. Among the possible explanations, an active sensitization through residual antigenic material in the peritoneal exudates seems rather improbable because a transfer was possible also with the exudate of animals in which the injection of dead tubercle bacilli and picryl stromata was made under the skin of the neck (using as a vehicle "Aquaphore" and paraffin oil, according to a method devised by Freund) [see Part 8/Freund, 1942]. This is further supported by the appearance of the sensitivity after a short interval, namely, 2 days after injection of sufficient material, and fading of the reactivity within a few days. Finally, there is preliminary evidence that moderate heating sufficient to kill the exudate cells abolishes the effect. Consequently one would be inclined to assume that the sensitivity is produced by an activity in the recipient of the surviving cells, if not by antibodies carried by these. Positive results were obtained with about 1.5 cc of sediment, which were given in 3 portions on successive days or all at one time; with the present procedure this necessitates the use of quite a number of donors.

Definite results have been obtained with an acyl-chloride, o-chlorobenzoyl chloride; the majority of experiments have been made with citraconic anhydride, one of the acid anhydrides shown by Jacobs et al., to produce a new and particular form of re-

*Landsteiner, K. and M. W. Chase. 1942. Experiments on transfer of cutaneous sensitivity to simple compounds. *Proceedings of the Society for Experimental Biology and Medicine* 49:688–690. [With permission of the Society.]

action (in animals), namely, urticaria-like reactions often with pseudopods appearing immediately after a scratch-test. Positive transfer in human beings had been mentioned briefly by Kern with serum from a patient sensitive to phthalic anhydride, suggesting further experimental study. We found that sera from highly sensitive guinea pigs which have received intensive treatment with intracutaneous injection of oil solutions of citraconic anhydride contain an antibody which upon intraperitoneal injection into normal guinea pigs render them sensitive. Upon scratch tests made through a drop of a solution of this incitant in dioxane, the recipients gave reactions similar to the immediate ones seen in actively but not highly sensitized guinea pigs. However, upon intracutaneous injection of potent sera (amounts of 0.15 to 0.05 cc were used) into normal albino guinea pigs, intense reactions were elicited within a few min-

utes in scratch tests made on the prepared site, consisting in swelling and a pinkish coloration, most often with pseudopods and extending over an area up to 3 cm in diameter. The color receded within an hour or so, whereas the swelling persisted for several hours more; the next day the reaction was no longer present. Such reactions occurred in the sensitized sites also when the scratch test was made elsewhere on the normal skin or an oil solution was injected subcutaneously. Furthermore, reactions, even stronger ones (e.g., 5 cm × 4 cm), were obtained at the prepared sites upon subcutaneous injection of a conjugate made with citraconic anhydride and guinea pig serum. The prepared areas were commonly tested after one or two days but are still well reactive after 3 days. Whether the immediate skin reaction described is attributable to an anaphylactic antibody is being investigated. . . .

The cellular transfer of cutaneous hypersensitivity to tuberculin

1945 • Merrill W. Chase

Comment

Landsteiner's co-author of the previous milestone and the sole investigator of this follow-up note, Merrill W. Chase, was first an undergraduate and later a doctoral student at Brown University, receiving his Ph.D. in immunology in 1931. The next year he became an assistant to Landsteiner at the Rockefeller Institute. Chase was concerned with the double sensitization of the animals, which received intraperitoneally both the chemical allergen and the tuberculin of the adjuvant. In the second report, he modified the procedure by injecting the mycobacteria intradermally and collecting the oil-stimulated peritoneal exudate, establishing that cells alone could transfer the property of delayed hypersensitivity. Chase remained at Rockefeller, rising to Associate Member in 1953, when he began collaboration with Rene J. Dubos, and then Professor in 1965.

The administration gave him his own laboratory in 1956. In 1976, Chase became an active Emeritus Professor.

These two classic reports led to the resuscitation of cellular immunology. Progress in biochemistry and ceaseless new technology would help the search for the immune cell and the identity of its sensitizing mechanism. The answers would not be simple. Metchnikoff, however, would have been pleased that the research pendulum again swung his way, even demonstrating a significant role in antibody production for his beloved macrophage.

For further information:

Chase, M. W. 1985. Immunology and experimental dermatology. *Annual Review of Immunology* 3:1–29.

Corner, G. W. 1964. *A History of the Rockefeller Institute 1901–1953. Origins and Growth.* Rockefeller Institute Press, New York. 635 p.

Heidelberger, M. 1969. Karl Landsteiner June 14, 1868–June 26, 1943. *National Academy of Sciences. Biographical Memoirs.* 40:177–210.

Turk, J. L. 1967. *Delayed Hypersensitivity.* North-Holland Publishing Company, Amsterdam. 252 p.

The Paper*

In studies on experimental drug allergy, it has been found that specific hypersensitiveness of the "delayed type" is transferable to normal guinea pigs by means of cells in exudates recovered from sensitized guinea pigs. Resemblances between the delayed type of reaction to drugs and the classical tuberculin reaction have prompted investigation as to whether cells from tuberculin-sensitive animals may likewise transfer tuberculin sensitivity. The experiments show that guinea pigs receiving such cells acquire for a limited time a skin hypersensitivity that exhibits the essential features of the typical tuberculin reaction.

Guinea pigs were rendered hypersensitive to tuberculin by subcutaneous injection of killed human tubercle bacilli suspended in paraffin oil, usually mixed with vaseline; each animal received 0.5 to 2.5 mg of dried tubercle bacilli in a total inoculum of 1 cc. Between 5 and 9 weeks later, the cutaneous reactivity to tuberculin then being pronounced, exudates were induced by the intraperitoneal injection of about 28 cc paraffin oil into each of the group of guinea pigs so sensitized. After 48 hours, the peritoneal cavities were washed out with heparinized Tyrode solution containing gelatin or normal guinea pigs serum. The washings were combined and the cells recovered from the aqueous layer by minimal centrifugation. The sedimented cells were resuspended in fresh washing fluid by gentle pipetting, and again spun down. A similar washing was made, using Tyrode solution mixed with 1/10 volume of normal guinea pig serum. The washed cells were then suspended in serum-Tyrode and immediately

*Chase, M. W. 1945. The cellular transfer of cutaneous hypersensitivity to tuberculin. *Proceedings of the Society for Experimental Biology and Medicine* 59:134–135. [With permission of the Society.]

injected into male albino guinea pigs. The yield of cells amounted to 0.1 to 0.15 cc per donor, and recipients were usually given the cells of between 2 and 10 donors. The cells were comprised of 15 to 30% of polymorphonuclear leucocytes, 20 to 35% of lymphocytes, and 50 to 65% of large mononuclear cells. The recipient animals were tested with Old Tuberculin, preferably freed by glycerine by rapid precipitation with cold alcohol, or special preparations containing tuberculoproteins of either the larger or small molecular variety; these were employed in the highest concentration that produced no reactions, or only trivial ones, in untreated control animals.

The latent period preceding the development of skin hypersensitivity varies according to the route of administration of the cells—2 to 3 days after intraperitoneal injection, and 20 to 36 hours after intravenous injection.

By way of illustration, in one experiment the cells of 9 sensitized donors were given intraperitoneally to a normal guinea pig, and the first test injections were made 2 hours later with 0.1 cc of 1:4 dilution of "deglycerinated" Old Tuberculin and with "deglycerinated" control broth in like amount; the testing was repeated on each succeeding day. Tuberculin hypersensitiveness became established in the cell recipient in about 48 hours, and exhibited maximal reactivity 72 to 96 hours after injection of the cells. . . .

In contrast to the reactions following upon the injection of washed cells, similar effects have not been obtainable with serum of the donors of active cells, or with cells from normal animals.

Of 17 experiments of the sort described, successful transfers have been obtained in 16 instances. The intensity of the transferred hypersensitiveness has varied in accordance with several factors—chiefly the amount of cells used, and the degree of sensitivity of cell donors.

It has been established that the cells became largely or entirely inactive upon being heated at 48°C for 15 minutes or upon freezing, and are markedly less active after being kept in the icebox over night. The duration of the transferred sensitivity appears to be brief. In addition to exudate cells from the peritoneal cavity, cells from the spleen or lymph nodes are capable of transferring hypersensitiveness to Old Tuberculin. The brief duration of sensitivity and the activity of cells from peritoneal exudates, spleen, and lymph nodes parallel our experiences in the transfer of drug allergy.

The bursa of Fabricius and antibody production

1956 • Bruce Glick, Timothy S. Chang, and R. George Jaap

Comment

The laboratory demonstration went awry, and the students made sport of their teaching assistant Timothy S. Chang (1925–   ). After he had performed a series of inoculations of heat-killed salmonella into chickens, some animals died and a simple, well-established test of antibody formation in the survivors failed. There was no antibody to detect. What could have gone wrong? Chang's fellow graduate student Bruce Glick (1926–   ), teased his friend about the foul fowl, but was struck with the aha!, jaw-dropping symptom of insight when he found out exactly which chickens Chang had used.

Glick had been making his own experimental stab at determining the function of the small sac called the bursa that opens into the cloaca of the avian digestive tract. For some 400 years since its discovery by Hieronymus Fabricius, zoologists had failed to find a single valid clue. In the course of his research, Glick had removed the organ from chickens of various ages, and observed in disappointment that they remained in apparent perfect health. He, therefore, returned the birds to the animal pool as surplus. For his classroom demonstration, Chang had chosen at random birds that had been bursectomized as a newly hatched chick. It was an especially fortuitous event, because Glick, who was responsible for teaching the section on immunity, had persuaded Chang to take his place.

The experimental steps were retraced, and with the assistance of R. George Jaap additional research was carried out to verify their discovery. Their brief note, which is in the next milestone, was initially sent to the prestigious journal *Science,* but the editors judged it to be, in the parlance of their regrettable form letter,

"of no general interest." The authors then submitted the report to a journal of their own specialty, *Poultry Science,* which although tactically useful for veterinary scientists just entering the career marketplace, was far afield from mainstream immunology. As Gregor Mendel's report was temporarily lost in obscurity, their contribution sat idle.

Then in 1959 the biochemist Harold R. Wolfe, a friend of Robert A. Good, encountered the article while investigating blood proteins of chickens. He relayed the information to Good, who was trying to explain the link between thymic tumors and broad immunodeficiency. Like the bursa, the thymus was a poorly understood organ. Good had tried thymectomy of rabbits to observe any immunological effect, but since he was using adult animals, immune responses remained normal. However, armed with Glick and Chang's model, which required neonatal bursectomy, Good repeated his experiments with newborn rabbits. This time he succeeded in demonstrating immunological deficiency. The thymus and the bursa thus seemed to be immunological organs, but the details of how these body parts operated were still unknown. Also all kinds of lymphocytes resembled each other, except for the highly reticulated, antibody-forming plasma cells. Immunology therefore had stumbled upon two mysterious body compartments that somehow functionally differentiate their morphologically similar contents.

Glick and Chang crossed the princely path of Serendip while at Ohio State University. Glick had previously earned degrees at Rutgers University and the University of Massachusetts. After receiving his Ph.D. in genetics and physiology in 1955 at Ohio State University, he continued at this university as Assistant and then Associate Professor. In 1959 Glick went to Mississippi State University as a professor of poultry immunology. Chang, who was born in China, had received a bachelor's degree at North Carolina State University. In 1953 he came to Ohio State University, completing his Ph.D. in avian microbiology in 1957. After a series of industrial research appointments with Rohm and Haas Company, Norwich Company, and Burroughs Wellcome Company, he joined Michigan State University in 1971, where he is Professor of Poultry Pathology and Avian Microbiology.

Glick could have chosen to investigate the thymus instead of the bursa, since birds have both organs. Six years later, bursectomized chickens were found quite capable of rejecting skin grafts; neonatal thymectomy would hinder it. The two classical divisions of immunological responses, humoral and cellular, now had respective organ correlates, at least for birds. The search for a bursa equivalent in mammals stirred anatomists and immunologists alike. Since the bursa emptied into the intestine, Peyer's patches, a cluster of lymph nodules near the ileum, were introduced as a plausible candidate in mammals. The tonsil and the appendix were also proposed. However, a great crush of research eventually established that no one organ can be assigned as functional analogue. Finally, bone marrow, the source of all the blood cells, was given the nod.

In the winter of 1969, Ivan Roitt, bedridden with influenza, coined the term B cells and T cells. B stood for bursa, and T for thymus. Although historically confusing, it is nonetheless convenient in mammalian situations to regard B cells as bone marrow-derived cells. Of course, after long and constant use the nomenclature has become function associated, losing its organ significance.

For further information:

Abdou, N. I. and N. L. Abdou. 1972. Bone marrow: the bursa equivalent in man? *Science* 175:446–448.

Good, R. A. 1973. The dual immunity systems and resistance to infection. *Medicine* 52:405–410.

The Paper*

The bursa of Fabricius is a structure peculiar to *Aves*. It is a blind sac connected by a small duct to the dorsal part of the cloaca. Often nicknamed "the cloacal thymus," the function of the bursa is believed to be similar to that of the thymus. There is no question that the bursa of Fabricius functions as a lymph gland during the first two to three months after the chicken hatches. Like the thymus, the bursa in birds is believed to have some endocrine function in relation to growth and sexual development.

Although reticular cells of lymph glands and lymphocytes may participate in globulin and antibody synthesis, suspicion regarding the importance of the bursa in antibody production arose in the folowing accidental manner. A source of chicken blood possessing a high titer of antibody for antigen O of *Salmonella typhimurium* was desired for other experiments. Seventeen and one-half ml of a 48-hour, heat inactivated, broth culture were injected intravenously during a 20-day period. Surplus 6-month-old females from an experiment designed to study the effect of bursectomy were used. To our surprise six females which had been bursectomized at 12 days of age died as a result of the injections. Three survived but produced no antibodies. The nonbursectomized females seemed unaffected and built up normal titers of antibodies in their blood.

To test whether the bursa of Fabricius was involved in antibody production, 85 out of 168 male and female chickens were bursectomized at two weeks of age. Twenty of these White Leghorns received 8.5 ml of *S. typhimurium* antigen per bird in six intramuscular injections at four-day intervals between the 3rd and 6th week after hatching. Blood samples taken one week after the last injection were tested by the homologous antigen-antibody reaction test at 1:25 dilution. Out of ten bursectomized birds antibodies to *S. typhimurium* were present in three individuals while eight of the ten normal controls developed antibodies.

The larger group composed of 74 White Leghorns and 74 Rhode Island Reds were each injected with

---

*Glick, B., T. S. Chang, and R. G. Jaap. 1956. The bursa of Fabricius and antibody production. *Poultry Science* 35:224–225. [By permission of the Poultry Science Association.]

17.5 ml of the suspension of *S. typhimurium* in six intramuscular injections at four-day intervals from the 13th to the 16th week after hatching. Their reaction to the test for antibodies at 17 weeks of age is given in the accompanying table.

Antibody titers were demonstrated for 63 out of the 73 controls. This is considered to be a normal result with the typhimurium antigen. Only 8 of the 75 bursectomized birds developed antibodies. These results demonstrate that the bursa of Fabricius plays a vital role in the production of antibodies to *S. typhimurium*. No information is available concerning the possible role of the bursa in the production of antibodies for other antigens.

The bursa of Fabricius reaches its maximum size as early as 4 to 5 weeks in White Leghorns and as late as 9 to 10 weeks in Rhode Island Reds. This rapid growth period for the bursa coincides with the period when chickens attain the ability to develop many antibodies to foreign proteins. Once the bird has developed the ability to produce antibodies this ability is maintained throughout life.

The bursae of White Leghorns begin to atrophy

TABLE 1.—*Number of chickens and antibody production resulting from injections of 0 antigen (S. typhimurium) between the 13th and 17th week after hatching*

	Bursectomized		Controls	
	Positive	Negative	Positive	Negative
Rhode Island Red	5	33	35	1
White Leghorn	3	34	28	9
Total	8	67	63	10

about 7 weeks after hatching. In Rhode Island Reds atrophy of the bursa begins later, about the 13th week. It is unlikely that the atrophic bursae of chickens between the 13th and 17th week after hatching could have a direct influence on antibody production. . . .

Immunological function of the thymus

1961 • Jacques F. A. P. Miller

Comment

With the coming of the 1960s immunology was on the march. While the immunochemists were taking apart the antibody, clinical and cellular researchers were engaging the lymphocyte and lymphoid tissue. By 1961 several captains of immunology around the world had focused their attention on the thymus: Robert A. Good at the University of Minnesota, working with rabbits, mice and hamsters; Byron H. Waksman at Harvard University, using rats; Sir Macfarlane Burnet at the Walter and Eliza Hall Institute in Melbourne, with embryonated hens' eggs; and the author of the following milestone, Jacques F. A. P. Miller (1931–   ), at the Chester Beatty Research Institute in London, operating on mice. Miller was the leader of the pack with the

first and most extensive contributions of the blizzard of research papers being published on the thymus around this period.

Miller was born in Australia and educated at Sydney University, receiving his Ph.D. in 1957. The next year he went to Royal Cancer Hospital in London to begin his immunopathological research. In 1965 he was appointed Reader in Experimental Pathology at the University of London, but a year later he was back in Australia. Miller is presently head of the experimental pathology unit at the Walter and Eliza Hall Institute of Medical Research at the Royal Melbourne Hospital. Fellowship in the Royal Society of London in 1970 is one of his many international honors.

The thymus presented an interesting and challenging problem. At birth its size is at its maximum relative to that of the body. It enlarges with the growth of the child, but begins to atrophy around age 10. By adulthood the organ is barely recognizable, and thymectomy at this time is harmless. Remarkably, up to the 1960s, no one knew what the thymus did. M. Falconer in 1777 and J. Beard in 1900 regarded the thymus as the source of the lymphocytes found throughout the body, but the function of these lymphocytes was pure conjecture. As late as 1959 some investigators thought that these cells were involved in nutrition or protein metabolism. The young thymus is so packed with lymphocytes, whose nucleoplasm-to-cytoplasm ratio is comparatively high, that the thymus was once the prime source of DNA, then called consequently thymonucleic acid, for chemical studies before its genetic importance was understood. Thymine, one of the two pyrimidine bases, reflects the organ from which it was initially isolated. The only clue that the thymus might have some role in infectious disease was that the organ in children would decrease in size with prolonged illness, its lymphocytes disappearing to sites unknown.

The work of Miller and others clearly demonstrated that the thymus was responsible in some manner for cell-mediated immune responses, such as so-called delayed hypersensitivity and rejection of transplanted tissues. However, these studies indicated that the thymus has a significant influence on antibody formation as well. B cells of neonatally thymectomized animals, or children born without a thymus (DiGeorge syndrome), were present, sometimes at normal levels, but their response to antigens was generally feeble. Transplantation of a thymus into a patient or laboratory animal would restore normal immunity.

Thymus transplantation itself brought some insight into what made the thymus so special. Most of the T cells of these treated subjects were of host, not donor origin. Furthermore, pregnant animals that had been previously thymectomized gained the capability of normal tissue rejection. The concept that the thymus was producing a diffusible agent was verified when a mouse thymus situated in a filter paper chamber to prevent cell contact was implanted in a thymectomized mouse. Soon the hormone thymosin, followed by thymulin, thymopoietin, and other protein or polypeptide agents were discovered. A minor component of the organ, the epithelioid cell meshwork, synthesizes these hormones, which cause immature bone marrow lymphocytes to differentiate into a variety of T cells. Thus, bursal or marrow lymphocytes enter the thymus *in utero* and shortly after birth, where they are processed, replicated, and stored for subsequent seeding of the various lymphoid tissues and also the bone marrow. The microenvironment of each tissue selects the most fitting lymphocyte population. Within lymph nodes and spleen one may also find specific zones of B and T cells, which initiate further generations of their kind. (The transplantation of compatible bone marrow in treating immunity-destroying radiation sickness will restore both T and B cells.) The thymus, having completed its mission, withers.

One particular question haunted the research on the thymus. Why would the removal of the organ alter the antibody response in such a strange way? After thymectomy some antigens could still readily elicit immunoglobulins, mainly IgM; other antigens were virtually ignored. Did the thymus secrete a special factor needed to activate the B cell? Or was the T cell somehow necessary? Whatever the mechanism, the simple dualistic formula of B cell = antibody and T cell = cell-mediated hypersensitivity would have to be revised. This matter is the subject of later milestones.

For further information:

Cooper, M. D. and A. R. Lawton III. 1974. The development of the immune system. *Scientific American* 231(5):59–72.

Marx, J. L. 1975. Thymic hormones: inducers of T cell maturation. *Science* 187:1183–1185; 1217.

Osoba, D. 1968. The regulatory role of the thymus in immunogenesis. In: *Regulation of the Antibody Response* (B. Cinader, editor). Charles C Thomas, Springfield, IL. pp. 232–275.

The Paper*

It has been suggested that the thymus does not participate in immune reactions. This is because antibody formation has not been demonstrated in the normal thymus and because, even after intense antigenic stimulation, plasma cells (the morphological expression of active antibody formation) and germinal centers have not been described in that organ. Furthermore, thymectomy in the adult animal has had little or no significant effect on antibody production.

On the other hand, there are certain clinical and experimental observations in man and other animals which suggest that the thymus may somehow be concerned in the control of immune responses. Thus, in acute infections, when presumably the need for antibody production is great, the thymus undergoes rapid involution; in patients with acquired agammaglobulinemia the simultaneous occurrence of benign thymomas has been described, and in fetal or newborn animals, at a time when responsiveness to antigenic stimulation is deficient, the thymus is a very prominent organ.

The apparent contradiction between these two sets of observations may be partly explained by recent work, which suggests that the thymus does not respond to circulating antigens because these cannot reach it owing to the existence of a barrier between the normal gland and the blood-stream. If the barrier is broken, for instance by local trauma, the histological reactions of antibody formation take place in the thymus.

In this laboratory, we have been interested in the role of the thymus in leukemogenesis. During this work it has become increasingly evident that the thymus at an early stage in life plays a very important part in the development of immunological response.

In the preliminary experiments mice of the C3H and Ak strains and of a cross between T_6 and Ak were used. The thymus was removed 1–16 hours after birth. Alternate littermates were used as sham-thymectomized controls, i.e., they underwent the full

operative procedure, including excision of part of the sternum, but their thymuses were left intact. Mice in another group had thymectomy at 5 days of age. Wounds were closed with a continuous black suture and the baby mice were returned immediately to their mothers. No antibiotics were administered at any time either to the operated mice or to the mothers.

Mortality during and immediately after the operation ranged between 5 and 15% (excluding deaths due either to neglectful mothers or to cannibalism). Mortality in the thymectomized group was, however, higher between the 1st and 3rd month of life and was attributable mostly to common laboratory infections. This suggested that neonatally thymectomized mice were more susceptible to such infections than even sham-thymectomized littermate controls. When thymectomized and control groups were isolated from other experimental mice and kept under nearly pathogen-free conditions, the mortality in the thymectomized group was significantly reduced.

Absolute and differential white-cell counts were performed on tail blood at various intervals after thymectomy. . . . In sham-thymectomized animals the lymphocyte/polymorph ratio rose progressively in the first 8 days of life to reach the normal adult ratio of 2.5 ± 0.08. In the animals whose thymus was removed on the 1st day of life the ratio did not increase significantly and was only $1.0 + 0.10$ at 6 weeks of age.

Histological examination of lymph-nodes and spleens of thymectomized animals at 6 weeks of age revealed a conspicuous deficiency of germinal centers and only few plasma cells.

At 6 weeks of age, groups of thymectomized, sham-thymectomized, and entirely normal mice were subjected to skin grafting, Ak mice receiving C3H grafts and vice versa, and $(AkXt_6)F_1$ mice receiving C3H grafts. The median survival time of skin grafts in intact mice, sham-thymectomized mice, and mice thymectomized at 5 days of age ranged from 10 to 12 days. In more than 70% of mice whose thymus was removed on the 1st day of life the grafts were established and grew luxuriant crops of hair. Most of these grafts were tolerated for periods ranging from 6 weeks to 2 months and some for even longer than 2 months. Thereafter they gradually diminished in size, lost their hair, and eventually disappeared. A small group of C3H mice thymectomized immediately after birth, which were 3 weeks later grafted with thymuses taken from C3H fetuses towards the end of the gestation period, did not tolerate Ak skin grafts for more than 15 days.

The above results indicate that thymectomy in the immediate neonatal period is associated with severe depletion in the lymphocyte population and serious

---

*Miller, J. F. A. P. 1961. Immunological function of the thymus. *Lancet* ii:748–749. [By permission of *The Lancet*.]

SURVIVAL OF ALLOGENIC SKIN GRAFTS IN MICE THYMECTOMISED IN THE
NEONATAL PERIOD

Group	Age at operation	Strain of mice	Skin graft	Number grafted	Number tolerant	Median survival time of graft (days)
Thymectomised	1–16 hours	C3H Ak (AkXT6)F$_1$	Ak C3H C3H	7 6 8	5 4 8	45 − 101● 41 − 90 ● 50 − 118●
Thymectomised	5 days	C3H	Ak	5	0	11 ± 0·7
Thymectomised and thymus-grafted 3 weeks later	5 hours	C3H	Ak	5	0	11 − 15
Sham-thymectomised	1–16 hours	C3H Ak	Ak C3H	6 3	0 0	11 ± 0·6 10 ± 0·8
Intact		C3H Ak (AkXT6)F$_1$	Ak C3H C3H	61 45 10	0 0 0	11 ± 0·6 10 ± 0·9 11 ± 0·1

● These figures apply to the tolerant mice.

immunological defects in the mature animal. Several hypotheses might account for these results. One is that the thymus, particularly in early life, regulates lymphocyte production, not only by being the main producer of such cells, but also by secreting a factor, such as Metcalf's lymphocytosis-stimulating factor, which, after birth, stimulates lymphopoiesis in other lymphoid organs. In mice thymectomized at birth, the deficiency of lymphocytes would simply weaken the host's immunological defense as a whole. Another hypothesis attributes to the thymus a more direct role in the development of immunological response. During embryogenesis the thymus would produce the originators of immunologically competent cells many of which would have migrated to other sites at about the time of birth. This would suggest that lymphocytes leaving the thymus are specially selected cells, and this might possibly be correlated with their epithelial (rather than mesenchymal) origin during embryogenesis. In accordance with elective theories of antibody formation, genetically distinct clones of cells might differentiate at various stages during thymic morphogenesis. In parallel with experience gained from experiments on classical immunological tolerance, one might predict that the originators of those cells capable of reacting with the more distantly related antigens would differentiate earlier in embryonic life than the originators of those cells concerned with more closely related antigens. . . .

Thymus-marrow cell combinations

*1966 • Henry N. Claman, Edward A. Chaperon, and
R. Faser Triplett*

Comment

Synergism has been defined as behavior of a whole system unpredicted by the behavior or integral characteristics of the parts considered separately, according to Buckminster Fuller, and as the holistic increase of activity over the sum of the parts taken independently, according to the more limited and particular Webster. Is synergy, by whichever description, not the very essence of society or any biological organization or system? Therefore, it would not be a surprise to find the T cell and B cell, lymphocytes of common origin with distinct but nevertheless related immunological function, interacting supportively in some fashion. This conception, however, went against the reductionist tendencies of mid-twentieth-century thinking. The first and easier presumption was to assign each phenomenon to a particular organ or cellular population.

In the report that follows, Henry N. Claman (1930–   ) and Edward A. Chaperon (1920–   ) began their investigation as a simple search for antibody-producing cells in the thymus. Immunological knowledge of lymphocyte function had passed the organ level and was focusing on the organ-derived or associated cells. Since thymectomy interferes with antibody formation, then such cells might be key constituents of the organ. They referred to them as immunocompetent cells, as if antibody production was the sole or primary function of the immune system! Their work helped to overthrow that hierarchical model.

Claman, a graduate of Harvard University, earned the M.D. in 1955 at New York University and completed his medical training at Massachusetts General Hospital. In 1962 he received an appointment in the Department of Medicine at the University of Colorado Medical Center, and in 1973 he was appointed a professor in medicine, microbiology, and immunology. Chaperon was a postdoctoral fellow between 1965 and 1968, also in the Department of Medicine, having attained his Ph.D. in zoology at the University of Wisconsin. In 1968 he became a professor of microbiology at Creighton University in Omaha, Nebraska. The two were assisted by R. Faser Triplett in the Department of Pediatrics at the University of Colorado.

Their research report is a milestone for providing, through an interesting and clever experimental design, the first evidence for T and B cell cooperation. The data were still inferential but unmistakable and strong. The surprising result launched a thousand papers. Their data meet the dictionary definition of synergy, but their conclusion especially fits Buckminster Fuller's definition.

The experiment required the X-irradiation of mice to destroy their immune system. It was not a matter of simply wiping the slate clean; the condition is permanent and life-threatening. However, applying the method developed by Playfair, Papermaster, and Cole after irradiation, the animals were seeded with active immune tissue and afterwards immunized. Antibody-forming foci in the spleen could then be analyzed. These previous workers transferred spleen cells only, which contain T and B cells in somewhat similar numbers; the Colorado team took the experiment further. They compared the antibody-forming capacity of thymus, a T cell organ; bone marrow, which is B cell dominant; and most importantly the mixture of their constituents. The small amount of antibody production in the individual sources, especially the thymus, was due to a small number of cells of the opposite type present in each organ. With few exceptions, the isolated B cell can not be triggered to manufacture antibodies, and the T cell, of course, lacks this capability. Therefore, the synergy hypothesized by the investigators was not like that noted with drugs, which are active alone, but more like the rainbow-forming combination of sunlight, prismatic rain, and the observant eye, which interacts individual external characteristics to release an implicit entity.

Science is a conservative endeavor. Once the tautology of axiom and definition is instituted, everything must be derived. Nothing else is accepted until proven, and even then it becomes merely operational and susceptible to undermining. Fortunately, science demands verification of the philosophically obvious, since there is always the chance that the epistemological construction may collapse as a house of cards. Furthermore, as this milestone demonstrates, all sorts of tangental information and questions, as well as occasional surprises, may arise from the experiment that tacitly attempts to affirm an underlying general principle. The authors of the report indicated cellular cooperation, but the data demonstrated cooperation only of organ-derived cells, a mixture of cell types that allows erroneous interpretations. Hence, the next step in the lymphocyte probe was to use isolated or differentially marked cells. Subsequent research soon substantiated by direct evidence which lymphocyte cell type is the effector, but the mechanism of interaction would remain a quandary for a few more years.

For further information:

Beveridge, W. I. B. 1980. *Seeds of Discovery*. W. W. Norton, New York. 130 p.

Katz, D. H. and B. Benacerraf. 1972. The regulatory influence of activated T cells on B cell responses to antigen. *Advances in Immunology* 15:1–94.

Miller, J. F. A. P., A. Basten, J. Sprent, and C. Cheers. 1971. Interaction between lymphocytes in immune responses. *Cellular Immunology* 2:469–495.

The Paper*

The source of potentially immunocompetent cells and the regulatory mechanisms involved in their maturation are unsolved problems of great interest. Recently considerable evidence has accumulated indicating that the thymus plays an important role in lymphocytopoiesis and in the development and maintenance of the immune system. Although small amounts of antibody are synthesized within the intact thymus, a more important role of this structure may be to provide potentially competent lymphoid cells which migrate to other lymphoid structures, such as the spleen and lymph nodes, there to differentiate into immunologically active cells. Data also exist showing that the thymus may produce a diffusible hormone-like product, influencing the multiplication and maturation of lymphoid cells in the peripheral lymphoid tissues. These two mechanisms are by no means mutually exclusive.

The experiments reported here sought to test for the existence of potentially immunocompetent cells in the thymus . . . by demonstrating discrete clones of active, antibody-producing cells arising from a unit number of nonsensitized progenitors which are transferred to irradiated hosts and stimulated with antigen. In the course of these experiments, we found that combinations of normal thymus and bone marrow cells were far more active in producing hemolysins than cells of either type alone. Graft vs. host activity of cells was eliminated since the donor and recipient cells were of the same inbred strain.

Nine- to twelve-week-old LAF_1 or CBA/J recipient male mice were given a single exposure to 650–750 r 250 kvp x-rays followed by intravenous injection of syngeneic cells (spleen, thymus, marrow or thymus plus marrow). . . . When mice received both thymus and marrow cells, the 2 cell populations were combined shortly before injection in a total volume of 0.5 ml. All recipients were injected within 2 hours following irradiation.

In the first group of experiments, the mice were injected iv with 0.2 ml of a 10% suspension of washed

---

*Claman, H. N., E. A. Chaperon, and R. F. Triplett. 1966. Thymus-marrow cell combinations. Synergism in antibody production. *Proceedings of the Society for Experimental Biology and Medicine* 122:1167–1171. [With permission of the Society.]

sheep erythrocytes on the first day following irradiation. Five days following irradiation, the mice were killed and their spleens removed, cut into fragments, and plated. . . . After 2 hours, incubation at 37°C, 2 ml of 33% guinea pig complement was added to each plate. The plates were incubated for 30 minutes more, fixed by pouring 10% neutral formalin over the surface, then coded and read as unknowns and scored by two methods. . . .

The spleen fragments with significant surrounding hemolysis were not randomly distributed but tended to occur in clusters or "active areas." Playfair et al. have shown that an active area is probably derived from a unit number of precursor cells, but when there are many active pieces, the delineation of discrete active areas is difficult since they tend to overlap. For this reason, the percentage of spleen pieces with hemolysis was also calculated and designated "specific activity." This was found to be linearly related to the number of active areas and permitted quantitative scoring of a larger range of activities. . . .

To determine the percentage of cells reaching recipient spleens, separate suspensions of CBA spleen and thymus cells were incubated for 6½ hours with H^3-thymidine. The cells were washed and the percent labeling determined by autoradiographs of aliquots. Irradiated recipients were injected iv with 10^6 thymus or spleen cells and were sacrificed one hour later. The recipient spleens were made into single cell suspensions and the total number of cells counted. Smears of measured aliquots were made and the number of labeled cells determined by autoradiography. The total number of labeled cells in the spleen was calculated to be 6.5% of those labeled spleen cells injected, and 2.9% of those labeled thymus cells injected. Assuming that the distribution of labeled cells reflected the distribution of all donor cells, roughly twice as many spleen as thymus cells reached the recipient spleens. . . .

When 5×10^6 spleen cells from non-immunized CBA/J donors were injected into irradiated syngeneic recipients, the mean number of active areas in the spleen 5 days later was found to be 2.5 times that found when 2×10^6 spleen cells were injected. Approximately 2.2×10^6 cells produced one active area in both cases. Five hundred thousand spleen cells from donors injected 3 days previously with sheep red cells (labeled immune) produced as many active areas as two million non-immune cells. Thymus cells from normal and immunized donors did not produce significantly more active areas than controls given no cells.

In the next group of experiments the x-rayed recipients received injections of antigen on days 1 and 4 and were sacrificed on day 8 following irradiation.

Some animals were given 10^7 syngeneic marrow cells either alone or together with thymus cells. Spleens of mice receiving 5×10^7 thymus cells plus 10^7 marrow cells had more and strikingly larger zones of lysis than animals receiving either cell type alone. Marrow alone showed no activity above background, but thymus alone at 8 days showed slight activity.

LAF_1/J were used in all subsequent experiments because of their greater resistance to x-rays. . . . [Data were pooled] from 6 experiments showing specific activity as related to the dose of thymus cells. When mice received 10^7 marrow cells, the response curve was linear at least through 5×10^7 thymus cells, with 5.5×10^6 cells producing one active area and 10% specific activity. Thymus cells alone were much less effective and approximately 4.3×10^7 cells were required to produce one active area (10% specific activity).

In the reciprocal experiment, the hemolytic response was evaluated as a function of the number of marrow cells injected. In the groups of mice receiving varying numbers of marrow cells plus 2×10^7 thymus cells, the response was linear between 2×10^6 and 2×10^7 marrow cells, but leveled out with higher doses of marrow. Recipients of marrow cells alone were never significantly more active than controls given no cells. . . .

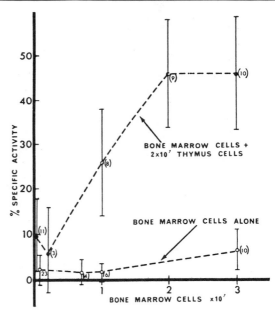

Figure 3 Percent specific hemolytic activity of recipient spleen fragments as related to number of marrow or marrow plus 2×10^7 thymus cells injected. Numbers in parentheses represent numbers of mice for each data point. Range indicates $\pm$ two standard errors.

Over the range tested, the mean number of active areas was directly proportional to the number of cells injected. Five $\times 10^6$ spleen cells produced more active areas in 8-day experiments than in 5-day experiments. Since 2.2×10^6 normal spleen cells produced one active area, and presumably contain one precursor cell, and since 6.5% of transferred spleen cells (labeled in vitro) appear in the recipient spleen, then one precursor is contained in 143,000 normal spleen cells. . . . Since a normal mouse spleen contains about 10^8 nucleated cells, it would contain 700 precursor cells. . . .

The thymus does not appear to contain similar potentially immunocompetent cells since thymus cells from normal or immunized donors did not produce significant hemolytic activity in recipient spleens at 5 days. At 8 days there was a small amount of activity in recipients of thymus cells, but none in recipients of marrow cells. The combination of thymus and marrow cells, however, produced more active areas and greater specific activity than can be accounted for by simple summation of the activities of the two donor populations.

The simplest interpretation is that one cell population contains cells capable of making antibody ("effector cells"), but only in the presence of cells from the other population ("auxiliary cells"). These data do not establish which cell suspension contains

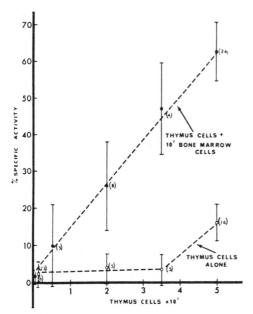

Figure 2 Percent specific hemolytic activity of recipient spleen fragments are related to number of thymus or thymus plus 10^7 marrow cells injected. Numbers in parentheses represent numbers of mice for each data point. Range indicates $\pm$ two standard errors.

either effector or auxiliary cells nor how these cells interact. . . .

The known antibody-producing activity of marrow from immunized donors together with evidence that marrow cells migrate through the thymus make it possible that the immunocompetence of transfered thymus from immunized donors is due to the presence of marrow-derived cells within the thymus. A growing body of data shows that the immunocompetence of marrow cells depends upon the presence of the thymus. On the basis of all these data, we feel that it is most likely that the effector cell in our experiments is marrow-derived, and that the thymus provides the auxiliary cells.

The role of thymic lymphocytes in the induction of tolerance

1970 • Richard K. Gershon and K. Kondo

Comment

Tolerance is the subject of the next milestone. It is an operative term referring to the absence of an immunological response to a given antigen. The response may be cellular-mediated or antibody-forming. Tolerance, thus, is a restricted condition compared with immunological deficiency disorders or that produced by irradiation or drugs, and may be temporary or capable of being broken. Various mechanisms can generate this state of unresponsiveness, such as the lack of an antigen-recognizing lymphocyte clone (see Part 5/Burnet, 1959), the presence of very low or very high concentrations of blocking antigen, and antibody to the antigen receptor on lymphocytes. The antigen may also be hidden from processing. The mother is naturally tolerant of the fetus as well as her own tissues. Inherent in the mechanisms of tolerance is the solution to the question, What turns the antibody machine on and off?

Tolerance is therefore a terminus of immunoregulation. The previous milestone concerned the contribution of the T cell in initiating antibody production by B cells. Other evidence suggested that the T cell could somehow be hindered from activating specific cellular immune responses. Could these thymus-derived lymphocytes, other than by their obvious absence, also be instrumental in suppressing the antibody response?

In his truncated career, Richard K. Gershon (1932–1983) helped determine that the T cell is not the monolithic entity as supposed. T cells are specialized in subsets: helper (T_H) cells to activate B cells; suppressor (T_S) cells to prevent or arrest antibody formation; cytotoxic (T_C) cells, which destroy tumors and grafts; and cells that secrete various cellular mediators called lymphokines, causing, for instance, the rapid replication of lymphocytes and alterations in macrophage behavior. Gershon, a Harvard University undergraduate in 1954, went to Yale University for his M.D., completed in 1959. Three years later he was in uniform for a two-year assignment at the 406th U.S. Army Medical and General Laboratory in Japan. He returned to Yale, rising in 1977 from an instructor to a professor of pathology and Director of the Cellular Immunology Laboratory.

His landmark work began in the late 1960s at the Chester Beatty Institute of Research in London as part of a collaborative investigation. It is a difficult study to follow, not by its organization, methods, or writing style, but by the multitude of experimental combinations. Sixteen players are on the field, and their game plan can be followed only by constantly referring to the score card. The result is worth the effort. The experimental design provided insight into the regulation of T cells and of T cell-independent and T cell-dependent B cells (an antigen-related distinction). Gershon was surprised by the results, since he set out believing that B cell tolerance was due to a direct antigenic effect. Instead, he found it to be an indirect result of T cell activity.

His next report yielded more unexpected information: the addition of normal T cells, B cells, or their combination could not break tolerance. Indeed, tolerant spleen cells conferred tolerance to normal B and T cells in their presence. The condition was antigen specific, since normal antibody production could occur against similar substances (sheep versus horse erythrocytes). Gershon speculated that a suppressive agent was secreted by the T cells.

Through several mechanisms, T cells interact with B cells, macrophages, and other T cells. The variety of specific idiotypic molecules on B cells and B cell-receptors on T cells form a regulatory network. The results of research attempting to determine these mechanisms were confusing, often contradictory, as multifaceted. For example, evidence for the secretion of soluble suppressors, as Gershon predicted, was offered, but other researchers observed cell-to-cell bridging. Both specific and nonspecific suppression by T cells were next described. Another point of controversy was whether a single receptor on the T cell recognizes both the foreign antigen and the self-histocompatibility molecule or whether two separate receptors are necessary. This question was resolved with the subsequent identification and isolation of the T cell receptor proteins: There was only one receptor.

The overwhelming data elevate the thymus to chief executive officer of immunity. Nothing occurs in immunity without regulatory control of its two T cell division presidents—helper and suppressor. The demoted B cell is director of production and the effector T cells are directors of marketing and sales. Immunology, Inc.

may be a peaceful alternative to the usual military analogy, but in any format immunity must not be regarded as a static table of organization and equipment. It is a process, a self-evolving system of interactions that intermesh with other body systems, so that boundaries are as artificial as the political lines on a topographical map.

For further information:

Beer, A. E. and R. E. Billingham. 1976. *The Immunobiology of Mammalian Reproduction*. Prentice-Hall, Englewood Cliffs, NJ. 240 p.

Marx, J. L. 1975. Suppressor T cells: role in the immune regulation. *Science* 188:245–247. Also: 1985. The T-cell receptor—the genes and beyond. 227:733–735.

Paul, W. E. and B. Benacerraf. 1977. Functional specificity of thymus-dependent lymphocytes. *Science* 195:1293–1330.

Rowley, D. A., F. W. Fitch, F. P. Stuart, H. Kohler, and H. Cosenza. 1973. Specific suppression of immune responses. *Science* 181:1133–1141.

The Paper*

Recent work has established that interactions between two types of lymphocytes play an important role in the production of antibodies to heterologous red blood cells in the mouse. These lymphocytes are distinguished by the fact that they enter the peripheral pool of cells from different source organs. Those that enter via the thymus (referred to as thymus-derived, or TD cells) have been shown to respond to antigenic stimulation by mitosis and protein synthesis. They do not, however, release significant amounts of circulating antibody.

It is not yet clear whether the other lymphocytes in the response, referred to as bone marrow-derived (BMD) cells come directly from the bone marrow or pass through another source organ, such as an equivalent to the bursa of Fabricius of avian species.

*Gershon, R. K. and K. Kondo. 1970. Cell interactions in the induction of tolerance: The role of thymic lymphocytes. *Immunology* 18:723–737. [With permission of Blackwell Scientific Publications.]

It is clear, however, that these are the cells that produce antibody in the response to sheep red blood cells (SRBC). Although it appears that a few BMD cells (mostly 19S producers) can make antibody without the assistance of TD cells, most require TD cell help, particularly in the primary response.

At present little is known about the role these cells may have in the induction of tolerance. Several investigators have presented evidence which suggests the TD cell may be made tolerant, but it has not yet been established whether the BMD cell may also be. The experiments reported below test this possibility by determining whether pretreatment with antigen can abolish the ability of the BMD cell to cooperate with normal thymocytes. In addition they test what role cooperation of TD cells might play in this event.

The general outline of the experimental plan is presented in Fig. 1. Each group studied has been given a number which is referred to when they are discussed in the text.

The role of the TD cell in the production of tolerance was tested by heavily pretreating two groups of mice; one deprived of TD cells and one with TD

cells present. Uninoculated animals in both groups served as controls.

To obtain mice without TD cells, adult CBA mice were thymectomized at 7–8 weeks of age. One week later they were lethally irradiated and given 5×10^6 syngeneic bone marrow cells, intravenously.

To obtain mice with TD cells the same procedure was carried out but 15×10^6 thymocytes were added to the bone marrow inoculum. . . .

Immediately after inoculation and on the next 2 days, half of each group was given 3×10^9 SRBC intraperitoneally. They were then given 4×10^9 SRBC/week for 4 weeks (in four weekly injections) making a total dose of approximately 2.5×10^{10} SRBC. The remaining mice were not injected with SRBC. Four days after the last injection, serum was collected from all mice and titrated against SRBC and horse red blood cells (HRBC). Half of each of the four groups were then given 15×10^6 normal thymocytes intravenously. The resultant eight groups were then immunized; half of each group with 5×10^8 SRBC and half with 5×10^8 HRBC as a specificity control. Thus, sixteen groups of mice were produced.

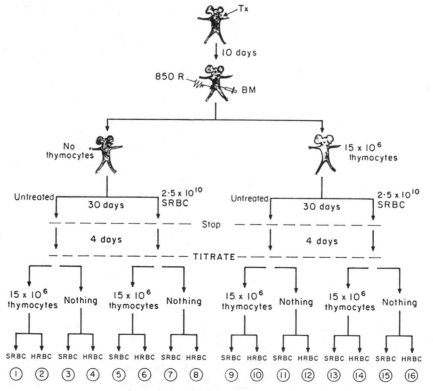

Figure 1   Plan of experiments. The figures in circles indicate the experimental group number and these numbers are referred to when the groups are discussed in the text.

The sera of these mice were then titrated for hemagglutinating antibodies against SRBC and HRBC on days 5, 7, 10 and 15 after immunization. A second injection of the homologous immunizing antigen was given on day 17. . . .

The thymus-independent response: Animals pretreated with SRBC (Group 7) did not respond to an immunizing injection of antigen. The non-pretreated controls (Group 3) made a small, transient response of 2-mercaptoethanol sensitive (MES) antibody. . . . Neither group responded to a second injection of antigen on day 17 (both groups responded to a third injection of antigen given 1 month after the second injection, in a typical primary fashion). . . .

The specificity of the suppression . . . was poor. Animals pretreated with SRBC (Group 8), except for day 5, made significantly less antibody in response to immunization with HRBC than did non-pretreated controls (Group 4). As above, neither group responded to a second challenge on day 17. . . .

These results suggest that antibody-making cells which do not require the assistance of TD cells to make antibody to SRBC may be paralyzed by antigenic overloading, and that TD cell cooperation is not required for this event to occur.

The thymus-dependent response: The addition of 15×10^6 thymocytes to pretreated animals (Group 5) did not significantly augment their immune response to SRBC on days 5 and 7 after challenge. However, by day 10 and thereafter a significantly increased antibody titer was produced as a result of the thymic cell inoculation. By comparing these animals with non-pretreated controls (Group 1) it [was evident] that their antibody titer was depressed on day 5 and day 7. From day 10 onward (up to 100 days) the groups had similar titers. . . .

One further experiment was performed with these groups. An additional three days was allowed to elapse between the termination of the pretreatment and the addition of thymocytes, to see if the recovery noted above on day 10 could be foreshortened. . . . [N]o significant recovery took place in the absence of thymocytes.

Specificity in this instance was quite good. No significant depression of antibody formation to HRBC was produced by pretreatment with SRBC (similarly in Groups 2 and 6). . . . [N]o suppression of the HRBC response was produced by pretreatment with SRBC in these animals.

SRBC pretreatment of mice in the absence of thymocytes does not impair subsequent cooperation between their MER antibody-making precursor cells and normal thymocytes. It does, however, temporarily diminish the response of MES-antibody making cells even after the addition of thymocytes. . . .

Antigen pretreatment in the presence of thymocytes; without the addition of thymocytes after pretreatment: No significant immune response either primary or secondary, occurred in pretreated animals (Group 15). On the other hand, non-pretreated controls (Group 11) responded in the same fashion as animals that received a single inoculation of 15×10^6 thymocytes on day -34 (Group 1) instead of on day 0. The depression of the antibody response produced by the pretreatment was statistically significant on day 7 and thereafter, when compared with non-pretreated controls (Group 15 versus 11).

The specificity of this depression was poor in the primary but improved in the secondary response. . . . [A]nimals pretreated with SRBC and given HRBC without thymocytes (Group 16) made a very poor response that was depressed all days of the primary response when compared with non-pretreated controls (Group 12). However, 7 days after a second immunization they made a significant response, although it was deficient in MER antibodies. . . .

The SRBC pretreatment of mice with thymocytes present, similar to its effect in mice deprived of thymocytes, leads to a state of unresponsiveness to further challenge. This paralysis lasts for more than 3 weeks.

Antigen pretreatment in the presence of thymocytes; with the addition of thymocytes after pretreatment: In giving a second injection of thymocytes to determine if an animal is tolerant, it is important to know if these cells can affect a non-pretreated control. . . . [T]he second inoculation of thymocytes produced a significant increase in antibody produced in both the SRBC (Group 9 versus 11) and the HRBC (Group 10 versus 12) systems. This was true in both the primary and secondary response.

Although the thymocytes were able to boost non-pretreated controls, they were without effect in the pretreated animals (Groups 13 versus Group 15). This was in sharp contrast with the results presented above in animals pretreated in the absence of thymocytes. The difference between the non-pretreated controls and test animals in this case was highly significant on all days of the primary response. Reimmunization of pretreated mice on day 17 resulted however, in a response that was significantly greater than that made by animals which had received the same pretreatment but had not been given a second inoculation of thymocytes (Group 13 versus Group 15). Although these animals responded to a second immunization, their response was significantly less than that made by non-pretreated controls (Group 9). It was in fact almost exactly the same as the response of non-pretreated animals which had received only a single inoculation of thymocytes, either on day −34 (Group 11) or on day 0 (Group 1). MER-antibody titers of these three groups were likewise similar.

The response to HRBC of pretreated animals was also somewhat depressed compared to non-pretreated controls (Groups 14 versus 10). This depression was statistically significant on days 5 and 7 but on days 10 and 14, although the response remained suppressed, the difference was no longer significant. The response of the two groups was very similar in the secondary response.

The SRBC pretreatment of mice with thymocytes present, in contrast to its effect in mice deprived of thymocytes, prevents the addition of thymocytes from restoring the immune response. The ability to respond partially recovers in less than 17 days but then is similar to the response of non-pretreated mice given only a single dose of thymocytes.

Before entering into a discussion of the effects of the various treatment schedules, it is important to consider the reasons for the lack of specificity noted in these experiments. In some of the groups studied, pretreatment with SRBC led to a significant suppression of the subsequent response to HRBC. It was however, always of lesser magnitude and duration than the effect on the response to the homologous antigen. Three possible explanations for these observations have been considered.

(1) A nonspecific immunosuppression, such as reticulo-endothelial blockade, produced by the noxious effects of the injection of large numbers of heterologous red cells. This explanation is unlikely as the injection of animals deprived of TD lymphocytes had no effect at all on the ability of thymocytes to restore the response to HRBC. Since the same injections given in the presence of TD cells depressed the HBRC response, even after the addition of more thymocytes, it would appear that the presence of TD cells was a causative factor.

(2) One mechanism by which TD cells could have acted is through antigenic competition. To test this possibility some non-pretreated animals were given only a single injection of SRBC 4 days prior to the inoculation of HRBC and thymocytes. Their response to HRBC was not impaired. This explanation is also weakened by the observation that antigenic competition does not occur in animals unresponsive to one of the competing antigens. . . . In the experiments reported above the response to HRBC was depressed in animals that made no response to SRBC. . . .

(3) A third possibility is that cross tolerance was produced even though the antibodies made in response to challenge with SRBC are not supposed to cross-react with HRBC. . . . [A]lthough we confirmed the reported absence of cross-reactions between SRBC and HRBC in the primary response prior to initiating these experiments, we have discovered more recently that hyperimmunization may lead to high titers of cross-reacting antibodies. This observation makes the possibility that we are observing cross-reacting tolerance more feasible. . . .

Whatever the explanation may be, since the cross-reacting suppression was dependent upon the presence of thymocytes, it is most likely that the basis for it was immunological rather than nonspecific. . . .

The basic question asked was whether tolerance to SRBC in the mouse was . . . thymus dependent. . . .

The results showed that the SRBC treatment in the absence of thymocytes could eliminate the small transient MES antibody response that mice without TD cells are capable of making. It could, however, influence the ability of added thymocytes to restore the MER antibody response.

On the other hand, the same pretreatment with antigen given in the presence of . . . thymocytes not only made mice unresponsive to further antigen injections, it also temporarily prevented the addition of thymocytes from having a restorative function. . . .

Thus, the interaction of SRBC and thymocytes had temporarily resulted in an abrogation of the ability of the BMD cells to cooperate with normal thymocytes. It is indeed possible that the BMD cells had been made tolerant. . . .

The loss of tolerance in less than 17 days can most simply be explained by regeneration of new cells from the bone marrow. These new cells, although probably also present in animals without a second inoculation of thymocytes, cannot respond in that case, as the only TD cells present are themselves tolerant. . . .

Before considering the mechanisms by which tolerance might have occurred, there is one other result that should be considered. This is the depressed response, on days 5 and 7, of animals pretreated in the absence of thymocytes and then given thymocytes. . . . [T]hose antibody making cells that could produce antibody without assistance from TD cells were tolerant and the addition of thymocytes could not restore their reactivity. The observation that the early depressed response of these animals was related in time to the addition of thymocytes and not to the termination of pretreatment indicates that the recovery noted at day 10 was not due to regeneration of new cells from the bone marrow. Thus, no indication that thymus-dependent BMD lymphocytes can be affected by antigen pretreatment in the absence of TD cells was found in these experiments.

Rather it would appear that most thymus-dependent BMD lymphocytes are incapable of reacting to antigen without some form of assistance; they previously have been shown to be incapable of making antibody and in this work they have been shown to be incapable of becoming tolerant. They appear to have both capabilities in the presence of TD cells. Thymus-independent BMD cells, on the other hand, have both capabilities in the absence of TD cells.

Two alternate mechanisms may be suggested for how the TD cell participates in the production of tolerance. It may act in the same fashion as it does in the production of immunity. That is it makes some substance which facilitates theinteraction of antigen and potential antibody making cell. . . . The other suggestion we might offer is that the TD cell not only makes a facilitating substance, but also a "shut-off" substance. . . .

Synergy among lymphoid cells mediating the graft-versus-host response

1970 • Harvey Cantor and Richard Asofsky

Comment

Individuality is correlated with histocompatibility antigens on tissue cells. T cell receptors recognize the configurations of these surface molecules as either friend or foe. Such antigens are carried by T cells themselves as well as by other immunological cells, and are of central importance in T and B cell interactions. Functioning internally as knotted intersections for network regulation and externally as territorial markers, histocompatibility antigens maintain biological order (see Part 7). Before these fundamental principles were known, experimenters in a wholly artificial design unintentionally created a situation that internalized the external. The researchers had introduced an immunological Trojan horse. The result was the graft-versus-host reaction.

In 1916 the phenomenon was first described but was unrecognized in James B. Murphy's experiment involving the introduction of spleen and neoplastic tissue in embryonated hens' eggs. In 1953 Morton Simonsen and W. J. Demster, working independently with dog kidney allografts, mistakenly deemed a similar manifestation as the graft-versus-host reaction. Finally, in 1956 Rupert E. Billingham and Leslie Brent correctly matched the interpretation with the condition. In order to allow mice to retain transplanted alien tissue, they attempted to induce tolerance by injecting spleen cells of donor type. With certain combinations of mouse strains and doses of spleen cells, the recipient mice would undergo inflammation, splenic enlargement, hemolytic anemia, atrophy, and finally develop into runts. The donor lymphocytes migrated to the recipient's spleen and lymph nodes, where they replicated into cytotoxic cells. Next spreading along the lymphatics, the donor cells defended their integrity against the surrounding foreign tissue. However, someone's freedom fighter is someone else's terrorist, and the recipient would have mounted a more virulent and certainly more massive campaign of search-and-destroy were it not for its tolerance to the antigen. Like the intoxicated and sleeping Trojan army, the recipient was immunologically incompetent to the active intrusive lymphocytes.

Thus, the graft-versus-host reaction occurs when the host is immunologically weak or deficient, when differences in histocompatibility antigens are great, and when the graft contains sufficiently high numbers of lymphocytes. The nature of the reactive lymphocyte was first examined in the following report by Harvey I. Cantor (1942–   ) and Richard M. Asofsky (1933–   ). Their milestone indicated the ability of T cells to interact, the old cooperating with the young.

Cantor, Professor of Pathology at Harvard University School of Medicine and Chief, Laboratory of Immunopathology at the Dana-Farber Cancer Institute, completed his undergraduate education at Columbia University in 1963, and four years later attained his M.D. at New York University. He interrupted the normal course of medical training by becoming a staff associate in the Laboratory of Microbial Immunity at the National Institute of Allergy and Infectious Diseases between 1968 and 1970. For the next two years, Cantor was an NIH Special Fellow at the National Institute for Medical Research in London. With this solid foundation in research, he went to Stanford University for his residency in medicine. In 1974 he joined the faculty of Harvard.

His associate Asofsky received his M.D. in 1958 from the State University of New York. After a residency at the New York University Medical Center, he joined the staff of the National Institute of Allergy and Infectious Diseases. Starting as an associate immunologist in 1963, he became Head of the Experimental Pathology Section in the Laboratory for Germ-free Animal Research two years later, and in 1972 became Chief of the Microbial Immunity Laboratory.

Their milestone was an outgrowth of an investigation on hemolytic anemia in mice. The disease was associated with an inability to support a graft-versus-host reaction. Their initial working hypothesis was that lymphocytes were being diluted by compensating hematopoietic cells. In the course of their experiments of injecting young spleen cells into the mice, they unexpectedly discovered that the graft-versus-host reaction could be synergistically modulated by two populations of lymphocytes, one from thymus tissue and the other from spleen or lymph nodes. Although T cells were involved, the thymus cells were still immature or progenitors, while the spleen and lymph node cells were more fully developed. The molecular distinctions between these cells and their mechanism of interaction are yet unknown. The subsequent separate treatment of thymus and lymph node cells with anti-Thy-1 (T cell common antigen) antibody and complement prevented synergy, ascertaining that only T cells were responsible.

For further information:

Elkins, W. L. 1971. Cellular immunology and the pathology of graft-versus-host reactions. *Progress in Allergy* 15:78–187.

Wolstenholme, G. E. W. and M. P. Cameron (editors). 1962. *Ciba Foundation Symposium on Transplantation*. J. & A. Churchill, London. 426 p.

The Paper*

The preceding paper describes an example of synergistic interaction between two cell populations that mediate a cellular immune reaction, the graft-vs.-host (GVH) reaction. Mixtures of spleen cells obtained from NZB/B1 mice at two different stages of an autoimmune disease were shown to produce GVH reactions far greater than could be accounted for by summation of the separate activities of either population. The demonstration that the GVH activity of a weakly reactive lymphoid cell population could be enhanced by addition of appropriate numbers of cells obtained from lymphoid tissues comparatively rich in GVH activity suggested that at least two cell types were required to effect a GVH reaction. This hypothesis would be strengthened considerably if synergy could be demonstrated using cells from mice without disease. To this end, the GVH activity of

---

*Cantor, H. and R. Asofsky. 1970. Synergy among lymphoid cells mediating the graft-versus-host response. II. Synergy in graft-versus-host reactions produced by Balb/c lymphoid cells of differing anatomic origin. *Journal of Experimental Medicine* 131:235–246. [By copyright permission of the Rockefeller University Press.]

different combinations of lymphoid cells from Balb/c mice were examined. . . .

In the present study, appropriate proportions of adult spleen and femoral lymph node cells are shown to act synergistically with thymus cells and with spleen cells from neonatally thymectomized animals. In one case, two populations of lymphoid cells that produced no detectable reactions when injected separately in large numbers were able to produce significant GVH reactions when combined. . . .

Spleen cells from 12-wk old Balb/c mice were injected intraperitoneally into litters of Balb/c × C57BL/6 F_1 hybrid recipients in doses of 2.5, 5, and 10 × 10^6 cells. Spleen indices were determined in recipient mice 9 days after inoculation and plotted against the logarithm of the number of cells inoculated. Recipient spleen indices were also calculated in litters that had received from 0.5 × 10^6 to 2.0 × 10^6 femoral lymph node cells and 5 × 10^6 to 20 × 10^6 thymus cells. Cells obtained from thymus tissue were found to contain substantially less GVH reactivity than either spleen or femoral lymph node cells; at any cell dose, thymus cells contained approximately 20% of the reactivity of spleen cells, and 5% of the reactivity of femoral lymph node cells.

0.5 × 10^6 femoral lymph node cells, able to initiate barely significant GVH reactions when injected alone, were combined with 4.5 × 10^6 thymus cells, which were inactive at this dose. Reactions equivalent to those produced with inoculation of 1.3 × 10^6 femoral node cells or 25 × 10^6 thymus cells were achieved with this mixture. When 1 × 10^6 femoral lymph node cells were added to 4 × 10^6 thymus cells, reactions were produced that were quantitatively similar to those seen with 3.0 × 10^6 femoral lymph node cells. Moreover, inocula of spleen cells that were too small to initiate significant GVH reactions were shown to confer reactivity on otherwise unreactive amounts of thymus cells (Fig. 3). Thus, 1 × 10^6 spleen cells combined with 4 × 10^6 thymus cells produced spleen indices in recipient F_1 hybrid mice that were usually seen after 2 × 10^6 spleen cells had been injected.

In order to test a population of lymphoid cells that possessed no inerent GVH reactivity, spleen and thymus cells were obtained from 1-wk old Balb/c mice. No significant reactivity was apparent when these "immature" cells were injected in F_1 hybrid litters in numbers as great as 35 × 10^6 cells. Although neither cell population could produce significant reactions separately, even when exceedingly large doses of cells were used, when 10 × 10^6 cells from each of these inactive populations were combined, recipients consistently evidence significant GVH activity. . . .

Spleen cells from 10-wk old Balb/c mice that had been thymectomized 3 days after birth were injected

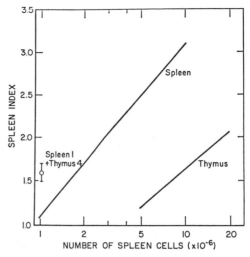

Figure 3 Graft-vs.-host reactivity of mixtures of spleen and thymus cells. The mean spleen index produced by inocula composed of 1 × 10^6 spleen cells and 4 × 10^6 thymus cells is shown; vertical bar indicates the limits of one standard error. Reference to the two standard curves shows that neither component of the mixture can produce significant reactions separately. The reactivity of this mixture is equivalent to that obtained with almost 2 × 10^6 spleen cells.

into F_2 recipient mice. These cells were approximately eight times less reactive than spleen cells from control, sham-thymectomized mice. Spleen cells from mice that had undergone sham-thymectomy were exactly as reactive as those from normal animals. When 4 × 10^6 spleen cells from thymectomized animals were combined with 1 × 10^6 control spleen cells, the mixture produced reactions equivalent to those that would have been obtained had the inoculum contained almost 3 × 10^6 control spleen cells or 22 × 10^6 spleen cells from the thymectomized mice. . . . When the proportions of spleen cells from thymectomized and sham-thymectomized mice in the mixture were reversed, no synergy was noted. Indices obtained from this mixture were identical to those usually produced using 4 × 10^6 spleen cells from sham-thymectomized mice. When only 1 × 10^6 spleen cells from sham-thymectomized mice were added to 1 × 10^6 cells from thymectomized animals, reactions were produced equivalent to those obtained with 2 × 10^6 control spleen cells from sham-thymectomized mice.

In another experiment, thymus cells from adult Balb/c mice were combined with spleen cells from neonatally thymectomized mice. When 1 × 10^6 thymus cells were combined with 4 × 10^6 spleen cells from thymectomized mice, reactions were produced that were similar to those obtained had the inocula been composed of 9×10^6 spleen cells from thymectomized mice. When the proportions between the two cell populations were inverted . . . the resulting mixture produce no significant GVH reactions. . . .

The importance of interaction among lymphoid cells in the development of humoral immune responses is well established. . . . The present study extends the foregoing to include the graft-vs.-host reaction, a form of cellular immunity.

Synergy was usually demonstrated by combining cells from tissues comparatively rich in GVH activity, such as femoral lymph node and spleen, with cells from tissues with much less activity, such as thymus and spleens from immature or neonatally thymectomized mice. Proper adjustment or the ratio between the cell populations studied was essential for the demonstration of this synergy. . . .

The observations may be explained by postulating that at least two cell types are required to mediate GVH reactions. The ratio between these subpopulations of GVH competent cells in different lymphoid tissues determines the degree of reactivity of that tissue. . . . This finding suggests that an important component in the ontogeny of GVH reactivity in such tissues as spleen might be the acquisition of cells derived from the thymus. . . . Further weight is given to this possibility by the observation that relatively small numbers of thymus cells from adult animals can restore reactivity to hypoactive spleen cells obtained from adult, neonatally thymectomized mice. . . .

In the case of cellular immune phenomena, the nature of the effector cells—those cells which cause damage to tissues without antibody synthesis—is not so precisely known, nor is the means of effecting the damage. Although the small numbers of cells from tissues rich in GVH activity that are required for synergy suggest that they might be important for the recognition part of the response, the present data do not discriminate between a cooperative action between two cells or a sequential action in reacting to allogeneic tissues. . . .

Cooperation of antigenic determinants and of cells in the induction of antibodies

1970 • N. Avrion Mitchison, Klaus Rajewsky, and R. B. Taylor

Comment

IgX. By convention, X represents the unknown, the tentative. Thus, when N. Avrion Mitchison (1928–   ) and Klaus Rajewsky (1936–   ) proposed in 1970 that a cell-bound immunoglobulin of T cells, "IgX," was crucial in antibody production, they effectively threw down the gauntlet. The hypothetical immunoglobulin, serving as an antigen receptor, was their answer to the carrier problem that arose from the research of Baruj Benacerraf and his associates P. G. H. Gell and Zoltan Ovary between 1959 and 1963.

Haptens, which are able to react with antibodies either alone or bound to a variety of carriers, lack the capacity to induce antibody formation; a carrier is required. Karl Landsteiner had clearly established this principle with his synthetic antigens. Ovary and Benacerraf wondered about the specificity of the carrier, and attempted to boost the antibody response to a hapten by inoculating an antigen consisting of the same hapten but a different carrier. The animal produced a primary response as if it had encountered the hapten for the first time. A subsequent experiment using spacer peptides to separate hapten and carrier discounted the possibility that the cellular receptor reached beyond the hapten to recognize a portion of the carrier. Two distinct receptors, one for hapten and the other for carrier, therefore, seemed to be necessary.

However, the concept of antibody-producing cells with two specific receptors undermined clonal selection, strained credibility, and countered all experimental evidence. By the clonal selection theory, as will be described in detail later (Part 5/Burnet, 1959), B cells are restricted to the synthesis of a single antibody type whose particular specificity is determined by random genetic recombination and mutation. Antigens select the appropriate line of B lymphocytes by binding to a corresponding cellular receptor (IgD), initiating the replication and maturation of the affected lymphocyte. A similar receptor on T cells would alleviate the heterodoxy but complicate antibody synthesis.

Rajewsky, working independently, reported at an international conference in 1968, that he had discovered a new twist to the carrier problem. Rabbits were first inoculated with the hapten bound to a carrier and with a second carrier alone. When hapten was reintroduced, this time bound to the second carrier, he found a typical secondary antibody response. Attending the presentation was Mitchison, who had also pursued the phenomenon. His evidence for a two-cell solution was based on transfer of two populations of spleen cells into irradiated mice, one from mice immunized to the hapten-carrier union and the other from mice immunized to a different carrier. The subsequent injection of hapten bound to the second carrier elicited enhanced antibody production. The data in both cases were preliminary and a little fuzzy along the edges.

It was obvious that the two should pool their efforts, and nine months later they presented their expanded study and hypothesis, which is the following milestone. They were joined by R. B. Taylor, who had been examining the influence of the thymus in determining antigenicity. In this collaboration, spleen cell studies were augmented with experiments using archetypal and less questionable thymus and bone marrow cells. By this time evidence was pouring

in from many laboratories on the synergistic and cooperative effects of T and B cells. Mitchison and colleagues now added their own confirmation at the antigen functional level.

Their mechanistic model of cell interaction was well received, spurring on research on T and B cell receptors. One of the first reports was by Martin C. Raff, who showed with the tool of anti-thymocyte antibody that the elimination of carrier-primed T cells could abolish the secondary response, while the removal of hapten-primed T cells had no effect. The T cell, therefore, carried the receptor for the carrier portion of the antigen; the B cell receptor specialized in hapten binding. This was the most reasonable organization, since B cells, the antibody-secreting cells, synthesize hapten-specific antibodies. As mentioned previously, the T cell receptor was eventually isolated; Mitchison and Rajewsky's hypothetical IgX was realized as a protein of two disulfide-linked chains of even greater functional complexity. The antigen-T cell-B cell complex is apparently a cozy arrangement with the T cell receptor joining the B cell indirectly via the antigen bridge and directly by the B cell histocompatibility antigen. This double-clamping, membrane-squeezing situation, which leads to antibody synthesis, bears resemblance to the dual IgE trigger of mast cells.

Mitchison's distinguished career began with his M.A. in 1949 from Oxford University. He remained as a Fellow of Magdalen College until 1952, when he went to Edinburgh University as a Lecturer. In 1961 he was appointed Reader. The following year he came to the National Institute of Medical Research in London, where he was Head of the Division of Experimental Biology. In 1970 Mitchison became Professor of Zoology at University College, London. He was elected a Fellow of the Royal Society in 1967.

Educated at the University of Frankfurt with specialty in chemistry and medicine, Rajewsky received his M.D. in 1962, and spent a year at the Pasteur Institute in Pierre Grabar's laboratory. Rajewsky joined the Institute of Genetics of the University of Cologne in 1964. Coming to Cologne as a research assistant, he soon became the head of the newly established immunology unit. In 1969 he took leave for work with Mitchison in London as a Senior Fellow of the European Molecular Biology Laboratory. The following year he was appointed Professor of Molecular Genetics at the University of Cologne.

For further information:

Marrack, P. and J. Kappler. 1987. The T cell receptor. *Science* 238:1073–1079.

Paul, W. E. and B. Benacerraf. 1977. Functional specificity of thymus-dependent lymphocytes. *Science* 195:1293–1330.

Rowlands, D. T., Jr. and R. P. Daniele. 1975. Surface receptors in the immune response. *New England Journal of Medicine* 293:26–32.

Sulitzeanu, D. 1971. Antibody-like receptors on immunocompetent cells. *Current Topics in Microbiology* 54:1–18.

The Paper*

This paper describes a conjunction between two fields of work with quite separate origins. We are so delighted that this has occurred, and so anxious to persuade others to share in the implied simplification of our thinking, that we feel bound to issue a warning: the evidence that carrier effects can be mapped onto the thymus-marrow interaction is still only flimsy.

One of us (R. B. T.) had been studying the role of the thymus in the response to protein antigens. . . . [Previous data on the effect of thymectomy] was at first (we believe) misinterpreted as evidence that the response proceeds in two steps, one

---

*Mitchison, N. A., K. Rajewsky, and R. B. Taylor. 1970. Cooperation of antigenic determinants and of cells in the induction of antibodies. In: J. Sterzl and I. Riha (editors), *Developmental Aspects of Antibody Formation and Structure. Proceedings of a symposium held in Prague and Slapy on June 1–7, 1969.* Volume II. Academia/Academic Press, New York. pp. 547–561. [Copyright 1970 by Academia, Czechoslovakia.]

of antigen recognition (by the thymus-derived lymphocyte) and the next of production without recognition (by the marrow-derived lymphocyte). We now believe, for the reasons outlined below, that both steps involve antigen recognition.

The others (K. R. and N. A. M.) had been studying carrier effects, at first independently and then in collaboration. We were led successively (i) to abandon the previously prevalent theory that carrier effects could be attributed to the local environment in which a determinant, typically as synthetic hapten, was situated on a carrier, and (ii) therefore to search for evidence of independent recognition of the carrier influencing the anti-hapten response. . . .

In a general way we hope to show that cooperation takes place between the two cell populations in the following manner. Specific receptors synthesized by the carrier-primed cells ("helper" cells) pick up the antigen via its carrier determinants (the "cooperative" determinants) and present the hapten determinants (the "inducing" determinants) to lymphocytes of the conjugate-primed population which bear the corresponding receptors ("inducible" cells); the latter cells are thereby stimulated to produce the anti-hapten antibody. We do not wish to imply that haptens will not serve as cooperative determinants or are in any way unique, although they tend to behave somewhat differently from protein determinants in these experiments. In the light of this working hypothesis we propose to redefine carrier effects in the following way (or at least explicitly confine our attention to the following category of carrier effects): A carrier effect operates when immunity to one determinant on a multi-determinant antigen enhances the immune response to another determinant.

We shall introduce evidence that the helper cells are thymus-derived lymphocytes. . . .

The following details were obtained with the mouse transfer system . . . and with hapten-carrier systems in rabbits.

1. Cooperation seems to be general. . . . Our best experiments so far have been obtained with NIP-OA-primed cells [4-hydroxy-3-iodo-5-nitrophenyl-acetic acid-ovalbumin] and BSA-primed helpers [bovine serum albumin], and this combination was used in the following experiments except where otherwise stated. In rabbits, human gamma globulin (HGG) or keyhole limpet hemocyanin (KLH) primed cells cooperate with hapten (sulphanilic acid) primed cells, and protein determinants cooperate with each other, as shown in the lactic dehydrogenase (LDH) system.

2. Cooperation occurs in the induction of both 7S and 19S antibodies. . . .

3. Cooperation can be obtained only in a restricted range of antigen dosage. Smaller doses of antigen do not stimulate even in the presence of helper cells, while larger doses may induce maximum stimulation without the need to add helpers. . . .

4. When due allowance is made for carrier proteins which are intrinsically more strongly antigenic (through some unknown mechanism), the carrier-effect can be entirely cancelled out by cooperation. . . .

5. Over part of the dose-response range, increase in antigenic stimulation causes an increase in anti-hapten antibody proportional to the increase in anti-carrier antibody. . . .

6. With increase in the number of anti-carrier cells, cooperation reaches a maximum earlier than antibody production by the same population. 10 to 20×10^6 spleen cells/host from well immunized mice may show optimum cooperation, while their antibody production continues to increase as up to 100×10^6 cells are transferred. This qualifies any putative evidence of differential suppression, tending to strengthen evidence for suppression of cooperation and to weaken evidence for suppression of antibody production.

7. Attempts to obtain cooperation with passively transferred antiserum, purified immunoglobulins, and heat-killed cells have invariably failed in both mice and rabbits.

8. The allotype of the hapten-primed cells is conserved: when BSA-primed cells of allotype Ig-$I^{a/b}$ cooperate with NIP-primed cells of allotype Ig-$I^{a/a}$, the anti-BSA antibody is a+b+, and the anti-NIP antibody is a+b−. . . .

9. In the sulph-carrier system in rabbits, the class (7S/19S) of anti-hapten antibody produced in the secondary response depends mainly on the dose of sulph-carrier complex, and not of secondary carrier, used for priming. . . .

10. The helper cells must interact with complete conjugate. NIP-OA-primed cells mixed with BSA-primed cells cooperate if stimulated with NIP-BSA pl HSA, but not if stimulated with BSA + NIP-HSA (vice versa if mixed with HSA-sensitive cells). Analogous results were also obtained in both the LDH- and the sulph-carrier system in rabbits. Thus the presence of the inducing determinant and of an antigen to which the helper cells are primed is not sufficient for cooperation to occur: the two have to be structurally linked.

11. Attempts to demonstrate cooperation in vitro have so far failed. . . .

12. Macrophage-rich cell populations are not particularly good at cooperating. . . .

13. Certain combinations of allogeneic or parental-F_1 donors and hosts result in antibody production on the part of the BSA-primed cells without this helper activity. . . .

14. Treatment of the donors of the helper cells with colchicine suppresses antibody production by their transferred cell population without apparently affecting helper activity; cellular immunity, it may be recalled, is little affected by irradiation, in its preproliferative phase. On the other hand, treatment with anti-lymphocyte serum, an agent thought to act differentially upon cellular immunity, suppresses helper activity.

15. Cells taken early after immunization are disproportionately good at cooperating, in relation to their ability to produce antibody. . . . The production of helper cells therefore has the rapid tempo characteristic of cellular immunity.

16. Cells taken from the spleens of lethally irradiated, thymocyte-repopulated, immunized donors can cooperate. . . .

17. "Carrier" priming can be replaced by priming with a second hapten. . . . DNA-primed cells can help NIP-primed cells to mount an anti-NIP response if the appropriate double conjugate is employed. . . . It may be noted that the effects observed are rather weak, as might be expected . . . based upon the premise that hapten-sensitive helper cells are normally in short supply. Analogous experiments in rabbits and rats have so far entirely failed.

18. Rabbits primed with one type of LDH subunit and challenged with a hybrid molecule consisting of both types of subunit produce antibodies also to the subunits to which they had not been confronted before. This effect is not mediated by circulating antibody and does not occur in unprimed animals. . . .

19. The addition of DNA-primed cells does not normally enhance the stimulation of BSA-primed cells by DNP-BSA, but does so if the BSA-primed cells come from anti-lymphocyte serum-treated donors. . . .

Cellular cooperation for an anti-protein response has been demonstrated in another way. Unprimed thymus and marrow cells were transferred, alone and in combination, to irradiated recipient mice. When these were challenged with BSA alum pertusis, the mice which receive both thymus and marrow cells made up to 10 μg/ml ABC, while the mice which receive either cell type alone made no more antibody than the mice which receive no cell transfer. This confirms the work of Claman, Chaperon and Triplett and Mitchell and Miller who showed the same phenomenon in the response of mice to sheep erythrocytes. It was no surprise that the place of bone marrow cells could be taken rather more effectively by spleen cells from mice thymectomized in adult life, irradiated and reconstituted by injection of bone marrow cells. Presumably the spleens of these mice contain larger numbers of mature marrow-derived lymphocytes than does marrow, rather as thoracic duct cells are richer in competent thymus-derived cells than is thymus. . . .

Both [marrow and thymus] cell types probably have a specific part to play in the response. The . . . conclusion can be drawn from paralysis experiments in which thymus grafts, thoracic duct cells, or thymus cells taken from donors treated with antigen in a form likely to induce paralysis failed to restore responsiveness to recipients deficient in thymus cells but adequately provided with bone marrow cells. . . .

The specificity of thymus cell paralysis was examined in another experiment, where donors were treated with either BSA or HSA, and various combinations of marrow and thymus were made. . . . The results clearly show specific paralysis towards the antigen used to treat the thymus-cell donors.

In none of these experiments was any significant paralysis detected in the bone marrow. . . .

An analogy may be drawn between paralysis in thymus-marrow cooperation and in the cooperation of anti-carrier and anti-hapten responses. Paralysis induced to the carrier protein usually induces prolonged unresponsiveness to its hapten conjugates. Hapten-specific paralysis has been less easy to demonstrate. . . . This apparent capacity of the heterologous carrier to "break" paralysis towards the hapten finds no obvious explanation. But . . . if thymus cells perform the function of carrier-recognition, then the presence of unparalyzed thymus cells might have "broken" bone marrow paralysis in the same way. . . .

Does cell-cell cooperation involve an antigen-bridge?

Some possible mechanisms of cooperation are illustrated in Fig. 5. Mechanism (i) involves the two cells binding, via their receptors, to antigen, deposited on a macrophage. Following binding, the thy-

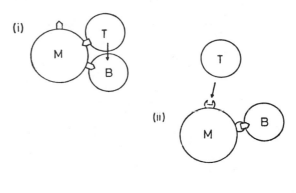

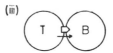

Figure 5 Possible mechanisms of cooperation. M = macrophage; T = thymus-derived lymphocyte; B = bone marrow-derived lymphocyte; pentagon = antigen.

mus-derived cell transmits a non-specific stimulus to the marrow-derived cell, which is thereby encouraged to initiate its response. Mechanism (ii) involves secretion by the thymus-derived cell of an antibody which has the special property of being taken up rapidly either by a third party cell, presumably a macrophage, or possibly the marrow-derived cell itself. This antibody then concentrates antigen and thereby makes it available to the receptor of the marrow-derived cell. Mechanism (iii) involves an antigen-bridge, in which the two cells bind to separate determinants of a multideterminant antigen.

Against mechanism (i) may be cited the finding listed as point 10. . . . Against mechanism (ii) may be cited the evidence listed as point 13. . . . Mechanism (ii), we note in passing, has a corollary: we do not know whether thymus-derived lymphocytes produce normal but non-secreted immunoglobulins, or whether alternatively they produce "IgX". . . . We lean toward mechanism (iii) on the present evidence, although with some hesitation.

How could an antigen-bridge lead to the response?

Here again a number of alternative ideas suggest themselves. One possibility is that antigen absorbed onto a cell surface (that of the thymus-derived cell) binds more efficiently to the receptor of another cell: the local-concentration hypothesis. Another is that the spatial arrangement of many molecules of antigen on one surface "meshes" with receptors on another surface. A third is that the antigen serves merely as a link, and that the essential element in triggering the response is the bringing of two lymphocytes together surface-to-surface. . . .

Natural killer cells in the mouse

1975 • Rolf Kiessling, Eva Klein, Hugh Pross, and
Hans Wigzell

Comment

In the years following Paul Ehrlich's morphological differentiation of white blood cells, biological explorers observed the natural history of these cell types, following their movements, probing their composition, testing their behavior to various stimuli, and determining exactly how they fit into the scheme of the body. Questions abounded. Functions of the phagocytes were nearly self-evident; the inflammatory connection of basophils and mast cells was soon established; but no one had the slightest clue about the role of the eosinophils or of the huge population of lymphocytes. When eosinophils could be correlated with allergy and parasitic infection, and when lymphocytes were finally linked with antibody production, a sense of order was reestablished. Even after the functional subtypes of lymphocytes, the cellular specialists of immunity, were distinguished, the consensus was that at least all the major classes of blood cells were discovered and categorized. Cells with slightly different morphology were merely natural variants. However, lurking among its lymphoid cousins was the natural killer (NK) cell.

What a name! Elie Metchnikoff called the various amoeboid murderers of microorganisms "phagocytes," meaning eating cells, since he regarded their activity as an evolutionary derivation of nutrition. The lymphocytic cellular assassins are referred to as cytotoxic T cells for the simple reason that they produce a lethal toxin, lymphotoxin. These poisoners, as other lymphocytes, have specific targets, acting against altered or foreign tissues rather than infectious agents. The natural killer cells, however, are not so discriminating, nor are they as impartial as the neutrophils. They take the mid-dle path. Their name reflects their normal aggressive and vigilant state.

The discovery of NK cells was not surprising, since they existed as a hypothetical entity to explain some anomalies in transplant rejection and in immunological studies of tumors, particularly those associated with viruses. F_1 hybrids of mice, which normally accept tissue of parental origin, destroyed such small grafts; the action was resistant to X-irradiation and required no prior sensitization. Other studies had established the presence of cytotoxic T cells against certain types of tumors in animals or human patients. What soon perplexed researchers was that normal subjects also possessed cells with anti-tumor cell activity. There is nothing like a consistent glitch in an experimental control to open new scientific territory. Antibody had no role in the destruction of the tissue. A few years later, these mysterious cells were shown to be especially deadly against virus-infected cells; subsequently interferon was deemed the enhancing agent. Interferon is a secreted protein that renders neighboring cells nonspecifically resistant to lethal viral multiplication (see Part 6/Isaacs, 1957).

Pieces of an infectious disease puzzle suddenly fell into place: before the specific antibody and T cell-mediated immune responses become effective, what defends host integrity against microbial assault, particularly against the agents first encountered? Bacteria are generally resisted by phagocytes with the later assistance of antibodies. Viruses present a far different problem. As noted above, interferon released from the infected cell can convey to adjacent cells some resistance, particularly to lysis, against the invading virus. Unless the viral disease itself is cytotoxic, the infected cell remains an active focus. NK cells, however, can kill the cell even before the virus replicates. Cells and secretory agents thus form effective teams against both bacterial and viral invaders.

What then are the physical characteristics of this natural killer? It appears to be a compromise between phagocytes and T lymphocytes: mid-sized, with a high proportion of cytoplasm to a slightly indented nucleus similar to macrophages, and nonphagocytic, but possessing receptors for the Fc portion of IgG. While lacking common antigens with thymocytes, it does express a macrophage marker as well as its own. Generally described as a large granular lymphocyte, long observed under the hematological microscope, and sharing with T cells the growth factor of interleukin-2, NK cells may form an intermediate family of blood cells with its own functional subgroups.

One mechanism for killing apparently is like that of cytotoxic T cells, eosinophils, and even complement-mediated cellular lysis: ring-shaped pore formation in target cell membranes. Complement component C9 and the proteins from all these cells that ring the hole are immunologically related.

No single report can be hailed as the discovery of the NK cell, for several laboratories had previously described the phenomenon and partially, but variably, defined the attributes of the active cells. However, the following milestone significantly helped to establish the uniqueness of natural killer cells. A collaboration originating with the Karolinska Institute and Hospital in Stockholm, comprised of Rolf Kiessling, Eva Klein, Hugh Pross, and Hans Wigzell, reached their somewhat controversial conclusion through a process of elimination.

For further information:

Herberman, R. B. and J. R. Ortaldo. 1981. Natural killer cells: their role in defenses against disease. *Science* 214:24–30.

Lotzová, E. and R. B. Heberman (editors). 1986. *Immunobiology of Natural Killer Cells.* Vol. 1 & 2. CRC Press, Boca Raton. 232, 272 p.

Marx, J. L. 1986. How killer cells kill their targets. *Science* 231:1367–1369.

Serrou, B., C. Rosenfeld, and R. B. Herberman (editors). 1982. *Natural Killer Cells.* Elsevier Biomedical Press, Amsterdam. 286 p.

The Paper*

Specific cytolytic or growth inhibitory activity has been ascribed to various effector cells derived from the reticulo-endothelial cell system. Thymus-derived lymphocytes have been shown to function as highly efficient killer cells, which recognize the target via its actively produced, antigen-specific surface receptors. Macrophages can be rendered selectively cytotoxic via a specific T cell factor. Monocytes and lymphocytes of yet undefined type have been found capable of cytolytic aggression towards IgG-coated target cells. Immune B lymphocytes were shown to be necessary in certain growth inhibitory assays in vitro. A variety of cells have thus been shown to be effective in various in vitro cytolytic or growth inhibitory test systems.

We would like to report another new cell type having selective in vitro cytotoxic behavior with unique functional as well as surface characteristics. This cell is found in normal mice, yet it displays specific cytolytic activity against certain mouse Moloney leukemia lines in vitro.

It will cause rapid lysis of such leukemic cells in the absence of added antibodies. As judged by surface markers and other characteristics it cannot be classified as a lymphocyte of B or T type nor as a monocyte. The distribution pattern with regard to age and organs will be reported, as well as its lack of known surface markers. . . .

The cytotoxic effect of normal spleen cells was found to be dependent on the age of the spleen donors. . . . [N]ewborn and 6-month-old CBA mice yielded less efficient killer spleen cells than mice between 3 weeks and 2 months of age. Similar age influence was found in A/Sn × C57BL/6 F_1 mice.

Various lymphoid organs were then analyzed for cytolytic activity. Spleen cells were always found to be most active; lymph node and bone marrow-de-

*Kiessling, R., E. Klein, H. Pross, and H. Wigzell. 1975. "Natural" killer cells in the mouse. II. Cytotoxic cells with specificity for mouse Moloney leukemia cells. Characteristics of the killer cell. *European Journal of Immunology* 5:117–121.

rived cells had significantly lower efficiency and thymocytes were not active at all.

In order to identify the killer cell we first used spleen cells from athymic nude BALB/c mice with control cells from littermates heterozygous for the nu gene. In three experiments performed the nude cells were either equal to more efficient than the control cells. Using a 50:1 killer-to-target cell ratio the mean % lysis by the nude cells was 51% (range 48–56), whereas the lysis by the control cells was 32% (range 17–50). As the nude spleen cells in other tests functioned as expected with regard to lack of functional T lymphocytes, we consider this a first, strong indication that the killer cells in this system do not involve conventional mature T lymphocytes.

Iron carbonyl powder treatment of the spleen cells did not influence the cytotoxic effect. Treatment with anti-θ serum plus complement compared to the effect of complement alone.

Passing the iron-treated cell suspension through a FCS [fetal calf serum] column did not change their efficiency. If, however, they were passed through an anti-Ig column a clear increase in cytotoxic activity was seen, as compared to untreated or control column (FCS) passed cells.

In order to eliminate both T and B cells, the iron-treated suspension was exposed to anti-θ serum plus complement and thereafter the supposedly T cell-free population was passed through the anti-mouse IgG column. The yield after such treatment was 1–5% of the original cell number. This combined effect increased the efficiency of the spleen cell population around 30 times.

The passage through a control column (FCS) did not cause any change in the reactivity compared to the population which had only been treated with anti-θ serum. This result would suggest that all the killer activity exerted by the total spleen cell population was present in the final yield of the original cell population left after anti-θ and anti-Ig column passage.

The efficiency of nude spleen cells in lysing YAC-1 target cells was not affected by treatment with iron powder. Nor was it affected by treatment with anti-θ serum plus complement or by complement alone. . . . [P]assage of the nude spleen cells through an anti-mouse IgG column resulted in a highly significant increase in activity, while passage through a control column (FCS) was without effect. It would thus seem clear that the killer cell in the present system is a non-adherent cell. It is neither a B or T lymphocyte as judged by surface markers or by existence in nude mice. Nor would it seem to be a monocyte, as they are normally removed by the above-described methods. . . .

The morphologies of such enriched cells . . . under the light microscope . . . were shown to consist

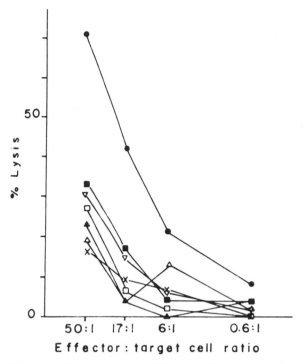

Figure 3 Various effector cell fractions from spleens of nu/+ BALB/c mice were tested against the YAC-1 in vitro line. Spleens from 15 mice were pooled. Effector cells were fractionated as follows: iron-treated (Fe) (x—x), Fe + complement (C) (△—△), Fe + anti-Θ serum + C (□—□) Fe + FCS column (▲—▲), Fe + anti-Ig column (■—■), Fe + anti-Θ+C + FCS column (△—△), Fe + anti-Θ—C + anti-Ig column (●—●).

of 95% of small lymphocytes with the remaining few being of undefinable nature. . . .

It is well known that interations resulting in both stimulatory or inhibitory effects can occur in cell-mediated immune reactions when mixed cell populations are used. As the A/Sn mice could be shown to provide the least efficient killer cells in the present system we tried to enrich for killer cells from low reactive A/Sn as compared to the more cytotoxic A/Sn × C57BL F$_1$ hybrid spleen cells. . . . A highly significant enrichment of killer activity was found in both populations after treatment with anti-θ serum plus complement plus passage through an anti-Ig column. The increase of Aa/Sn cells, however, did not reach the activities of the purified A/Sn × C57BL F$_1$ cells and we thus failed to prove any existence of suppressor cells in A/Sn spleens. Thus, A/Sn spleens would seem to contain the same kind of killer cells as in other mouse strains, but with lower cytolytic activity. Whether this is due to a lower frequency of killer cells or to a lower killer capacity per cell is unknown.

Chicken red blood cells coated with rabbit anti-chicken antiserum are lysed by effector cells from normal unimmunized mice, where the effector cells are neither of T or B lymphocyte nature, but behave rather like adherent cells with monocytic characteristics, having receptors for Fc of IgG molecules and with some surface Ig. The effector cells in this antibody-dependent lysis were compared to the effector cells which lyse the YAC-1 target cells. In a parallel study each cell population was tested either against the YAC-1 target cells or against CRBC in the antibody-mediated lysis system. Efficiency in this system was drastically reduced by the passage of cells through either a control column coated with FCS or through a column coated with anti-mouse IgG.

Anti-θ serum plus complement decreased the cytotoxicity to some extent, but a similar decrease was found using complement alone. Cells which have been treated both with anti-θ serum plus complement followed by passage through anti-IgG column are also highly inefficient in this kind of lysis.

These results clearly show that the majority of the spontaneous killer cells which lyse the YAC-1 target cells must be different from those that effectuate the lysis in the antibody-mediated CRBC system. . . .

Part 5
Theories

A theory has only the alternative of being right or wrong. A model has a third possibility: it may be right, but irrelevant. —Manfred Eigen

The great tragedy of Science: the slaying of a beautiful hypothesis by an ugly fact. —Thomas H. Huxley

The formal scientific method presented to students in their first high school science class is a creation of philosophers who looked over the shoulder of researchers. From afar. The sequence generally given—problem formulation, historical review, hypothesis development, tactical testing, result evaluation—publication (if possible), and revision or advancement—makes a nice series of subject headings. Closer inspection, however, dispels any beliefs in a rigid doctrine of methodology; each situation, the personality of the investigator, the specific problem, and the available technology evokes a unique approach or strategy. Otherwise scientists would be technicians or engineers and the field reduced at best to a craft. In fact, the practitioners of the scientific arts proceed almost intuitively. A fair number of discoveries arise entirely unintentionally out of unrelated pursuits. Some researchers, depending on their training and talents, will be apt to conduct systematic experiments, amassing details about the subject from one or several perspectives; others may leapfrog the nearby obstacles to strike at the heart of the problem. At times the insight of such a bold hypothesis, or proposition, matures into a fundamental, phenomenon-encompassing theory, or an explanatory principle. Every experiment has a hypothesis, but immunology has had only a few great theories. Immunology may also be contributing to a revolution of thought, a new general paradigm.

A paradigm, which in principle is a model or pattern with overtones of metaphor and myth, is in practice the current standard framework of reality. Paradigms embody a variety of mechanisms and disciplines. Examples of paradigms are Charles Darwin's conception of evolution and the Copenhagen consensus of Niels Bohr and colleagues on the interpretation of quantum mechanics. Paradigms, which arise from collections of theories, temper the investigative process by defining the limits of scientific domains in which theories may arise. In short, paradigms define orthodoxy. Theories, which typically are created to explain experimental paradoxes and consistent anomalies, may also engender validating hypotheses. Indeed, good theories are readily or foreseeably testable. Hypotheses, theories, and paradigms are thus stages of significance as well as development. Together they shape science. They are the experimenter's raison d'être, the justification of research.

The following group of milestones focuses on the contribution of theory to immunology, beginning with a report by the founder of immunology, Louis Pasteur. It is the first of three papers to be presented that explain immunity in terms of nutrition. Pasteur proposed a very simple explanation of acquired immunity: the invading microorganisms deplete a key nutrient that is both necessary and specific for a given species. Since in 1880 not everyone was convinced that bacteria were causative agents of disease, Pasteur's nutrition concept was not universally or enthusiastically acclaimed. Pasteur's idea did not survive long. Knowledge gained on the rapid turnover and replacement of body cells and chemicals, experiments demonstrating an acquired lethal inhibitor in the serum, and immunity to toxins blasted this first theory apart. His model was inadequate.

George H. F. Nuttall's report, while not presenting a formal theory, serves as a founding and influential representative of the humoral school of immunity. Four years before Nuttall's paper, Elie Metchnikoff provided evidence that phagocytes engulf and destroy living microorganisms in Darwinian combat. Evidence was lacking, however, for acquired immunity as might result from the activation or adaptation of populations of phagocytes. Nuttall's data for microbial killing by serum, whose effect could be prevented by heating but enhanced by immunization, clearly established the presence of humoral immune factors. Nuttall offered no opinion on mechanism. Theory, which depends on specific data for its inception, does not need to supply specifics; it merely presents a uniting principle.

Paul Ehrlich's side-chain theory of antibody formation was also a theory based on nutrition, since the function of the cell receptors was thought to involve the uptake of food substances. Thus, the haptophore atomic groups of toxins, being accidental analogs of nutrients, were thought to block the side chains and trigger the nucleus to produce replacements. According to the law of overcompensation, the membrane would become saturated, so to speak, throwing off the excess protein into the surrounding fluids as antitoxins. With great creativity and insight, Ehrlich formulated the first molecular theory that included cellular selection, specific functional domains of antigens and antibodies, and the existence of natural or innate antibodies. It lent support to the humoral side of immunology, but was also compatible with the cellular theory. Unfortunately, Ehrlich's theory was too advanced and encompassing for the time. Methods and technology were not yet available to test its proposals. Attacks on the weaker, more specific components of the theory overshadowed the merits of its significant biological principles. Core features of the side-chain theory are continually being rediscovered with the advance of the science.

The evolutional proposal of Elie Metchnikoff is next considered. His phagocyte theory was first conceived in 1883, but the included milestone is the text of the lectures he gave in 1891 on the phylogenic development of the inflammatory response. It is a well developed, broadly fashioned analysis. It is also the third theory averring the nutritional origin of immunity and it can be summarized as follows: Phagocytes at the bottom of the evolutionary tree are digestive and nutrient-dispersing cells. In more advanced animals they are involved as well in metamorphosis and tissue repair. These cells in still more evolved creatures also defend against parasites. Whatever their function, phagocytes are fundamentally digestive, and inflammation is not a disease, but an expression of normal, health-maintaining processes. While making a case for comparative zoology in understanding human diseases, Metchnikoff employed the phagocyte theory to emphasize the continuity, union, and development of immunity from the primitive metazoan to the conscious mind of humans. The theory was sound, but the serologists were not listening.

Sir Almroth E. Wright did not precipitate much controversy with his minor but reconciling theory. Wright found that both phagocytes and serum factors taken individually are effective destroyers of bacteria, but their activity is variable with the particular pathogen and experience of the host. However, united as a team, they act synergistically. The concept is narrow in scope, which perhaps is why it was successful. The key serum factors are opsonins, which allow in some cases and enhance in others phagocytosis of the microorganism. Wright found a common ground for cellular and humoral theories; he did not, however, merge them.

The next three milestones continue the path of Ehrlich in dealing with the mechanism of antibody formation. Linus Pauling's paper was the ultimate and most developed of the chemical proposals under the banner of direct template instructional theories. His concept was supported by the latest knowledge of chemical bonding, to which he himself had much contributed. Pauling's theory was a humoralist's dream, because it did not involve cells, except to secrete an undifferentiated immunoglobulin. Pauling called for the antibody to fold its chain around the antigen template, the tertiary protein structure thus being stabilized with hydrogen bonds. The idea was seriously flawed because it did not consider immunobiological facts. The model, however, was too elegant to dismiss easily. Advancing technology and new molecular genetic principles soon permitted testing of Pauling's conception. Although his template idea was invalidated, his principles of molecular structure survive.

Sir Macfarlane Burnet with Frank Fenner authored an intermediate theory which still was dependent on a template or instructional signal. However, it was biological in concept. Antibody specificity was impressed on the genetic machinery; it required the elimination of self-reactivity; and specificity was thereafter passed on to replicated cells, permitting immunological memory.

More significant, Burnet and Fenner offered an explanation of tolerance to "foreign" antigens and a mechanism of distinguishing "self" and "nonself" through patterns of antigenic "self markers." The theory was vague but a fundamental improvement, nonetheless. A new genetic paradigm was needed to open the antibody-synthesizing black box, and James D. Watson and Francis Crick supplied the crowbar.

Neils K. Jerne, one of most creative theoreticians of immunology, recognized the role of randomness in the generation of specific antigen receptors on cells, and published a theory of natural antibody selection. Burnet incorporated Jerne's ideas in his own, more developed clonal selection theory of antibody formation. No longer was the cell a clean slate awaiting imprinting of the antigen. Antibody specificity was predetermined by genetic recombination and somatic mutation. The theory was tested thoroughly, and result after result seemed to be consistent with it. Clear, and with established mechanisms, Burnet's theory, his fourth attempt, has become dogma.

Theories, however, are first or second order approximations that organize an agenda for additional, refining experiments. The last milestone of the series, which reflects both new data and a new approach, is by Jerne. His network theory concerns the regulation of the antibody response by system recognition of both antigen and immunoglobulin (antibody and cellular receptor) idiotype. Highly inventive, abstract, and holistic, it is leading to a new context of immunological organization whereby all the antigenic patterns external to the host also lie within it or, to be more precise, are constituent configurations.

For further information:

Beveridge, W. I. B. 1980. *Seeds of Discovery*. W. W. Norton & Company. New York. 130 p.

Bruni, C. G. Doria, G. Koch, and R. Strom (editors). 1979. *Systems Theory in Immunology. Proceedings of the Working Conference.* (Lecture Notes in Biomathematics. Volume 32.) Springer-Verlag, Berlin. 273 p.

Cunningham, A. J. 1978. "Gestalt immunology": a less reductionist approach to the subject. In: *Theoretical Immunology* (G. I. Bell, A. S. Perelson, and G. H. Pimbley, Jr., editors). Marcel Dekker, New York. pp. 45–61.

Silverstein, A. M. 1979. Cellular versus humoral immunity: determinants and consequences of an epic 19th century battle. *Cellular Immunology* 48:208–221.

Silverstein, A. M. 1985. A history of theories of antibody formation. *Cellular Immunology* 91:263–283.

On virulent diseases, and in particular the disease commonly called fowl cholera

1880 • Louis Pasteur

Comment

Louis Pasteur, the grand patriarch of immunology, did not provide the first theory of immunity, which may come as a surprise from what we have encountered of his research. Pasteur did, however, propose the first theoretical framework of immunology, the scientific discipline. The difference between the two stages of theoretical development is the comparatively recent maturation of the formal science of immunology; notions about disease and its recovery or avoidance may be found in the earliest chronicles of civilization.

The view that a person's resistance to disease is the will of a god or demon can not be regarded as theory. This, rather, is a matter of religious speculation and belief. A person's emotional profile within a religious perspective, however, can influence immunity. Since most Eastern religio-philosophies are introspective, psychoanalytical, and self-experimental, one may find merit in their theories of immunity based on the mental control of stress. Disease, after all, is dis-ease. Theory traditionally arose with the assignment of agency to the material astrological world of planetary and stellar orbs. While astrology was a step toward scientific analysis, certainly in astronomy, it lacked any medical merit beyond the obvious meteorological-environmental correlates. The intermediate conception of a miasma was simultaneously one step forward and one back, for it approached the idea of contagion but postulated a diffused and ethereal agency. Immunity-exemption, in contrast to active resistance, hence was due to the absence of the untoward event.

Girolamo Fracastoro, a gentleman of Verona, published in 1546 his treatise on contagion by the dissemination of specific seeds of disease. In addition to the advance in the development of germ theory, this work also brought forward some interesting concepts, indeed theories, of immunity. Selective affinities and conditions of host and agent explained natural resistance, and acquired immunity was said to be a result of cleansing supposed tainted, congenitally infused menstrual blood. Susceptibility thus was related to a predisposition; subsequent resistance resulted from the removal of that characteristic.

The idea of changing an internal constituent itself is probably of greater fundamental importance to immunology than the germ theory. We should not forget that immunological surveillance of any aberrant tissue or alien structure and homeostasis are also attributes of immunity. The theory that disease can occur when the body elements are out of balance, to use the Taoist or classical Greek models, long predated the discovery of microbial life. During the late Renaissance, with the development of the scientific method of experimentation and the advances in chemical and physical knowledge, changes were not the cause, but the effect of illness. The concept of immunity through disease-induced changes in blood took on a mechanical flavor. Blood was transformed, rendering resistance to the etiological agent.

Next was a focus on the nature of the conversion. In its various guises by eighteenth-century authors, a depletion theory took root, but it was only slightly more developed than that advanced by Fracastoro. Here a favorable but unknown substance necessary for the function of the germ is consumed by a previous encounter. Experimentation was lacking, ideas were vague, and the fabled germ had yet to be discovered. The theories and notions of immunity of this and earlier centuries were empty and idle, merely conjecture constructed on untestable foundations. Since, whatever the era, mechanistic conceptions are generally modeled on familiar technological principles—analogies, for instance, with the seed often needed in crystallization; the influence of heat in transforming water from solid through liquid to gas; the implicit spectrum in white light divulged by a prism; and the penetrating ability of electromagnetic fields to move the point of a compass—early thinkers were limited to fundamental examples in physics and chemistry to explain biological phenomena.

Enter Pasteur. He gave us experiments, his ideas were developed from data, and the isolated germ, a clearly observable microorganism, was his very tool. After demonstrating acquired immunity in chickens to fowl cholera (with, as we recall, a good deal of help from Emile Roux), Pasteur quickly formulated an opinion on its mechanism. His version of the nutrient depletion theory, which follows, was a noble attempt. He showed through in-vitro studies, that each microorganism has unique food requirements, and that the exhaustion of a key substance by one bacterium does not preclude the growth of a second. In a follow-up report, he proposed that the body is analogous to a culture medium, since whether he injected the pathogen into the muscle, a vein, or by way of the digestive tract, immunized animals survived while normal chickens perished. As in the earlier test tube studies, he ascertained that these resistant chickens were susceptible to other diseases.

Pasteur, nevertheless, was astute enough to offer an alternative explanation as well. The second proposal served as a clay pigeon: having tossed it into the air, he then proceeded to shoot it down. He granted the possibility that the initial infective bacterium, whether of a natural or an attenuated vaccine strain, could leave a fermentative product inhibitory to its further growth. However, when he evaporated an old culture in the cold and replenished its volume with fresh medium, he observed subsequent growth. Despite this failure, the theory of a retained inhibitor specific to each microorganism, first proposed in 1879 by M. von Nencki, survived until the rise of the humoral theory of immunity.

For further information:

Dubos, R. J. 1955. Second thoughts on the germ theory. *Scientific American* 192(5):31–35.

King, L. S. 1982. *Medical Thinking. A Historical Preface.* Princeton University Press, Princeton. 336 p.

Lindenmann, J. 1981. Immunology in the 1880s: two early theories. In: *The Immune System. Vol. 1* (C. M. Steinberg and I. Lefkovits, editors). Basel, S. Karger. pp. 413–422.

Pasteur, L. 1880. Sur le choléra des poules; étude des conditions de la non-récidive de la maladie et de quelques autres de ses caractères. *Comptes rendus l'Académie des Sciences* 90:952–958.

Silverstein, A. M. and A. A. Bialasiewicz. 1980. A history of theories of acquired immunity. *Cellular Immunology* 51:151–167.

The Paper*

Before going any further, may the Academy permit me to digress on a matter highly worthy of interest. Resulting from that which preceded, the affliction indicated by the name of fowl cholera can be easily produced in chickens without death being a necessary consequence of the disease. . . . Let us consider a chicken very well vaccinated by one or several previous inoculations of the attenuated virus. Let us now reinoculate this chicken. What will happen? The local lesion will be, so to say, relatively insignificant to that produced by the first inoculations. This first one especially initiated an alteration in the muscle so great that enormous sequestra [necrotic separations] were perceived merely by touch. The cause of the difference in the effects of these inoculations

---

*Pasteur, L. 1880. Sur les maladies virulentes, et en particulier sur la maladie applée vulgairement choléra des poules. *Comptes rendus l'Académie des Sciences* 90:239–248. [With permission.]

seems to reside entirely in the great ease in growth of the microbe following the first inoculation, in contrast to the latter in which growth was, as it were, none or very slight and then promptly arrested. The consequences of these facts, so to say, leap before your eyes. The muscle that had been diseased becomes, after healing and repair, powerless, so to speak, to support the cultivation of the microbe, as if the latter, by prior culture, had removed from the muscle some principle that the body could not restore and whose absence stops the development of the small organism. In my thinking, this explanation, to which the most evident facts take us, could probably become generally applicable to all virulent diseases.

The explanation that I gave on resistance to the disease of fowl cholera appears all the more plausible when after three or four days from seeding the microbe in a culture medium, one filters the latter in the cold to perfect clearness and reinoculates it for several days of testing of its limpidity at a temperature of 33°C: all cultivations have become impossible. However, the amount of the microbe formed at the start was unweighable. Remarkably, this now sterile filtered liquid is far from being able to maintain this sterility with respect to other microscopic organisms, for example, the anthrax bacterium. This allows us to understand how an organism in which a virulent disease does not recur is nevertheless capable of contracting a virulent disease of another nature. It would be easy to give anthrax to chickens vaccinated for fowl cholera. . . .

Experiments on the antibacterial influence of animal substances

1888 • George H. F. Nuttall

Comment

During the first four years after proposing his conception of immunity-providing phagocytosis, Elie Metchnikoff had only to defend its novelty and distinction from previous observations of amoeboid cell activity. Beginning in 1888, however, the opposition to his theory was based on fundamental theoretical differences. Phagocytosis, according to the new contenders, was a secondary phenomenon; immunity was chiefly a result of humoral bactericidal factors. The leading author of the challenge was George H. F. Nuttall (1862–1937), whose opening salvo is the next milestone.

The son of a San Francisco physician, Nuttall gained his general education in England, France, Germany, and Switzerland. He returned in 1878 to the United States for his M.D., awarded in 1884 by the University of California Medical School in San Francisco. After a year at the Johns Hopkins University, Nuttall made a second sojourn to Europe in 1886, this time to the universities at Breslau and Göttingen. He obtained his Ph.D. at Göttingen under the guidance of Carl Flügge. Back again at Johns Hopkins University in 1891, Nuttall became an associate of William H. Welch, and participated in the isolation of *Clostridium perfringens*, the gangrene bacillus. Since the university was instituting its own center of hygiene, Nuttall was sent to the Institute of Hygiene at the University of Berlin to further his training. While so doing, he conducted some pioneering studies of germfree animals. However, instead of returning to Baltimore, he accepted an appointment in 1899 as Lecturer in bacteriology and preventive medicine at Cambridge University. He stayed in England for the rest of his life. In 1906 he received an endowed chair, as the first Quick professor of biology at Cambridge University. By this time, Nuttall's research interests had shifted, eventually leading to his directorship of the new Molteno Institute of Research in Biology and Parasitology at Cambridge. Nuttall was elected a fellow of the Royal Society in 1904.

The degeneration of bacteria described in Nuttall's report contrasts with both the bacteriostasis of Louis Pasteur's original nutrient depletion idea and the toxic retention view, since these theories were related to acquired immunity and Nuttall observed a lethal action in normal blood, although activity was generally enhanced in immune sera. Furthermore, Nuttall found variation among animal blood, with some totally lacking killing power. The thermolability of the bactericidal agent and its instability after prolonged storage reminded him of fermentative enzymes rather than simple chemical antiseptics. The question of heat inactivation confused and stymied immunologists for decades. Nuttall declined to interpret his findings in a grand theory. Indeed, the paper takes a moderate, compromising stand by admitting a significant role for the phagocytes. Still, something in blood had destroyed the tested microorganisms before they were engulfed by the white cells. Nuttall had not excluded the possibility that the agent was secreted by the phagocytes—a deficiency that Metchnikoff would exploit in his counterattack—probably because the precedent of toxic secretions was only then being presented by Emile Roux and Alexandre Yersin in their discovery of diphtheria toxin.

What distinguished Nuttall's work from previous armchair speculation was the extensive experimentation. It was far more, for instance, than the parenthetical notes of Moritz Traube, who in 1874 commented on the resistance of stored blood to putrefaction even after he obtained it from rabbits previously injected with bacteria. Nuttall also went further than Joseph Fodor, who emphasized in 1886 the defensive function of blood fluid and in 1887 recorded the reduction of viable anthrax bacilli in clotted blood cultures. Nuttall's use of defibrinated blood escaped the criticism applied to Fodor

that the decreased bacterial colony counts on gelatin were an artifact of the organism's entanglement in the clot.

Nuttall's report much impressed the bacteriological community, and many built their own investigations on this foundation. Unfortunately, at this early period Metchnikoff took a highly defensive posture, and his foes, looking for a good alternative explanation, used Nuttall's work to emphasize, and then elevate and ennoble the humoral factor. Results, however, varied so greatly with each test system that a simple universal principle could not be attained, short of the agency of cell-free serum or plasma. Not all bacteria were susceptible, and the same blood sample might affect one species but not another. Immunized animals, compared to normal controls, typically but not always manifested superior killing power.

Ambiguity ceased with the studies of Shibasaburo Kitasato and Emil Behring in 1890, demonstrating passively acquired protection to tetanus through neutralization of the toxin (see Part 1/Behring, 1890). The evidence of antitoxin was immediately hailed as incontrovertible. It was a consistent, specific, and easily testable effect. While the results had no direct bearing on the destruction of microorganisms nor on natural immunity, they did establish that serum, not cells, could render an animal immune to an infectious disease. However, tetanus and diphtheria were special cases, since they are noninvasive diseases due to the action of toxins. When in 1894 Richard Pfeiffer dramatically exhibited the dissolution of cholera vibrio in vivo and in vitro by immune serum (see Part 6/Pfeiffer, 1894), he gravely wounded the cellular theory of immunity. The humoral theory would reign for the next sixty years.

For further information:

Graham-Smith, G. S. and D. Keilin. 1939. George Henry Falkiner Nuttall, 1862–1937. *Obituary Notices of Fellows of the Royal Society* 2:493–499.

Mazumdar, P. M. H. 1972. Immunity in 1890. *Journal of the History of Medicine and Allied Sciences* 27:312–324.

The Paper*

Metchnikoff has in the last few years tried to establish the principle that phagocytic activity, in which bacteria are taken up and destroyed, is responsible for protecting the animal against infectious disease and developing acquired immunity. The experimental foundation of Metchnikoff's theory, other than his observations on Daphnia, is supported by experiments with anthrax bacilli in frogs and rabbits and on examinations on the behavior of anthrax bacilli and leucocytes of different animals outside the body on a heated microscope stage. . . .

Rabbits were used for experiments on warm-blooded animals. Metchnikoff placed capillary tubes containing attenuated anthrax bacilli under the skin of the ear of an animal. He then broke the tubes, and under the microscope he could ascertain that the arising pus contained many leucocytes in which the anthrax bacilli had been absorbed. Virulent bacilli were not engulfed by susceptible animals, but they were ingested in large numbers by immune animals. . . .

Because of the importance of the question concerning the causes of immunity, on one hand, and the inadequate evidence by Metchnikoff, on the other hand, I was more than pleased to follow Professor Flügge's request to report these experiments.

I wanted mainly to find out if the phagocytes really engulf living bacilli and if they alone are capable of destroying bacilli. If there is a chance that absorption into the cells is limited to only a certain fraction of bacilli and that a further fraction not touched by cells is killed by other influences of the living body, then the functional meaning of the phagocytes would become doubtful, and it would even be possible that they are only capable of engulfing those bacilli that have already degenerated by other influences.

I repeated Metchnikoff's experiments on frogs. Then I carried out a couple of comparative experiments with attenuated and virulent anthrax bacilli in the ear of a rabbit. Finally I was able to make

---

*Nuttall, G. H. F. 1888. Experimente über die bacterienfeindlichen Einflüsse des thierischen Körpers. *Zeitschrift für Hygiene und Infektionskrankheiten* 4:353–394. [With permission of Springer-Verlag, Heidelberg.]

controlled observations on the relationship between leucocytes and bacilli using the heated stage of a microscope. . . .

A survey of the results on frogs confirms Metchnikoff's statements that when placed under the skin of frogs, fragments of organs containing anthrax bacilli accumulate leucocytes, and that these leucocytes engulf large numbers of the bacilli. Also confirmed was that the engulfed bacilli are destroyed within the leucocytes. My own findings in this last regard deviate from those of Metchnikoff, since I observed the same amount of bacilli, if not more, degenerating outside the leucocytes as within. I also found living, virulent anthrax bacilli in the inoculated fragment after 16 days of its placement under the frog's skin. As far as I could verify, the still active bacilli were not attenuated. . . .

That phagocytic activity is the most important protective measure must be weighed against the fact that anthrax bacilli under the skin of frogs are destroyed in large amounts outside phagocytes as well. It is clear that Metchnikoff's experiments suffer considerably by this finding. . . .

As the previous experiments already suggested, the destruction of the bacilli in the living body is not only caused by the leucocytes; other influences must also cause degeneration. In the living animal only certain phases of the mutual relationship of bacilli and leucocytes can be verified. I hoped to get a better insight by observing the behavior of leucocytes toward bacilli in microscopic preparations. By this manner it might be more exactly established whether leucocytes engulf the bacilli immediately or after a delay, and whether virulent and attenuated bacilli behave differently in this regard. Such observations also promised to give an answer to if and to what extent degeneration of the bacilli occur in animal fluids.

This method seemed especially appropriate, since Metchnikoff himself had used it. He found that, when bringing together anthrax bacilli with frog lymph on the heated stage, only the bacilli in the leucocytes showed degeneration, and that leucocytes of anthrax-susceptible animals in analogous experiments showed less capacity to engulf bacilli that those of totally or partly immune animals.

My own experiments in this regard showed remarkable results, such that a further extension seemed desirable. Therefore, I have one after another carefully examined the behavior of anthrax bacilli and other bacteria in blood, in lymph, and in several other tissue fluids of different animals species. . . .

A drop of fluid to be tested was placed on a cover slip and an inoculum of virulent anthrax bacilli was placed at the edge of the drop. The cover slip was

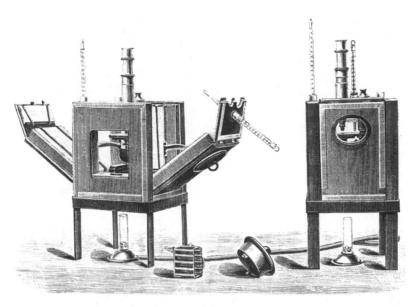

Warming cabinet for microscopy.

then applied to a concave slide and sealed with paraffin. . . . When observations were performed at the temperature of warm-blooded animals, the microscope was enclosed in a specially insulated and humidified heated chamber. The slide could be manipulated through an oval opening normally covered with a fitted lid. . . .

Two free bacilli observed constantly at 15°C showed after 4 hr clear signs of decomposition. . . . The changes consisted of the protoplasm of the bacillus becoming granular and the countour acquiring a more irregular boundary. Later, either the granular structure disappeared, the contour sharpened, and the bacillus itself became paler, almost disappearing to the eye, or the granulation of the protoplasm increased until the bacillus disintegrated. . . . Degeneration of bacilli in leucocytes was more difficult to observe. . . . After staining the preparation, decomposition of the bacilli could be observed readily. For staining, a weak alkaline methylene blue solution was used. . . .

In the following experiments with mammalian blood, a drop from a little wound or small blood vessel was aseptically put on a cover glass as described above. The preparation was then placed immediately into the chamber of the microscope, which was heated to the blood temperature of the animal in question and then observed. . . .

Since the blood on the cover glass coagulated after a few moments, serum collected at the rim of the drop. The anthrax bacilli were inoculated at the edge of the drop in order to keep them surrounded by

the liquid thoughout the examination and not trapped by the coagulum. . . . Coagulation did not abolish the antibacterial activity. Later we learned from other experiments that defibrinated blood also contains antibacterial attributes.

One or two of the preparations was constantly observed under the microscope. . . . Other preparations were monitored periodically. The experiments demonstrated that some of the bacilli are engulfed by leucocytes, but most of the bacilli remain free and degenerate to a smaller extent. With respect to the engulfment of bacilli by leucocytes and the rapidity and extent of degeneration of free units, the blood samples of different animal species showed remarkable differences. . . .

Degeneration occurs the fastest in human blood, in one case after 45 minutes, but generally after 1 hr and 45 minutes. . . . After 4 hr, normal bacilli again appeared. . . . Many bacilli were engulfed by leucocytes, but most of them remained free. A greater proportion of the free bacteria was degenerated than that found within the leucocytes.

Degeneration appeared almost as fast in immunized sheep blood as in human blood. After 1 hr it reached maximal degeneration. After 24 hr degenerative forms were still present, while after 26 hr growth could be detected. . . . In nonimmunized sheep blood, maximum degeneration was observed after 1½ hr, and growth observed sooner. . . .

Bird blood seems weakly bactericidal. . . . The absolute amount of degenerated free bacilli was still quite remarkable. . . . Much slower but much more complete was the degeneration of bacilli in the blood of rabbits. In general, the maximum was reached in about 5 hr, and almost all bacilli were involuted. Growth appeared after 28 hr. I noted leucocytes engulfing bacilli shortly (30 minutes) after mixing. . . . Therefore, I can not confirm Metchnikoff's statement that rabbit leucocytes on the heated stage are as incapable of engulfing virulent anthrax bacilli as the living animal. Without exception, almost no degeneration appeared in mouse blood. Engulfment by leucocytes was very slight.

Other tissue fluids were now examined, especially those with few cellular elements, in order to learn if leucocytes are in some way causing the degeneration of the bacilli. Aqueous humor seemed to be very suitable, having, as Metchnikoff noted, very few leucocytes. Pericardial fluid was similar in appearance. Both fluids were highly bactericidal. . . .

I also examined the length of time that blood preserves its antibacterial properties outside the body. . . . After 4–16 hr at 37°C, blood from immunized rabbits showed no degeneration but, instead, immediate growth.

Without attempting to explain the antibacterial attributes of animal fluids, we can conclude with certainty that the destruction of the bacilli is not caused by the activity of the leucocytes. . . . It seems that the bacilli absorbed by leucocytes are not in their normal condition, and that the antibacterial agency is found in the surrounding liquid. The parallelisms, which in most of the experiments consist of the rapidity of the degeneration and the ingestion by leucocytes, support my assumption. The faster the degeneration appears, the faster the bacilli are taken up by leucocytes. If the degeneration is slow, the life energy of the leucocytes becomes lame and fades, and engulfment is only possible in very small amounts.

Comparing humans and rabbits, where differences in phagocytosis are the most distinct, the leucocytes never stay alive more than 2½ hr. While the degeneration of the bacilli in rabbits reaches it climax after about 3 hr, in human blood it is complete after 1 hr. Therefore the engulfment of bacilli in human blood is greater than in rabbit blood. . . .

Experiments with the hanging drop could not ascertain . . . if the degenerated bacilli are truly dead. . . . Professor Flügge asked me to find out by culture experiments. . . . The culturing procedure determined the number of bacilli at the outset and over various intervals during which the bacilli were in contact with blood. . . . The blood from an artery or a vein was put into a sterilized bottle which also contained a little fine, sterilized sand. The bottle had been kept at 38°C. . . . After the necessary amount of blood (about 25–30 cc) was in the bottle, it was shaken several times to defibrinate the blood. Defibrination was necessary [for thorough contact of bacilli and fluids and facilitate sampling for cultures]. . . . Samples of about 0.5 to 1 cc were removed from the defibrinated blood with help of a sterilized pipette and placed into little preheated culture tubes. . . . For the inoculum, I placed in a sterilized solution of NaCl a thin suspension of spleen from a mouse recently killed by anthrax. A platinum loop was used to transfer the solution to the blood. About the same number of bacilli was added each time. . . . [Nutrient gelatin was the culture plate medium for colony counting. . . .]

In the blood of an immunized sheep, the number of anthrax bacilli decreased in one instance in 3½ hr from 4578 to 185 and from 4872 to 283, and in another case from 11,046 to 427 and 9,245 to 665. In the blood of nonimmunized sheep the number decreased in 3 hr from 7938 to 6664 and 8330 to 4782. . . . Considerable variation occurred in bactericidal activity. In one case of rabbit blood, 90,000 bacteria were destroyed, while in another experiment, about 45 to 153 bacilli survived from an inoculum of 7,000. The blood of a nonimmune sheep gave similar results. . . .

An important fact is that the bactericidal power of the blood decreases after some time, and then the blood becomes a good nutritive medium for the bacilli. The antibacterial attributes are not credited to a fixed disinfecting substance in the regular sense. . . . The antibacterial agent can only be very fragile or extremely unstable, easily decomposed by other components of the blood, or it is (which is quite possible) a development of fermentation. A further experimental series supports this last thought. I subjected blood to temperatures of 50°C and 55°C before adding the bacteria. It showed that dog blood, which had been heated to 52°C for 10 and 30 minutes, lost its bactericidal effect, as did rabbit blood after heating for 45 minutes at 55°C. Heating blood for 10 minutes to 48°C to 55°C did not completely abolish the disinfecting power of blood. The temperatures (19° and 38°C) at which the blood samples are kept after inoculation do not seem (on rabbit blood) to have any influence on the bactericidal attributes. . . .

It now seemed desirable to observe other bacteria and saprophytes to see if they, too, would be victims of the bactericidal power of blood. For this reason I chose *Bacillus megaterium* and *B. subtilis*. Twelve-hr old spore-free broth cultures were used for the inocula. *B. subtilis* was always totally destroyed after 2 hr. *B. megaterium* showed a considerable decrease, but only disappeared totally in one instance. The blood did not have any effect on *Staphylococcus aureus*. . . .

Results gained through microscopic observations verify that in all cases animal fluids have a negative effect on anthrax bacilli and other microorganisms independently of the leucocytes. . . . Culture experiments exclude the idea that engulfment of bacilli by leucocytes has anything to do with their degeneration. From all the results of my experiments I can state that Metchnikoff is wrong by claiming that the destruction of the bacilli in the living body is caused only by phagocytic activity. Only after another large number of experiments will it be possible to say more about the quality and quantitative fluctuation of this strange antibacterial mechanism.

On immunity with special reference to cell life

1900 • Paul Ehrlich

Comment

A theory built upon theories has a precarious foundation. If, however, the glue is strong and the design is masterful, then even toothpicks can form the imposing, efficient edifice of a geodesic dome. Paul Ehrlich was such a master architect and craftsman. In the milestone that follows, which was a purely theoretical study, not just an aside to an experimental report, Ehrlich presented his fully developed ideas on the nature and formation of antitoxins. It is the first theory of the humoral school proposing definite objects, functions, and mechanisms. Although it was attacked from every side, no one was able to produce as thorough a conceptual model for nearly a half-century. It was especially difficult to come up with a suitable alternative when so many of Ehrlich's insights were correct at their core.

The side-chain idea was derived from Eduard Pflüger's rather bizarre image of an extraordinarily massive molecule of protoplasm the size of the cell. This antique nineteenth-century model called for a central portion responsible for generic cellular functions and numerous side chains having the specialized physiological activity of kidney, muscle, stomach or other cell. Pflüger was a physiologist, and his theory generally found favor with other medically trained physiologists; organic chemists quickly discarded it. Both groups talked about chemical nuclear regions and side chains, but the difference in scale was almost like comparing the flagellum of a protozoan with the leg of an ant. Ehrlich accepted Pflüger's theoretical structure, since he was familiar with it from medical school and since he refused to accept the view that the cell was merely a bag of homogenously dispersed chemicals. Side chains per se were not crucial to Ehrlich's theory; however, they conveniently allowed membrane receptors that could somehow elicit from the executive center of the cell responsive actions.

Ehrlich's theory had a second foundation, which was both necessary and more plausible. In 1873, Ehrlich's cousin Carl Weigert and a small gathering of friends were discussing his new conception of pathology, which reminded them of the Hindu diety Shiva, whose attribute is change through destruction. Weigert published the Shiva theory shortly afterwards. It challenged Rudolf Virchow's theory, which postulated that inflammatory irritants passively trigger cells to replicate. For Weigert, pathological processes, particularly cellular proliferation, are active internal responses to a change in physiological equilibrium, a dynamic state. These activities were hence thought to be normal to host regulatory function as in repair or replacement. Tissue injury, of course, would upset the balance, but normal aging and trauma of cells would also cause a loss in population. Cellular replication, Weigert declared, resulted from the transformation of potential bioplastic energy to the kinetic form. Overproduction is normal, but enhanced in pathological situations. With age or certain conditions, underproduction may occur, leading to death. Ehrlich developed his immunological theory around the principles of his cousin's Shiva theory. The joining of the haptophore portion of the toxic antigen to the side-chain receptor would send a signal to the nucleus to manufacture replacements, which would be overproduced and then shed as a secretion. We know now that B cell receptors are immunoglobulins to haptens, which, together with T cells, signal the manufacture and secretion of numerous other immunoglobulins. Ehrlich's insight is astonishing, all the more so considering the paucity of chemical and physiological scaffolding he had available on which to shape a theory.

As previously discussed, Ehrlich's separation of chemical substances into unique, functional atomic groups was indeed correct, as was his lifelong focus on the stereochemical specificity of molecular coupling. His view that toxins are accidental analogs in cellular metabolism was keenly advanced for its day. Many antigens are more than mere stimulants of antibody production; receptor competition can influence kinetics of immunological reactions. The absence of cellular receptors, as observed by Ehrlich, does contribute to natural immunity. For instance, a bacterium lacking an appropriate surface component that matches any possible tissue receptor—for it works both ways—is ecologically disadvantaged, and being unable to anchor itself to host cells, is apt to be washed away by water or host fluids.

Ehrlich's classic diagrams depicting his side-chain theory have at times been more of a hindrance than an aid. When scanning electron microscopy was developed and turned upon B and T cells, activated cells displayed surface features highly analogous to Ehrlich's figures.

Some authors of recent review articles and textbooks have pointed out the similarity without noting that Ehrlich indicated in his lecture that his figures were purely representative. Indeed, even in his day many people asked whether the receptors can be seen in the microscope. "The stupid people think I really imagine that it looks that way," he once lamented.

For further information:

Bendiner, E. 1980. Ehrlich: immunologist, chemotherapist, prophet. *Hospital Practice* November:129; 133; 138–139; 145–146; 150–151; 154–157.

Morrison, H. 1924. Carl Weigert. *Annals of Medical History* 6:163–177.

Parascandola, J. 1981. The theoretical basis of Paul Ehrlich's chemotherapy. *Journal of the History of Medicine* 36:19–43.

Witebsky, E. 1954. Ehrlich's side-chain theory in the light of present immunology. Paul Ehrlich Centennial. *Annals of the New York Academy of Sciences* 59:168–181.

The Paper*

Honored President, my Lords and Gentlemen: It is to me the very greatest honor that I have been summoned here by your most highly esteemed Society, which for more than two centuries has represented and still represents the center of the scientific life of England, in order that I may deliver the Croonian Lecture. . . .

[T]he toxin was characterized by the possession of two different combining groups: one, which may be designated *haptophore,* conditions the union with antitoxin, while the other group, which may be designated *toxophore,* is the cause of the toxic action. . . .

If we now designated a toxin molecule, of which the toxophore group is destroyed, but its haptophore group retained, as *toxoid,* then the above-de-

*Ehrlich, P. 1900. On immunity with special reference to cell life. *Proceedings of the Royal Society, London.* Biology. 66:424–448. [With permission of the Society.]

scribed process will represent the quantitative progress of the conversion of the toxin molecules into toxoid molecules. Such a toxoid molecule has the same quantitative combining affinity for antitoxin as the original toxin molecule, in spite of the disappearance of toxicity to the animal body. In other words, the affinity of the haptophore group for the antitoxin is absolutely independent of the existence of a toxophore group. . . .

The separation of the characteristic atom groups of the toxin molecule into a haptophore and toxophore group, afforded not merely a satisfactory chemical explanation of the process of neutralization: the possession of the knowledge of the existence of these groups yielded us, at the same time, the key to the nature of the toxic property of toxins, and to the mystery of the origin of the antitoxins themselves. . . .

[O]ne was obliged to come to the conclusion that the union between the toxin and the tissues, which could only be overcome by means of a specific chemically related antagonizing agent, must itself depend on a chemical combination. One was therefore forced to accept the idea that the central nervous system, that is to say certain ganglion cells in it, possessed atom groups resembling those of the antitoxin, in having a maximum affinity for tetanus poison. The predilection of the nervous system for tetanus toxin,

the rapid union of the toxin with the nervous tissue, the gradual onset of the symptoms and their long duration could only be explained by the existence of such toxophile groups. . . .

We now come to the important question of the significance of the toxophile groups in organs. That these are in function specially designed to seize on toxins cannot be for one moment entertained. It would not be reasonable to suppose that there were present in the organism many hundreds of atom groups destined to unite with toxins. . . .

One may therefore rightly assume that these toxophile protoplasmic groups in reality serve normal functions in the animal organism, and that they only incidentally and by pure chance possess the capacity to anchor themselves to this or that toxin. . . .

We are obliged to adopt the view, that the protoplasm is equipped with certain atom groups, whose function especially consists in fixing to themselves certain food-stuffs, of importance to the cell-life. Adopting the nomenclature of organic chemistry, these groups may be designated *side-chains*. We may assume that the protoplasm consists of a specific executive center in connection with which are nutritive side-chains, which possess a certain degree of independence, and which may differ from one another according to the requirement of the different cells. And as these side-chains have the office of at-

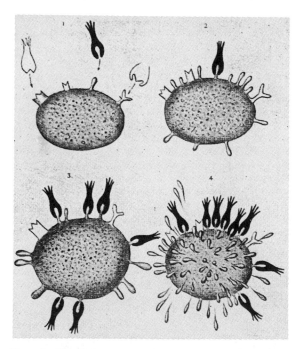

Plate I Diagrammatic representation of the side-chain theory.

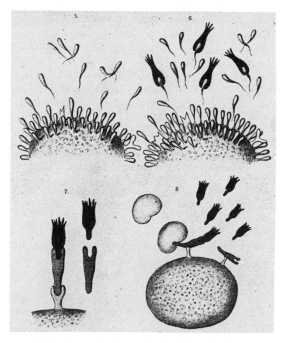

Plate II Diagrammatic representation of the theory of the formation of antitoxins.

taching to themselves certain food-stuffs, we must also assume an atom-grouping in these food-stuffs themselves, every group uniting with a corresponding combining group of a side-chain. The relationship of the corresponding groups . . . must be specific. The groups must be adapted to one another, e.g., as male and female screw (Pasteur), or as lock and key (E. Fischer). From this point of view, we must contemplate the relation of the toxin to the cell. . . .

[T]he relation between toxin and cell will cease to be shrouded in mystery if we adopt the view that the haptophore groups of the toxins are molecular groups, fitted to unite not only with the antitoxins but also with the side-chains of the cells, and that it is by their agency that the toxin becomes anchored to the cell. . . .

[T]here is sufficient evidence that the toxophile side-chains are the same as those which have to do with the taking up of the food-stuffs by the protoplasm. . . .

If the cells of these organs lack side-chains fitted to unite with them, the toxophore group cannot become fixed to the cell, which therefore suffers no injury, i.e., the organism is naturally immune. One of the most important forms of natural immunity is based upon the circumstance, that in certain animals the organs essential to life are lacking in those haptophore groups which seize upon definite toxins. . . .

The theory above developed allows an easy and natural explanation of the origin of antitoxins. In keeping with what has already been said, the first stage in the toxic action must be regarded as being the union of the toxin by means of its haptophore group to a special side-chain of the cell protoplasm. This union is . . . a firm and enduring one. The side-chain involved, so long as the union lasts, cannot exercise its normal, physiological, nutritive function—the taking up of definite food-stuffs. It is as it were shut out from participating, in the physiological sense, in the life of the cell. We are therefore now concerned with a defect which, according to

the principles so ably worked out by Professor Carl Weigert, is repaired by regeneration. These principles, in fact, constitute the leading conception in my theory. If, after union has taken place, new quantities of toxin are administered at suitable intervals and in suitable quantities, the side-chains which have been reproduced by the regenerative process are, in turn, taken up into union with the toxin, and so again the process of regeneration gives rise to the formation of fresh side-chains. In the course of the progress of typical systematic immunization . . . the cells become, so to say, educated or trained to reproduce the necessary side-chains in ever-increasing quantity. As Weigert has confirmed by many examples, this, however, does not take place as a simple replacement of the defect; the compensation proceeds far beyond the necessary limit; indeed, overcompensation is the rule. Thus the lasting and everincreasing regeneration must finally reach a state at which such an excess of side-chains is produced that, to use a trivial expression, the side-chains are present in too great a quantity for the cell to carry, and are, after the manner of a secretion, handed over, as superfluous ballast, to the blood.

Regarded in accordance with this conception, the antitoxins represent nothing more than the sidechains, reproduced in excess during regeneration and therefore pushed off from the protoplasm—thus coming to exist in a free state. With this explanation the phenomena of antitoxin formation lose all their strange, one might say miraculous, characters. I have deemed it advisable to represent, by means of some purely arbitrary diagrams, the views I have expressed regarding the relations of the cell considered in the manner I have been describing. Needless to say, these diagrams must be regarded, quite apart from all morphological consideration, as being merely a pictorial method of presenting my views on cellular metabolism, and the method of toxin action and antitoxin formation during the process of immunization. . . .

Comparative pathology of inflammation

1892 • Elie Metchnikoff

Comment

"Self-nonself" recognition is a property of cellular immune responses, and antibody formation is an auxiliary mechanism. Such views in 1890 would likely receive a stinging rebuttal from the humoral immunological community, which would reverse the order. The protest, however, would be unwarranted, as any earthworm would vouch were it able. Earthworms? Edwin Cooper presented an utterly astonishing work on transplantation of epidermidis among annelids, creatures lacking antibodies but quite able to cast off grafts from worms of the same species. They could even manifest enhanced and accelerated tissue rejection with a repeated grafting of tissue from worms of different species. The reception of these investigations was enchantment, even for those expressing incredulity. Having constantly examined immunology from the anthropocentric standpoint, researchers first regarded Cooper's data and photographs as totally new, when in fact their scientific foundation was as old as the science itself. It had the stamp of Metchnikoff.

Inflammation was once regarded as a harmful or disease process, not a normal protective response. The associated heat, pain, and discomfort might cause an affected person to agree. However, Elie Metchnikoff placed the process in its correct biological position by a careful series of phylogenic studies establishing its origin and evolutionary development. Immunity and inflammation came together or, from the reverse perspective, originated with the mesodermal phagocyte. However immune mechanisms may vary among orders and phyla, the phagocyte is the common denominator. Indeed, aside from the controversial and limited antitoxins, these cells were the only general immune mechanism known when Metchnikoff presented his lectures summarizing the research from his and other laboratories. Through its positive and negative chemotaxis and its digestive granules, be it of sponge, frog, or rodent, the phagocyte was described as an active destroyer of living invaders, all obeying the evolutional laws of variation and natural selection. All other subsequently developed inflammatory activities of tissues were quasi-independent adjuncts.

Metchnikoff returned from the August 1890 meeting of the International Congress of Medicine in Berlin unshaken by the reports on specific bactericidal serum. The challenge of the December 1890 reports on serum antitoxins, however, needed a reply. (He first discounted their significance in vivo, since tetanus and diphtheria do not produce serous exudates.) To solidify his position and educate others in his zoological approach, Metchnikoff published his well-received lectures as a book, from which the following milestone is excerpted. The focus was on inflammation. A full treatment of the phagocyte theory, a treatise of 600 pages, appeared in 1901: *Immunity in Infective Diseases.*

The phagocyte theory of immunity is appropriately linked with Metchnikoff, but he was not alone in thinking along these lines. For instance, as early as 1874, the epidemiologist Peter L. Panum suggested the protection afforded by white blood cells that could ingest bacteria. The American pioneer bacteriologist General George M. Sternberg issued by far the most specific theory of the forerunners, making some preliminary and highly speculative opinions in 1881, and publishing a fine synopsis, worthy of Metchnikoff himself, in 1884. No other scientist, however, developed his conceptions as extensively nor defended them as vigorously as Metchnikoff, who, however, never sought credit of priority. These earlier reports indicate that Metchnikoff's theory was not as radical as his critics implied.

Today, comparative immunology is continuing its contribution to our understanding of immunity and of the biochemical recognition of "self." The development of immune mechanisms, like most other biological systems, did not evolve in a straight line, and can not be properly examined in isolation from the anatomy and physiology—indeed the life—of the organism. Existent animals are but the blossoms of the phylogenetic tree; their ancestors are not available. Cells of the most primitive metazoans have the capacity of recognition and the ability to segregate in mixtures. Specific cellular immunity, as manifested by graft rejection, appears in its crudest form with the hydra. Lower animals may possess inducible humoral opsonins, agglutinins, lysins, or bactericidins, but they are nonspecific. When immunoglobulins first arose with the evolution of the vertebrates, they were probably of the IgM type, as suggested by its lone existence in hagfish, a very primitive fish. It is interesting, indeed a phylogenic recapitulation, that humans produce IgM before IgG when first encountering a given antigen. The antigen receptor on the surface of the hagfish lymphocyte is monomeric IgM. Hagfish also have T cells, but they lack the typical vertebrate thymus.

In his last lecture Metchnikoff completed his survey by considering immunity in humans. Seeing the concomitant and united evolution of all biological components of the organism, and with bold, sure mental brush strokes as in Zen calligraphy and painting, Metchnikoff merged immunity, neurons, and consciousness 35 years before his student Serge Metalnikov (see Part 9). Metchnikoff regarded the phagocyte as akin to a protist, the most rudimentary organismal mind-system, the anchor that leads across the aeons to the consciousness-mind of humans. He, therefore, accepted mind and consciousness as matter-dependent and emer-

gent. For Metchnikoff, the evolutionary path of immunity spans from the phagocyte, the most primitive mechanism, to human-created applied medical science, the most advanced.

For further information:

Bibel, D. J. 1982. Sternberg, Metchnikoff, and the phagocytes. *Military Medicine* 147:550–553.

Cooper, E. L. (editor). 1974. *Invertebrate Immunology (Contemporary Topics in Immunobiology. Vol. 4.* Plenum Press, New York. 299 p.

Cooper, E. L. 1976. *Comparative Immunology.* Prentice-Hall, Englewood Cliffs, NJ. 338 p.

Manning, M. J. and R. J. Turner. 1976. *Comparative Immunobiology.* Blackie & Son, Glasgow. 184 p.

Metchnikoff, E. 1905. *Immunity in Infective Diseases* (F. G. Binnie, translator). Cambridge University Press, Cambridge. 591 p.

The Paper*

As the comparative anatomy of former times treated only of man and the higher animals, so medicine has hitherto excluded all the pathological phenomena which occur in the lower animals. And yet the study of these animals, affording as they do infinitely simpler and more primitive conditions that those in man and vertebrata, really furnishes the key to the comprehension of the complex pathological phenomena which are of special interest in medical science.

If we examine the processes of inflammation from this point of view, we shall be able to form a more complete and definite idea of their real significance. . . .

Inflammation makes its appearance only in the animal kingdom and undergoes a slow evolution, which begins in the organisms that have a mesoderm. At first it cannot be distinguished from a simple intracellular digestion, effected by amoeboid and

*Metchnikoff, E. 1892. *Lecons sur la Pathologie Comparée de l'Inflammation Faites à l'Institute Pasteur en Avril et Mai 1891.* Masson, Paris. 239 p. (English translation by F. A. Starling and E. H. Starling. *Lectures on the Comparative Pathology of Inflammation.* Kegan Paul, Trench, Trübner & Co., London, 1893. 218 p.; Dover, 1968). [With permission of Dover.]

phagocytic cells of the mesoderm. Thus in the Sponges the digestive and the inflammatory functions are still united; but as soon as the endoderm becomes definitely separated from the mesoderm, the two functions diverge. The endoderm now acts exclusively as a digestive organ, while the mesoderm alone retains the power of protecting the organism against injurious agents by digesting them when possible. The mesodermic phagocytes preserve their property of intracellular digestion; this they effect either by fusing into plasmodia or by collecting to form capsules around the parasites or other foreign bodies. The phagocytic reaction is displayed by all the mesodermic phagocytes. In this process the prominent part is played in some cases by the connective tissue cells, in others by the perivisceral fluid or of the blood. In all these cases it is the phagocytes which war against the aggressor by devouring, englobing and digesting it.

It is apparent that the inflammation of vertebrates, in which the defending phagocytes emigrate from the vessels to proceed against offending bodies, is distinguished only quantitatively from the analogous phenomena in invertebrates and must therefore be also regarded as a reaction of the organism against deleterious agents. We must conclude that the essential originating factor, the primum movens of inflammation consists in a phagocytic reaction on the part of the animal organism. All the other phenomena are merely accessory to this process, and may be regarded as means to facilitate the access of phagocytes to the injured part.

The morbid phenomena properly speaking, such as the primary lesion or necrosis, as well as the processes of repair, do not form part of the inflammation and must not be confounded with it. . . .

Leucocytes which, by virtue of their chemiotaxis, are attracted at a distance by microbes and other particles, move towards these bodies and on coming in contact with them englobe them owing to their tactile sensibility. The ingested particles are now acted on by the leucocyte. It is an old observation that red corpuscles, when enclosed by leucocytes, partially dissolve, leaving a pigmented residue. It is also very easy to follow the changes undergone by pus-corpuscles in the interior of leucocytes, where they gradually lose their staining power and are finally converted into scattered granules which are partially dissolved. These changes are carried out by the protoplasm of the leucocytes, and must be looked upon as an act of intracellular digestion. This view is justified by the discovery of ferments in leucocytes. . . .

It is easy to follow the digestion of many other microbes within the leucocytes. Vacuoles are often seen to form around the bacteria that have been swallowed, just as we have noticed in the digestion of nutrient material by the protoplasm of the Protozoa and the Myxomycetes. . . . We are at present ignorant of the precise manner in which this digestive and destructive action is accomplished, and do not even know whether the substance which kills the microbes is a ferment or not. The fact that the ferments of the higher animals, such as pepsin and trypsin, do not kill bacteria, is no reason for assuming that there may not be other ferments which are capable of exercising a bactericidal action. . . .

It is undeniable then that leucocytes possess digestive power, and that in particular they are able to digest microbes. But it does not therefore necessarily follow that these cells kill and digest all the microbes they englobe. In certain diseases the leucocytes take in a number of bacteria, such as tubercle bacilli or the bacilli of swine erysipelas or mouse septicemia, a few of which may be digested while the others resist the digestive action of the leucocytes, multiply in the cells and finally invade the whole organism. . . .

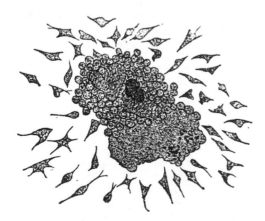

Figure 32 Collection of phagocytes round a splinter. *Bipinnaria asterigera.*

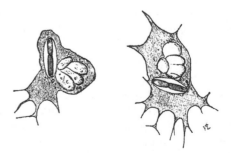

Figure 54 An anthrax bacillus stained by vesuvine, in a leucocyte of the frog. The two figures represent two phases of movement of the same cell.

I need not insist at length on the fact that the migration of the leucocytes through the vascular wall is due to their own active movements. In spite of all Cohnheim's endeavors, in spite of the general desire to refer all vital phenomena to mechanical causes, the view that the emigration is effected by the amoeboid power of the leucocytes has now found almost unanimous acceptance. This fact must strike anyone who compares the ease with which leucocytes transverse the vascular wall with the purely passive diapedesis of the red blood-corpuscles. . . .

In the very act of the passage of the leucocytes through the vessel-wall, a certain chemiotactic or physiotactic influence is manifested. . . .

The study of inflammation from the point of view of comparative pathology proves first of all that this phenomen is essentially reactive in its nature. The organism, threatened by some injurious agency, protects itself by the means at its disposal. Since, as we have seen, even the lowest organism, instead of passively submitting to the attacks of morbid agents, struggle against them, why should not the more highly developed organisms, such as man and mammals, act in the same manner? We must conclude then that the invaded organism fights against the injurious cause, but in what way? As the evolution of inflammation shows, it is this phenomenon itself which is both the most general and the most active means of defense among the members of the animal kingdom. . . .

All these cases of intravascular inflammation without diapedesis, as well as the inflammatory phenomena in the young larvae of Axololotls and Tritons (where it is the migratory cells that collect at the seat of injury), in fact the whole series of reactive phenomena in so many of the invertebrates, prove clearly that the essential and primary element in typical inflammation consists in a reaction of the phagocytes against a harmful agent. If the latter be in the general body-cavity, which is filled with blood, the phagocytes will collect here; if in the interior of the vessels, as in recurrent fever or in intravascular tuberculosis, the phagocytes will assemble in the blood itself; if on the contrary the injurious agent is outside the body-cavity or outside the vessels, the phagocytes will emigrate towards the threatened spot—an emigration without diapedesis in the invertebrata and young larvae of Urodela, or with diapedesis in the vertebrata. . . .

There is one more form of sensibility that we must mention, namely that of the nervous system, which aids the phagocytic and vascular mechanism in their reaction against deleterious agents. . . .

It has been often thought that the leucocytes which are gathered together in an inflamed area may only serve to effect the absorption of dead cells and microbes, and they have been looked upon as simple "scavengers" of the organism. We have already seen that this hypothesis is not justified by facts. . . .

In mammals the real "scavengers," that is to say the phagocytes which carry out the work of absorption, are the macrophages, especially the mononuclear leucocytes. The latter cells play an important part chiefly in the chronic inflammations, such as tuberculosis, while in the acute inflammations it is mainly the microphages, or neutrophile polynuclear leucocytes, that are involved. . . .

This biological theory has often been considered too vitalistic in its tendency. . . . The sensibility of the phagocytes is not a hypothesis that can be admitted or rejected at will, but an established fact, which cannot be ignored. . . . Whether they possess powers of thought and volition . . . is quite beside the question, though we are justified in considering that they possess a germ of these qualities and that their sensibility, like that of various vegetable and animal unicellular organisms represents the lowest stage in the long series of phenomena which culminate in the psychical activities of man. . . .

It is equally erroneous to attribute a teleological character to the theory that inflammation is a reaction of the organism against injurious agencies. This theory is based on the law of evolution according to which the properties that are useful to the organism survive while those which are harmful are eliminated by natural selection. . . .

But the curative force of nature, the most important element of which is the inflammatory reaction, is not yet perfectly adapted to its object. The frequency of disease and the instances of premature death are a sufficient proof of this. The phagocytic mechanism has not yet reached its highest stage of development and is still undergoing improvement. In too many cases the phagocytes flee before the enemy or destroy the cells of the body to which they belong. It is this imperfection in the curative forces of nature which has necessitated the active intervention of man.

The defense of the organism against deleterious agencies, which is at first confined to the phagocytic mechanisms and the somatic system of nerves, by and by spreads to and is undertaken by the psychical nervous apparatus. With the nervous cells which direct the contraction and dilatation of the vessels become associated other cells which control thought and voluntary actions. One function of these psychical cells has been to develop a complete science for the defense of the organism against hostile influences. By its means, methods for assisting the curative inflammation have been devised. . . . The application of agents which set up inflammation . . . is the conscious continuation of the defensive measures which have been unconsciously evolved by the long series of animals in their struggle for existence. . . .

An experimental investigation of the role of the blood fluids in connection with phagocytosis

1903 • Sir Almroth E. Wright and Stewart R. Douglas

Comment

The grand polemic of rival immunological theories (humoral versus cellular) collapsed after fifteen years, almost as much from the fatigue of its combatants as the weight of some experimental evidence. Humoral agents were conceded to be products of some unknown immunological cells, perhaps including macrophages, and whether microbial killing was intra- or extracellular became a minor controversy. In 1903 Elie Metchnikoff had already published his book summarizing his researches, and now was taking on bacteriological studies, particularly animal models and the therapy of syphilis. Few were willing to pick up the cellular sword; the exciting immunological research was with precipitins, agglutinins, and complement. Although differences in opinion, of course, remained, there was no lingering rancor. The English translation of Metchnikoff's masterwork was being prepared with the help of George H. F. Nuttall, who, as noted earlier (see Part 5/Nuttall, 1888), was among the first to dispute the phagocyte theory. Furthermore, Metchnikoff and Emil von Behring had become friends, and five years later Metchnikoff and Paul Ehrlich would share the Nobel Prize for their immunological advances. As if to finally and fully intertwine or consolidate the opposing theories, Sir Almroth Wright and Captain Stewart R. Douglas (1871–1936) introduced the opsonic model.

"Opsonin is what you butter the disease germs with to make your white blood corpuscles eat them," wrote George Bernard Shaw in 1906 in his satirical play on medical practices, *The Doctor's Dilemma,* based on Wright and his work. Shaw and Wright were cordial friends, whose relationship survived on wit, love of language, lively creativity, and wholly divergent opinions on almost everything. They were sparring partners. Shaw never understood immunology and the opsonic method, thinking that a person's immunological state is cyclic. (There is some truth to this, but not to the degree that Shaw imagined.) According to the confused dramatist, an immunization given in the negative phase may be harmful. Such an incident occurs in the play, and when this point was reached, Wright, who attended the opening performance, walked out in disgust.

Wright, who displayed a photograph of Metchnikoff in his laboratory and who included Ehrlich among his close friends, agreed that phagocytes, with rare exception, are necessary to destroy invasive bacteria. He also knew that specific humoral globulins react against these same microorganisms. In examining the two components separately and together, using his famous capillary tube techniques, he discovered the existence of opsonins. These humoral substances facilitate the ingestion of bacteria by the white cells. The initial report of his series of investigations on this phenomenon is the next milestone.

Wright had asked Stewart Douglas, who was commissioned in the Indian Medical Service in 1896, to join him at St. Mary's Hospital in London. They had met at the Army Medical School at Netley and later in India, when Wright was a member of a plague commission. Douglas continued as a distinguished researcher at Wright's laboratory until 1920, when he became Director of the Department of Bacteriology and Experimental Pathology of the Medical Research Council. Ten years later he rose to Deputy Director of the National Institute for Medical Research at Hampstead. He was elected Fellow of the Royal Society in 1922.

Wright and Douglas assumed incorrectly that phagocytes are equally active in normal and ill patients. This flaw, plus the awkward technology they used, thwarted the acceptance of the diagnostic and prognostic opsonic index of serum, a measurement of phagocytosis standardized to a "normal" person. Nevertheless, it was clear that phagocytes and humoral factors did cooperate. Wright and Douglas's milestone contained several ambiguities, since they believed that they were dealing with a single entity. Opsonins, however, are of two independent varieties: specific, thermostable immunoglobulins and nonspecific, thermolabile complement protein. The specific human opsonins are chiefly IgG subclasses 1 and 3; their Fab hapten receptors bind the bacterium and their Fc portion adheres to the receptor on the macrophage membrane. For instance, the pneumococcus, which resists phagocytosis in nonimmune subjects, is engulfed after interaction with anti-capsular antibodies. The complement component, which is generally present in normal as well as immune sera, is C3b. Proteases of bacterial or host origin split this substance from C3. The complement agent also serves as a bridge, being affixed to the bacterium's membrane and to the C3b receptors on the macrophage. Metchnikoff's macrophage, a versatile cell, is one of the host sources of opsonin precursor C3. The antibody opsonins are more effective than the complement product; however, taken together, which is the normal situation, they act synergistically.

Wright's hopeful role as mediator between the rival cellular and humoral camps was a lost cause. Opsonins did demonstrate that cell and humoral agent were integral team members, but with the continuing research focus on antibodies and complement, immunologists once more regarded the macrophage as a mere scavenger or at best an effete predator. Only with the return of the biological approach, with interest in delayed hypersensitivity and antibody-forming cells, has the macrophage regained fundamental importance. However, the status of this phagocyte is no longer viewed in opposition to antibodies and other humoral immune agents. Instead, the macrophage is now considered a member of the cellular team, including the B lymphocyte and the T cell family (see Part 4/Mitchison, 1970). Rankings and functional distinctions have actually become obsolete, for immunity must be considered as an undivided system. As indicated by Wright and Douglas, cells and their secretions are in the body a natural whole and in the test tube synergistic components.

For further information:

Allen, R. W. 1908. *The Opsonic Method of Treatment. A short compendium for general practitioners, students, and others.* P. Blakiston's Son & Company, Philadelphia. 138 p.

Colebrook, L. 1954. *Almroth Wright. Provocative Doctor and Thinker.* William Heinemann. 286 p.

Stossel, T. P. 1974. Phagocytosis. *New England Journal of Medicine* 290:717–723; 774–780; 833–839.

The Paper*

It is still a matter of uncertainty whether the blood fluids perform any role in connection with phagocytosis.

Certain facts suggest that the role of blood fluids, if it comes into consideration at all, is very subordinate. The facts we have in view are, on the one hand, the facts brought forward by Metchnikoff to show that bacteria may be ingested in the living condition, and on the other hand those brought forward by one of us . . . which show that the human serum exerts absolutely no bactericidal action on the staphylococcus pyogenes, the micrococcus Melitensis and the plague bacillus.

These facts are, however, not conclusive. They are not inconsistent with the idea that the blood fluids,

*Wright, A. E. and S. R. Douglas. 1903. An experimental investigation of the role of the blood fluids in connection with phagocytosis. *Proceedings of the Royal Society, London.* Biology. 72:357–370. [With permission of the Society.]

apart from actually killing the particular pathogenic bacteria here in question, may in some way co-operate in their destruction.

What are required for the resolution of the problem are experiments in which the phagocytes are tested apart from the blood fluids.

The experimental methods which we now pass on to describe enable these crucial experiments to be made. . . .

In the procedure described by [W. B. Leishman] equal volumes of a bacterial suspension of appropriate density and of blood drawn from the finger are measured off in a capillary tube, mixed on a slide and covered in with a cover-glass. The blood and bacterial culture are then left in contact for fifteen minutes in an incubator standing at bloodheat. After this interval the cover-glass is, if necessary, loosened from the side by a drop of physiological salt solution, and the slide and cover-glass are drawn apart by a sliding movement.

The films thus obtained are stained by Leishman's modification of Romanovski's stain, and are subjected to examination under an immersion lens. By enumerating the bacteria ingested in a number of polynuclear white blood corpuscles and dividing, an average is obtained. This average is taken as the measure of the phagocytic power of the blood. It is compared, when comparative experiments are made, with the phagocytic power of a normal blood.

We have modified this method for our purposes (a) by conducting the phagocytosis in capillary tubes, making afterwards film preparations in the ordinary way; (b) by decalcifying the blood with citrate of soda, thus avoiding the complications introduced by blood coagulation, and making it possible to separate the white corpuscles from the blood fluids by centrifugation, decantation and washing.

Three different procedures, varying only in details, were employed in our experiments.

Procedure No. 1, employed where nothing more than a comparison between bloods from different sources or blood subjected to different conditions is required. . . .

Procedure No. 2, where we desire to elicit separately the role of the white corpuscles and the blood fluids in phagocytosis, and to study the effect produced by experimental modification of one or other of these elements separately. . . .

Procedure No. 3, employed where we desire to obtain citrated serum for comparison with the citrated plasma furnished by Procedure No. 2. . . .

These experiments show that we must ascribe an important role to the blood fluids in connection with phagocytosis.

For the alternative assumption, the supposition, to wit, that inhibiting elements are developed in the serum during the process of heating, is rebutted by the results of a series of control experiments, which showed that the phagocytes display no greater activity in a medium of physiological salt solution than in a medium of heated serum.

It is further rebutted by the circumstance that the activity of phagocytosis falls off at the same rate when the unheated serum is diluted with salt solution as when it is diluted with heated serum. . . .

Do the Blood Fluids co-operate in Phagocytosis by exerting a Direct Stimulating Effect upon the Phagocytes, or by effecting a Modification in the Bacteria?

The following experiments were instituted with a view to elucidating the problem as to the nature of the activating influence exercised by the blood fluids. It will be seen that a comparison is in each case instituted between serum inactivated (by heating) before it came in contact with either bacteria or white corpuscles, and serum inactivated after it had come in contact with the bacteria, but before it had come in contact with the white corpuscles. . . .

We have here conclusive proof that the blood fluids modify the bacteria in a manner which renders them a ready prey to the phagocytes.

We may speak of this as an "opsonic" effect (opsono—I cater for; I prepare victuals for), and we may employ the term "opsonins" to designate the elements in the blood fluids which produce this effect.

Does the Unheated Serum contain, in addition to Elements which render the Bacteria more liable to Phagocytosis (Opsonins), also Elements which directly stimulate the Phagocytes (Stimulins)?

We have sought to elucidate this question by three separate methods.

In the first series of experiments, we experimented with staphylococci which had been exposed to high temperatures (115°C) with the design of rendering them insusceptible to the opsonic power of the blood fuids. Our expectations from this method—expectations based on the fact that we had noticed that typhoid bacilli acquired, when heated to over 70°C, a resistance to the bacteriolytic effect of the blood fluids—were unrealized. We found that the quantitative difference between the phagocytosis in heated and unheated serum respectively were not less in the case of staphylococci which had been exposed to the temperature of 115°C, than in the case of staphylococci which had not been subjected to high temperatures.

In a second series of experiments we substituted for suspensions of staphylococci suspensions of particles, which we assumed would be uninfluenced by the opsonic power of the blood. The results of these experiments, conducted both with carmine particles and with Indian ink, were inconclusive by reasons of the circumstance that we were not able to obtain any satisfactory enumerations. An impression was, however, left on our minds that phagocytosis was in every case more active in unheated than in the heated serum.

A third method of experimentation was then resorted to. In a first operation we mixed and digested together at blood heat a suspension of staphylococci and unheated serum. After allowing what we supposed would be a sufficient interval for the exhaustion of the effect of the serum upon the bacteria, we divided the mixture into two portions. While the first of these portions was mixed with corpuscles without undergoing any further treatment, the other was heated to 60°C, and cooled before it was so mixed. In each case the phago-cytic power exerted was greater in the case where the heating was omitted, and the differences were not less marked where the serum had been digested with the bacteria for fifty minutes and one hour respectively than in the case where it had been digested with these only for fifteen minutes.

These results are ambiguous. . . .

In conclusion we would briefly refer to the following points:

The opsonic power of the blood fluids disappears gradually on standing, even when the serum is kept in a sealed capsule sheltered from the light.

After five or six days we have found the opsonic power of the serum kept under these conditions to stand at little more than half of what it was originally.

The opsonic power of the blood fluids is but little impaired by the action of heat until temperatures above 50°C are arrived at. . . .

The opsonic power of the blood fluids is diminished while the phagocytic capacity of the W.B.C. is preserved when the blood fluids and corpuscles are separately digested with Daboia venom. . . .

Lastly, a fact which has a practical importance in connection with the study of immunity may be adverted to. It will be manifest that we have not exhausted a study of a condition of immunity when we have measured the phagocytic power of the white corpuscles, and the agglutinating, bacteriolytic, and bactericidal power of the blood fluids. We must, in connection with these last, take into consideration also the opsonic effect. . . .

A theory of the structure and process of formation of antibodies

1940 • Linus Pauling

Comment

Linus Pauling (1901–   ) turned his speculative eye to immunology in 1940. Whatever field he entered, be it chemistry, international politics, or preventive medicine, whether he was eventually proved on target or amiss, Pauling put on an exciting good show. He brought quantum mechanics to chemistry (1931), and discovered the alpha helix of proteins (1948). He determined that sickle cell anemia results from a defect in hemoglobin (1949). Pauling also spearheaded the campaign to stop atmospheric testing of atomic weapons. He received the Nobel Prize in chemistry (1954) and the Nobel Peace Prize (1963). In the instance of his theory on antibody formation, however, the conception was brilliant, but totally wrong.

Why then is his proposal considered a milestone? No single reason suffices. It was the first truly modern development of the problem; no other available alternative could match it. It was the virtual limit to an approach begun thirty years earlier. It held reign for some twenty years, despite its many recognized flaws. It was the first attempt to understand the tertiary protein configuration of antigen receptors.

Pauling entered the scientific path at age eight. His father, a pharmacist, did not influence him, but in short order Pauling read all his father's books and manuals and organized a home chemical laboratory. At 15, he entered Oregon State Agricultural College with the goal of becoming a chemical engineer. He soon set his sights on more theoretical subjects. After graduation in 1922, he began work on his Ph.D. at the California Institute of Technology, studying the molecular structure of crystals. His dissertation in 1925 was a fusion of his already published researches. In 1926 Pauling received a Gugenheim fellowship to visit the laboratories of Max Born, Werner Heisenberg, and Niels Bohr to soak in the wonderful weirdness of quantum theory. He also met Robert Oppenheimer. On his return in 1928 to the California Institute of Technology, Pauling became Assistant Professor of Chemistry, and soon tackled the problem of atomic configurations in molecules. He borrowed quantum concepts to develop the model of resonance, postulating that atoms share electrons. In 1931 he wrote a book called *The Nature of the Chemical Bond;* it shook the foundation of chemistry. He soon was engaged with studies on the architecture of molecules, developing the famous three-dimensional, electron space-filling, atomic "tinker toy" models. Crystallography, development of line spectral analysis, and binding of ions would have taken him to mineralogy, but instead he found himself within biochemistry. As Pauling observed, granting agencies can influence the progress of science. The Rockefeller Foundation with its biomedical bent came to the rescue when the Geological Society of America denied a grant request.

Politics also can regulate science. A nation barring a scientist from leaving to attend a conference or receive an international award is engaging in a crime against humanity. Hitler forced Gerhard Domagk to decline the Nobel Prize for the discovery of sulfa antimicrobial drugs. The Soviet Union prevented Andrei Sakharov from collecting his Nobel, and, indeed, segregated him from any scientific contact for many years. The United States between 1952 and 1954, the era of Senator Joseph McCarthy, prevented Pauling from leaving the country.

Whether he could have beat James Watson and Francis Crick in determining the three-dimensional structure of DNA is moot; when the Department of State withdrew Pauling's passport, he could not attend a critical conference in London, and thus was unable to inspect Rosalind Franklin's x-ray diffraction photographs of DNA. This handicap effectively put him out of the race. Pauling also would not have been able to receive his Nobel Prize were it not for a last moment policy reevaluation by the State Department, which issued his temporary passport two weeks before the award ceremonies. What had Pauling done to deserve this treatment? He advocated, along with Albert Einstein and notable others, the elimination of atmospheric testing of nuclear weapons to prevent radioactive fallout.

In 1964 Pauling resigned his professorship at the California Institute of Technology for successive positions at the Center for the Study of Democratic Institutions, University of California at San Diego, and Stanford University. In 1969 he helped found the Linus Pauling Institute of Science and Medicine, where he turned to prophylaxis of viral and oncogenic diseases with large doses of vitamins, particularly vitamin C.

Pauling's interest in the antibody began after a meeting with Karl Landsteiner at the Rockefeller Institute in 1936. The extraordinary number of specific antibodies, including those against artificial antigens, defied the genetic origin originally propounded by Paul Ehrlich. A somatic, custom-made template mechanism seemed more logical. The idea first came to Oskar Bail in 1909, who tried to synthesize antibody molecules in vitro. Between 1930 and 1932 Felix Haurowitz; W. W. C. Topley; Stuart Mudd; and Jerome Alexander all proposed variations of the direct template model. Their concepts were well outlined, but the actual means by which the polypeptide structure of the antibody molded itself around the antigen was obscure. Pauling, the authority on bonding and molecular structure, provided the answer through folding and coiling a preformed, presumably undifferentiated immunoprotein chain stabilized by hydrogen bonds. Cells were ignored.

Pauling's model required the antibody chain to fold over the antigen at different locations, hence at different haptenic groups; however, precipitation data indicated that the receptors of each antibody had the same specificity. None of the template theories could explain the secondary or booster reaction, nor the continuing occurrence of antibody production in absence of antigen. Of course, the unique sequences of amino acids in proteins were unknown, as was its code in the nucleic acids. Contemplating the nature of antibody in the absence of genetic mechanisms was as if wearing a blindfold.

For further information:

Bendiner, E. 1983. The passions and perils of Pauling. *Hospital Practice* April:210–243 [with interruptions].

Pauling, L. 1946. Molecular structure and intermolecular forces. In: *The Specificity of Serological Reactions*. Revised edition (K. Landsteiner). Harvard University Press, Cambridge. pp. 275–293.

The Paper*

During the past four years I have been making an effort to understand and interpret serological phenomena in terms of molecular structure and molecular interactions. The field of immunology is so extensive and the experimental observations are so complex (and occasionally contradictory) that no one has found it possible to induce a theory of the structure of antibodies from the observational material. As an alternative method of attack we may propound and attempt to answer the following questions: What is the simplest structure which can be suggested, on the basis of the extensive information now available about intramolecular and intermolecular forces, for

*Pauling, L. 1940. A theory of the structure and process of formation of antibodies. *Journal of the American Chemical Society* 62:2643–2657. [Reprinted with permission; copyright 1940 American Chemical Society.]

a molecule with the properties observed for antibodies, and what is the simplest reasonable process of formation of such a molecule? Proceeding in this way, I have developed a detailed theory of the structure and process of formation of antibodies and the nature of serological reactions which is more definite and more widely applicable than earlier theories, and which is compatible with our present knowledge of the structure and properties of simple molecules as well as with most of the direct empirical information about antibodies. This theory is described and discussed below.

When an antigen is injected into an animal some of its molecules are captured and held in the region of antibody production. An antibody to this antigen is a molecule with a configuration which is complementary to that of a portion of the antigen molecule. This complementariness gives rise to specific forces of appreciable strength between the antibody molecule and the antigen molecules; we may describe this as a bond between the two molecules. I assume, with Marrack, Heidelberger, and other investigators, that the precipitate obtained in the precipitin reaction is a framework, and that to be effective in forming the framework an antibody molecule must have two or more distinct regions with surface configuration complementary to that of the antigen. The rule of parsimony (the use of the minimum effort to achieve the result) suggests that there are only two such regions, that is, that the antibody molecules are at the most bivalent. The proposed theory is based on this reasonable assumption. It would, of course, be possible to expand the theory in such a way as to provide a mechanism for the formation of antibody molecules with valence higher than two; but this would make the theory considerably more complex, and it is likely that antibodies with valence higher than two occur only rarely, if at all. . . .

The effect of an antigen in determining the structure of an antibody molecule might involve the order of the amino-acid residues in the polypeptide chains in a way different from that in the normal globulin, as suggested by Breinl and Haurowitz and Mudd. I assume, however, that this is not so, but that all antibody molecules contain the same polypeptide chains as normal globulin, and differ from normal globulin only in the configuration of the chain; that is, in the way that the chain is coiled in the molecule. There is at present no direct evidence supporting this assumption. The assumption is made because, although I have found it impossible to formulate in detail a reasonable mechanism whereby the order of amino-acid residues in the chain would be determined by the antigen, a simple and reasonable mechanism, described below, can be advanced whereby the antigen causes the polypeptide chain to assume a configuration complementary to the antigen. The number of configurations accessible to the polypeptide chain is so great as to provide an explanation of the ability of an animal to form antibodies with considerable specificity for an apparently unlimited number of different antigens, without the necessity of involving also a variation in the amino-acid composition or amino-acid order.

Let us assume that the globulin molecule consists of a single polypeptide chain, containing several hundred amino-acid residues, and that the order of the amino-acid residues is such that for the center of the chain one of the accessible configurations is much more stable than any other, whereas the two end parts of the chain are of such a nature that there exist for them many configurations with the same energy. Four steps in our postulated process of formation of a normal globulin molecule are illustrated on the left side of Fig. 1. At stage I the polypeptide chain has been synthesized, the amino-acid residues having been marshalled into the proper order, presumably with the aid of polypeptidases and protein templates, and the two ends of the chain, A and C, each containing perhaps two hundred residues, have been liberated with the unstable extended configuration. (The horizontal line in each drawing separates the region, below the line, in which the polypeptide chain is not able to change its configuration from the region, above the line, where this is pos-

sible.) Each of these chain ends then coils up into the most stable or one of the most stable of the accessible configurations (stage II) and is tied into this configuration by the formation of hydrogen bonds and other weak bonds between parts of the chain. The central part B of the chain is then liberated (stage III) and assumes its stable folded configuration (stage IV) to give the completed globulin molecule.

There are also indicated in Fig. 1 six stages in the process of formation of an antibody molecule. In stage I there are shown an antigen molecule held at a place of globulin production and a globulin molecule with its two ends A and C liberated with the extended configuration. At stage II each of the ends has assumed a stable coiled configuration. These stable configurations A′ and C′ are not, however, identical with those A and C assumed in the absence of the antigen. The atoms and groups which form the surface of the antigen will attract certain complementary parts of the globulin chain (a negatively-charged group, for example, attracting a positively-charged group) and repel other parts; as a result of these interactions the configurations A′ and C′ of the chain ends which are stable in the presence of the antigen and which are accordingly assumed in the presence of the antigen will be such that there is attraction between the coiled globulin chain ends and the antigen, due to their complementarity in

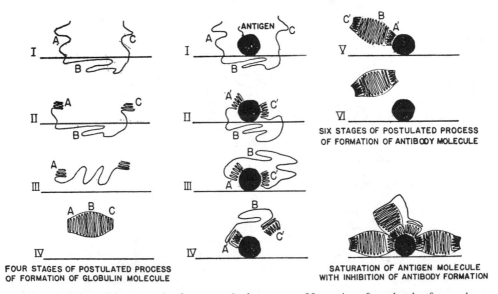

I

II

III

IV

**FOUR STAGES OF POSTULATED PROCESS
OF FORMATION OF GLOBULIN MOLECULE**

I

II

III

IV

V

VI

**SIX STAGES OF POSTULATED PROCESS
OF FORMATION OF ANTIBODY MOLECULE**

**SATURATION OF ANTIGEN MOLECULE
WITH INHIBITION OF ANTIBODY FORMATION**

Figure 1   Diagrams representing four stages in the process of formation of a molecule of normal serum globulin (left side of figure) and six stages in the process of formation of an antibody molecule as the result of interaction of the globulin polypeptide chain with an antigen molecule. There is also shown (lower right) an antigen molecule surrounded by attached antibody molecules or parts of molecules and thus inhibited from further antibody formation.

structure. The configuration assumed by the chain end may be any one of a large number, depending upon which part of the surface of the antigen happens to exert its influence on the chain end and how large a region of the surface happens to be covered by it.

When the central part B of the globulin chain is liberated from the place of its synthesis (stage III), one of two processes may occur. If the forces of attraction between the antigen and the portions A′ and C′ are extremely strong, they will remain bonded to the antigen for an indefinite time, and nothing further of interest will happen. If the forces are somewhat weaker, however, one will in time break away—dissociate from the antigen (stage IV). Then the portion B of the chain will fold up to achieve its normal stable configuration (stage V), making a completed antibody molecule. In time this will dissociate from the antigen and float away (stage VI). It is possible that an auxiliary mechanism for freeing the active ends A′ and C′ from the antigen molecule comes into operation. . . .

The middle part of the antibody molecule thus produced would be like that of a normal globulin molecule, and the two ends would have configurations more or less complementary to parts of the surface of the antigen. These two active ends are effective in different directions, so that, after the antibody is completely formed, only one of them at a time can grasp a particular antigen molecule.

The antigen molecule, after its desertion by the newly formed antibody molecule, may serve as the pattern for another, and continue to serve until its surface is covered by very strongly held antibodies or portions of antibodies or until the concentration of antibodies becomes so great that even with weak forces operating the antigen is combined with antibodies most of the time (as illustrated in Fig. 1), or until the antigen molecule is destroyed or escapes from the region of globulin formation. . . .

The production of antibodies

1949 • Sir Macfarlane Burnet and Frank Fenner

Comment

The template instruction theory of Linus Pauling lacked biological sense, although the model was handsome. Pauling, after all, was foremost a structural chemist, and his immunological knowledge largely came from several intensive sessions with Karl Landsteiner, an immunochemist. Pauling managed some refinements in 1942 in collaboration with a newly arrived professor at the California Institute of Technology, Dan H. Campbell, who had zoological and bacteriological training. Campbell's assistance, however, made little difference; the template theory was a vestige of the humoral school of immunity. It took another biologist to forge the next conceptual advance in understanding the nature of antibody formation. Well grounded first in bacteriology, virology, and infectious disease and then in immunological tolerance, Sir Frank Macfarlane Burnet (1899–1985) helped return the focus of immunity to the cell.

Burnet attended Geelong College and the University of Melbourne (Ormond College) for his undergraduate and medical degrees, the M.D. awarded in 1924. While working as a pathologist at the Royal Melbourne Hospital, an institution that remained the center of his career, he was designated a candidate researcher and administrator of the fledgling clinical research unit, the Walter and Eliza Hall Institute of Medical Research. To gain the necessary skills in bacteriology, he went to London as a research fellow at the Lister Institute, earning his Ph.D. from the University of London in 1928. In 1934 he was appointed Assistant Director and in 1944, Director of the Hall Institute in Melbourne. Between these dates,

Burnet was again in London, at the National Institute for Medical Research as a fellow in virus research. In 1942 he was elected a Fellow of the Royal Society, and in 1960 he shared the Nobel Prize with Sir Peter Medawar for his work in immunological tolerance. Burnet retired in 1965, but continued until his death as Research Fellow in the Department of Bacteriology at the University of Melbourne.

Although a physician, Burnet examined infectious disease from an encompassing ecological perspective. His book, *Biological Aspects of Infectious Disease,* later retitled *Natural History of Infectious Disease,* became a classic with four editions between 1940 and 1972. Burnet's immunological interests began in 1928 with his discovery and study of staphylococcal toxin and the development of antitoxins in the serum of patients. His later discoveries of strain variation among poliomyelitis and influenza viruses, his observations that bacteria and viruses were subject to mutation and selection, and his recognition that a bacteriophage could harmlessly replicate in tandem with the genome of bacteria over generations (lysogeny) provided a genetic background to his holistic thinking.

Elements from this wide experience began to connect. Burnet became fond of weaving diverse phenomena into general theories. In his small monograph of 1941, which reviewed the literature on antibody production, he offered a different scheme of template instruction: The antigen did not directly serve as a mold on which proteins are shaped; it instead impressed itself, through some sort of transformation, onto "adaptive" enzymes, which would then bring the amino acids together into the proper configuration. The concept of adaptive enzyme was the early interpretation of enzyme induction by a substrate, later related to derepression and exposure of the associated gene to messenger RNA. Somewhat Lamarckian, Burnet's theory required the inheritance of this acquired characteristic in progeny. Immunological memory and augmented responses were thus explained.

In 1944, while visiting the United States, Burnet met Pauling. In the ensuing conversations on antibodies, Burnet felt himself a tyro in matters of chemistry, but the immunochemical arguments did not persuade him to change his course. Meanwhile, intriguing developments were occurring in transplantation and in the induction of tolerance. After ruminating on mechanisms of self-nonself recognition, Burnet was ready in 1948 to revise his book on antibody production. He was assisted by Frank Fenner (1914–   ).

A fellow Australian and noted virologist, Fenner attained his degree in medicine from the University of Adelaide in 1938. After military service during and following the World War, he worked at the Hall Institute between 1946 and 1948. He next went to the Rockefeller Institute for training under the guidance of Rene Dubos. Thereafter, he joined the John Curtin School of Medical Research, Australian National University, first as Professor of Microbiology and then in 1967 as its director. Between 1973 and 1979, he served at the Center for Research in Environmental Studies. He continues his association with the Australian National University as a Fellow. In 1958 the Royal Society asked him to join its ranks.

Burnet and Fenner's book, excerpted in the following milestone, is significant more for its introduction of sets of "self markers," which antigenically describe individuality, and for a theoretical approach to tolerance, than for its described mechanism of antibody production. The opus marks the best reasoning prior to the dawn of the DNA paradigm. The adaptive enzyme notion was fading from favor, and the authors now took the instructive signal from the enzyme to the genome. Furthermore, they planted the germ of the selection theory by imprinting antibody specificity at uterine and neonatal stages. The patterns of self-antigens, which were first recognized at this time, would somehow be excluded from the adaptive machinery and maintained upon cellular replication. Nonreactive clones hence would prevent autoimmune reactions and vaguely explain the tolerance of foreign antigens introduced at birth. Burnet ascertained this firsthand. In 1947 he was unable to immunize chicken embryos against influenza virus antigens; these antigens were accepted as indigenous. This tolerance also includes the phenomenon described in 1946 by Ray D. Owen in which fraternal bovine twins, which shared the same placenta, carry each other's erythrocytes along with their own.

Mechanistically, the indirect template theory was admittedly nebulous, current scientific knowledge being simply inadequate to offer any plausible genetic or chemical agency. Its cellular and ontogenetic principles, however, had merit. Burnet and Fenner took immunological theory to the cusp of the new paradigm; later a catalyst from Denmark would drive it to clonal selection.

For further information:

Burnet, F. M. 1969. *Changing Patterns. An Atypical Autobiography.* American Elsevier Publishing Company, New York. 282 p.

Nossal, G. J. V. 1969. Burnet and science—an appreciation. *Australian Annals of Medicine* 4:311–315.

Stephenson, M. 1949. *Bacterial Metabolism.* Third edition. Longman, Green and Company, London. pp. 287–312.

The Paper*

Our own approach to the problem of antibody production is predominantly biological and is based essentially on a consideration of the survival value of immunological reactivity as part of the protective mechanism against infectious disease. . . .

The first step is almost universally regarded as the ingestion by macrophage-type cells of the antigenic particle, which may be either the living or dead microorganism or a product of its secretion or autolysis.

Ingestion and disintegration of microorganisms is not the sole function of reticulo-endothelial cells.

---

*Burnet, F. M. and F. Fenner. 1949. *The Production of Antibodies.* 2nd ed. Macmillan, Melbourne. 142 p.

Equally important is the part they play in dealing with effete or damaged body cells, the most important physiological examples of which are the taking up of red cells by the macrophages of the spleen and the phagocytosis of lymphocytic nuclei in the germinal centers of lymph nodes. . . . The failure of antibody production against autologous cells demands the postulation of an active ability of the reticulo-endothelial cells to recognize "self" pattern from "not-self" pattern in organic material taken into their substanace. The first requirement of an adequate theory of antibody production is to account for this differentiation of function by which the natural entry of foreign microorganisms or the artificial injection of foreign red cells provokes an immunological reaction while the physically similar autologous material is inert.

Any interpretation of antibody production along biological lines must consist essentially of a demonstration of analogies with biological phenomena in other fields. . . . Antibody production represents a change in physiological response induced by a chemical stimulus. We have given cogent evidence that the changed capacity to respond is transmitted to cells descended from those in which it was induced. There is not the slightest evidence of chromosomal inheritance of acquired immunity. The fields in biology then, in which useful analogy may be sought, are those similarly concerned with circumstances in which a chemical stimulus can permanently or semi-permanently modify the reactivity of a cell and its descendants. The formation of adaptive enzymes by microorganisms and the processes of embryonic differentiation as controlled by organizers immediately comes to mind. . . .

It is important not to press the analogy with known adaptive enzymes too closely. . . . If according to current usage one confines the term enzyme to the agent responsible for some chemically defined action on a particular aspect of the substrate molecule, it is inappropriate to refer to the postulated changes initiating antibody production as the formation of an adaptive enzyme. . . . It may well prove more correct to suggest that what we are considering is a reorganization within the cell of a rather complex mechanism which functions as a preliminary to a series of enzymic actions on the antigen substrate. . . . The essence of our hypothesis is that, irrespective of whether it is legitimate or not to call it an adaptive enzyme, a new self-replicating system is now present in the cell which can be caused to multiply by the appropriate stimulus. From the nature of the phenomenon of the accelerated secondary response to an antigen it seems highly probable that the function of first antigenic contact is to produce the adaptive modification while subsequent contacts stimulate its replication and the eventual liberation of partial replicas into the blood stream. The hypothesis also demands that when cells carrying the adaptive enzyme multiply, the descendant cells will also carry the new character. . . .

Circulating antibody of the classical type, i.e., antibody responsible for in vitro aggregation reactions with appropriate antigenic molecules or particles, is regarded as a partial replica of the intracellular enzymic system in the sense of carrying the specifically modified adsorptive pattern of the enzyme but lacking both enzymic activity as such and also the capacity to replicate itself. . . .

The macrophages are responsible for taking up the antigenic molecules or particles and in them the initial stages of antibody production take place. The plasma cell is a cell in which rapid production of antibody (or possibly in some circumstances, nonspecific or pathological) globulin is taking place. . . .

[W]e feel that the lymphocyte's part may be to maintain the slow liberation of antibody that goes on for years after the antigenic stimulus has ceased. If we take a lymph node subjected to an intense antigenic stimulus so that virtually all macrophages lining sinuses take up the antigenic particles, our interpretation would picture the transfer of a potential antibody-producing stimulus from such macrophages to most or all of the stem cells in the node. Many of these would proliferate and develop toward plasma cells from which most of the acutely produced antibody would derive. Others would give rise to lymphocytes in which cytoplasmic activity was much less marked. Still others would remain quiescent or give rise to cells like themselves. We can conceive no way in which antibody-producing power can persist far beyond the individual life of the "end-cells" which produce it unless the capacity is in some way implanted in the mother cell type from which the expendable cells are descended. . . .

In the first section of this discussion the importance of a means by which the same functional system of cells could react in two sharply different ways toward effete and damaged body constituents on the one hand and of foreign organic matter on the other was stressed. In a recent review of the relations between immunology and genetics the implications of this necessity were analyzed and the hypothesis put forward that differentiation is based on the existence of a small number of marker components in the expendable body cells. . . . [O]nly a limited number of recognizable components need be postulated. There may be 5 or 10 marker components in a red cell but probably not many more. . . . It is our contention that the primary units on which antibody production is based are modifications of enzyme systems primarily adapted to specific adsorption to one another of the self-marker components of the body cells. . . .

On general biological ground one would presume that the antigen most effective in antibody production would have a determinant pattern distinctively, but not too distantly, removed from the marker pattern. A very minor difference might not act as a stimulus to adaptation and too remote a resemblance might make adaptation impossible. . . .

It is of considerable interest that fetal mammals and chick embryos are incapable of producing antibody and the full capacity to do so develops only slowly in the young free-living animals. This raises the suggestion that the process by which self-pattern becomes recognizable takes place during the embryonic or immediately post-embryonic stages. The hypothesis of antibody production that we have developed can readily be adapted to such a possibility. Taking the red cells as the typical expendable body cell we may assume that in embryonic life phagocytosis and disintegration of worn out cells is actively taking place. During this phase appropriate intracellular enzyme systems are being adapted to deal effectively with those components which need to be broken down for reintegration into the metabolic activities of the body. . . . An adaptive enzyme specifically uniting with and initiating the destruction of the component is brought into being in the cells that destroy erythrocytes. This newly patterned enzyme becomes stabilized as part of the inheritable structure of these cells and is transmitted indefinitely to their descendants.

With the development of the free-living state this lability of intracellular enzymes is lost, the patterns engraved during embryonic life harden as it were and become permanent possessions. In such a process we have envisaged something essentially similar to the process of antibody production except that the subsequent steps leading to the appearance of free antibody do not occur. . . .

If in embryonic life expendable cells from a genetically distinct race are implanted and established, no antibody response should develop against the foreign cell antigen when the animal takes on independent existence. . . . What is at present a unique natural example of such a circumstance has been described. In the course of detailed studies of blood groups in cattle and their inheritance, Owen and his colleagues studied examples of multiple births in which there had been a common placental circulation although the embryos were of multiovular origin. In these instances the normal segregation of blood group character did not occur. Two calves from the same birth would each show two coexisting serological types of cells when by ordinary genetic rules each should have one only. . . .

It would also be expected that following a generalized non-fatal infection by a pathogenic microorganism of the embryo in utero, the animal after birth would be incapable of responding with antibody production to injection or infection with the same microorganism. In nature such occasions are naturally rare or at least unrecognized, but the condition is known to occur in certain strains of mice infected with lymphocytic choriomeningitis virus. . . . No clinical evidence of illness was apparent and the mice were quite resistant to intracerbral challenge with virus. No neutralizing antibody could be detected in the blood nor any complement fixing antibody. . . .

These phenomena are obviously complex but there is the development of a tolerance to the foreign microorganism during embryonic life which is in line with the present hypothesis.

The clonal selection theory of acquired immunity

1959 • Sir Macfarlane Burnet

Comment

Act 1, Scene 1: London, April 25, 1953. The double helix model of DNA by James Watson and Francis Crick appears in *Nature*. With this publication the entire realm of biological science and natural philosophy is changed, but at the time only a few people realize its extraordinary significance. Although Oswald Avery's team in 1944 and Alfred Hershey and Martha Chase in 1952 provided evidence that DNA is the hereditary substance, the absence of a molecular mechanism made the concept an abstract fuzzy ball. Watson and Crick's work removes this deficiency; work on deciphering the genetic code commences.

Scene 2: Melbourne, Summer 1955. In light of the advances in immunology and biochemistry, Sir Macfarlane Burnet decides to again revise his book on antibody formation. However, the results of his creative urge to theorize goes awry. He extends the discussion to enzymes and viruses in hope of a unified mechanism around the principle that the essence of life is to replicate a specific pattern. RNA is designated the template as well as the coded sequencer of amino acids in synthesizing viral capsids, antibodies, and the so-called adaptive enzymes. Burnet suggests that proteins transform their patterns onto RNA: Assuming RNA to have an inadequate binary code, he has the protein fold the linear nucleic acid in such a way as to produce a mathematical code-enhancing matrix. He also proposes that the carriage of antibody specificity to the next generation of cells is mainly through cytoplasmic distribution of the RNA template. The new biology is thus hung with the albatross of an obsolete model.

Burnet has grave misgivings about the manuscript. It contains too many inconsistencies and loose ends. The field is in rapid flux, and he is fearful that a new discovery will instantly sink his theoretical schemes.

Act 2, Scene 1: Pasadena, Summer 1955. In Max Delbrück's laboratory at the California Institute of Technology, Niels K. Jerne examines antibody reactions to bacteriophages, since bacterial virology is a hot field and immunology is not. Jerne recalls his evening walk in Copenhagen in March 1954, when he conceived a selective cellular approach to antibody formation. He now continues his speculations, and asks the opinions of Linus Pauling and James D. Watson. They reject the idea without hesitation. Colin M. McLeod and Wendell M. Stanley, however, encourage Jerne to publish. Jerne drafts his manuscript, and in early September, Delbrück places it in the mail.

Scene 2: Washington, D.C., November 15, 1955. Jerne's natural selection theory of antibody formation appears in the *Proceedings of the National Academy of Sciences*. Based on the discovery of low levels of natural antibodies to a bacteriophage, he suggests that all immunoglobulin specificities are originally constitutive. Having been produced by some cellular mechanism, apparently somatic, that involves the random generation of unique antigen receptors, these secreted immunoglobulins are then selected by the introduced antigen. The immune complexes are taken up by macrophages, which eliminate the antigen and by some manner transfer the structural information of the immunoglobulin to lymphoid cells whose specificity is unrestricted. Consequently, the normal constitutive antibodies are replicated in mass. Without giving details, Jerne requires that natural antibodies to self-antigens be eliminated. Jerne's proposal resembles Paul Ehrlich's side-chain theory, which also depends on selection and permits the formation of natural antibodies. Burnet in Melbourne reads the article, but is not impressed.

Scene 3: Geneva, 1956. Burnet and Jerne meet at the World Health Organization. Jerne criticizes Burnet's newly published book for creating vague metaphysical processes, and fails to convince him that the antibody selection thesis is superior. Burnet, however, finds something attractive about Jerne's concept. What it is, he is unsure.

Act 3, Scene 1: Melbourne, Summer 1957. Studying the proliferating immunological cells in graft-versus-host responses in hen's eggs, Burnet suddenly realizes that it is not antibodies that are selected but cells, indeed clones of particular immunocompetent lymphocytes. He proposes that somatic mutation during embryonic life generates the random specificities, that cells possess concordant antigen receptors, and that cells to self-antigens are killed.

In September, Burnet publishes his theory in the *Australian Journal of Science* to hedge his bet. Priority is thus ensured, and should the theory fail, few would have read the obscure journal. Despite initial good reviews, his new book no longer is relevant. It would be reprinted in 1958, nonetheless. Burnet fears another embarrassment, although he is confident of the soundness of his proposal.

Scene 2: Melbourne, December 1957. Joshua and Esther Lederberg visit the Hall Institute. With Gus J. V. Nossal, they test the clonal selection theory: introducing two antigens (from bacterial flagella) into animals and then segregating harvested antibody-producing cells, they find individual plasma cells are able to produce antibodies only against one or the other antigen, not both. Joshua Lederberg, a geneticist, in 1959 would explain the variety of antigen specificity through the lifelong random and somatic mutation of a certain nucleotide sequence.

Scene 3: Nashville, May 1958. Burnet delivers the Abraham Flexner lectures at Vanderbilt University, presenting a more thorough analysis and stronger framework of clonal selection. These lectures are published as a book from which the following milestone is excerpted. A concurrent symposium at Nashville allows Burnet to explain the theory to a representation of the immunological community. The audience is skeptical.

Act 4, Scene 1: Cold Spring Harbor, June 1967. After years of frustration and difficulty marketing clonal selection, Burnet is the introductory speaker at the symposium on antibodies. Gerald Edelman's work establishing Bence-Jones proteins as clonal-specific immunoglobulins from myelomas was the key to general acceptance of the theory.

Scene 2: One of many university classrooms, October 1967. The new gospel of clonal selection is taught to students of immunology.

For further information:

Burnet, F. M. 1967. The impact on ideas of immunology. In: *Volume 32. Antibodies.* Cold Spring

Harbor Symposia on Quantitative Biology, Cold Spring Harbor. pp. 1–8.

Jerne, N. K. 1966. The natural selection theory of antibody formation; ten years later. In: *Phage and the Origins of Molecular Biology* (J. Cairns, G. S. Stent, and J. D. Watson, editors). Cold Spring Harbor Laboratory of Quantitative Biology, Cold Spring Harbor. pp. 301–312.

Wood, T. J. 1969. Burnet and medicine. *Australian Annals of Medicine* 4:301–309.

Wood, I. J. 1970. Burnet of Australia. *Postgraduate Medical Journal* 46:175–181.

The Paper*

In 1955 Jerne published a new and strikingly different conception of antibody production in which, for the first time since Ehrlich, natural antibodies were seriously considered in relation to "true" antibodies. Jerne discarded altogether the view that antibody production was a direct result of the entry of an antigen into body cells. He held that the gamma globulin molecules of the plasma represent a population comprising carriers of all the reactive sites needed to unite with any potential antigenic determinant except those already existing in accessible components of the body. The function of the antigen which enters the body from without is to act as "a selective carrier of spontaneously circulating antibody to a system of cells which can reproduce this antibody". It is assumed that once antibody is taken into cells of the antibody-producing system, replicas of this natural antibody will be produced. With the liberation of this crop of new antibody a second injection of antigen will find many more antibody-producing cells and give a stronger "secondary" stimulus to antibody production. . . .

The great contribution of Jerne's theory was that it drew attention to the theoretical possibility that the recognition of self from not-self could be achieved in another fashion than by the recognition of "self-markers". As Talmage (1957) points out, Ehrlich's side-chain theory was in many ways the logical equivalent of Jerne's concept. The side-chain theory was

quietly shelved as evidence accumulated of the vast variety of antibodies that could be produced, some against nonbiological determinants such as arsanilic acid. . . . Nevertheless, if Jerne is correct that a comprehensive range of molecules corresponding to all organic patterns other than those of body components is present in the gamma globulin population, this would be an effective and much more elegant way of accounting for the differentiation of self from not-self.

The outstanding difficulty in accepting Jerne's theory is the claim that when a given type of natural antibody molecule is brought to a cell by antigen, the cell then proceeds to make more natural antibody molecules of the same type. . . . Talmage (1957) pointed out that it would be more satisfactory if the replicating elements essential to any such theory were cellular in character ab initio rather than extracellular protein which can replicate only when taken into an appropriate cell. . . . Our own view is that any tenable form of Jerne's theory must involve the existence of multiple clones of globulin-producing cells, each responsible for one genetically determined type of antibody globulin. This immediately poses the question of how the antibody-antigen complex can reach the cells, which are genetically determined to produce the corresponding type of antibody molecule. Clearly it would simplify matters a great deal if the antigen were in a position to react with natural antibody or a pattern equivalent thereto on the surface of the cell which produced it.

This is the crux of the clonal selection hypothesis. It assumes that in the animal there exist clones of mesenchymal cells, each carrying immunologically reactive sites corresponding in appropriate complementary fashion to one (or possibly a number of) potential antigenic determinants. This provides a population of cells which, when an appropriate stage of development has been reached, are capable of producing the population of globulin molecules which collectively provide the normal antibodies. When an antigen is introduced it will make contact with a cell of the corresponding clone, presumably a lymphocyte, and by so doing stimulate it to produce in one way or another more globulin molecules of the cell's characteristic type. The obvious way of achieving this is to postulate that stimulation initiates proliferation as soon as the cell in question is taken into an appropriate tissue niche, spleen, lymph node or subacute inflammatory accumulation. . . .

The antibody-producing cells of the body make up a mobile population of mesenchymal cells constantly undergoing physiological and mutational change. It is composed of large numbers of clones from which subclones are constantly arising as a result of somatic mutation.

---

*Burnet, [F.] M. 1959. *The Clonal Selection Theory of Acquired Immunity.* Vanderbilt University Press and Cambridge University Press. 209 p. [With permission of Vanderbilt University Press; copyright Sir Macfarlane Burnet 1959.]

Individual clones prosper or dwindle in accord with their experience of contact with the corresponding antigen determinants. The result of such contact will depend on a variety of physiological considerations of which the most important is probably the age of the individual concerned. . . .

How clones to cover all possible antigenic determinants can arise must be left for later discussion. We assume simply that this does take place at some stage in embryonic life and that mesenchymal cells, presumably lymphocytes, begin to circulate with the characteristic pattern on their surface but do not liberate antibody-type globulin. In the Burnet-Fenner theory, any potentialities of antibody production against body components were eliminated by the development of tolerance. In the present theory they are more readily disposed of by assuming that—at this particular stage of embryonic life—contact with the corresponding antigen pattern results in the death of the cell. . . . Self-not-self recognition means simply that all those clones which would recognize (that is, produce antibody against) a self component have been eliminated in embryonic life. All the rest are retained.

To obtain such a result a fairly complex developmental sequence must be postulated. The first point to be considered is how a complete sequence of globulin patterns capable of reacting with all possible determinants could be established. . . . [I]f at a certain stage of embryonic development certain synthetic elements in mesenchymal cells were "randomized", the possibility might well emerge of producing all the 10,000 or more patterns required.

Suppose that at the appropriate stage of development of a limited genetic determinant carrying the coding responsible for globulin pattern releases control in such a fashion that purely random arrangements are allowed which will be different at each replication. Then at a later stage control is reestablished and the various random sequences are sta-

bilized as the guides to the genetic control of globulin synthesis by the cell lines concerned. This is still during embryonic life when gamma globulins are not liberated into the blood and are produced only to the extent necessary to bring their specific patterns to the surface of the cell. It is at this stage that contact with any determinant associated with a body component or any foreign determinant artificially introduced results in the elimination of cells carrying such sites, and if all such clones are eliminated full tolerance is established.

The next phase is the gradual change in the response to contact with antigenic determinant. From the lethal effect seen in the early stage it changes, perhaps with an intermediate phase of damage and partial recovery, to stimulation of protein synthesis and, in the appropriate tissue environments, active proliferation to produce plasmacytoid cells and lymphocytes with active antibody-liberating capacity. . . .

The approach can, I think, be legitimately called an evolutionary one. . . . Irrespective of what field we are considering, as the environment changes the nature of the population changes, and in the present state of our knowledge the changes are best understood in terms of mutation and selective survival.

It is universally accepted that the phenomena of immunity are based on the functional activity of populations of mesenchymal cells within the body. The chief novelty of the clonal selection theory is its concentration, not on what happens in an individual cell, but on the way cell populations are modified by the presence of antigenic determinants in their environment of the body fluids. It is a Darwinian approach which, pressed to its logical conclusion, demands that immunological specificity is based on a special type of differentiation occurring in embryonic life plus a high subsequent potential for somatic mutation in that region of the genome concerned with immunologically significant pattern. . . .

Towards a network theory of the immune system

1974 • Niels K. Jerne

Comment

Sir Macfarlane Burnet in 1968 called Niels K. Jerne (1911–   ) the most intelligent immunologist alive. Sixteen years later a share of the

Nobel Prize was presented to Jerne not for some experimental discovery, indeed not for any particular body of laboratory research, but for his powerful, far-reaching immunological theories. This award was an extraordinary occasion, for while theoretical contributions in physics and chemistry have been frequently so lauded, biomedically related theories have not had this distinction. Burnet's clonal selection theory, of course, was built upon Jerne's foundation, and additional but more narrow propositions of Jerne followed. In the early 1970s Jerne formulated a bold new theory that concerned the spatial relationship of antigen receptors and antibody idiotypes and their role in regulating the immune response. It was a theory, produced concurrently with other advances in cybernetic and systems analysis, that was entirely and radically holistic in approach. It was alien to traditional immunological thinking, although the fundamental concept of natural anti-antibodies originated with Paul Ehrlich.

When Jerne, still developing this network theory, as it is termed, presented his concept at various universities, it frequently soared over the head of most of the audience. Complex and lacking tangibility, the theory generally received only polite applause from the somewhat perplexed gathering of researchers and students. Like Burnet, when he first encountered Jerne's natural selection model, many intuitively felt that something excellent lay within, if they could manage to fathom it. Evidence was fairly circumstantial; however, a good theory can predict experimental results, and eventually Jerne's did. Rarely, however, is a theory perfect as conceived. Variations and modifications of the network theory have been developed and continue to arise.

Born in England of Danish parents, Jerne received his college education first at the University of Leiden and then at the University of Copenhagen. He earned his M.D. in 1951. Between 1943 and 1954, he worked at the State Serum Institute in Copenhagen. The following year, as mentioned earlier, took him to the California Institute of Technology. Jerne next traveled to Geneva for a staff position with the World Health Organization. From 1960 to 1962, he was also Professor of Biophysics at the University of Geneva. For the next four years, he was back in the United States as professor and chairman of the Department of Microbiology at the University of Pittsburgh. In 1966 he became the Director of the Paul Ehrlich Institute at the University of Frankfurt, and in 1969 he was appointed Director of the Basel Institute for Immunology, where he finally rested from his trans-Atlantic sojourns. In 1980, when he was elected a fellow of the Royal Society, he retired from the Swiss post, spent a year as a professor at the Pasteur Institute, and now resides in France.

Jerne's network theory had popped up in skeletal form in several reviews prior to the publication of the paper presented here. He suggested the term eigen-behavior, "eigen" being German for *peculiar to* or *characteristic* and long used by physicists in similar expressions. The theory did not provide any details; that is the task of consequent experimentation. It could, however, explain, since they were its wellspring, certain peculiar results from previous investigations. Foremost was Jacques Oudin and Pierre-Andre Cazenave's paradoxical finding of identical idiotypes on antibodies directed against distinct, noncross-reacting epitopes of an antigen. Furthermore, Oudin and Cazenave noted that some of the induced antibodies having the same idiotype did not react with the antigen. Since idiotypes were associated with the hypervariable region of antibody receptors, the experiment implied a shared variable domain located elsewhere, and, as Jerne suggested, a cross-reactivity of tertiary antibodies, anti-(anti-antibodies), bearing an "internal image" of the idiotype of the primary anti-epitope antibodies. Trying to grasp the previous sentence, the reader perhaps can empathize with the mind-boggling feeling experienced by the uninitiated in Jerne's seminars!

Remarkably, tests of the theory did indeed demonstrate that anti-anti-antibodies could react with the initial antigen. Clarification of the suppressor role of the T cell and the discovery of its idiotypic antigen receptor have supported the proposal. Anti-idiotype antibodies have also been found to differ, being directed against all the variable domains of the immunoblogulin as predicted, not just the hypervariable antigen-combining region, although it dominates. Thus, all anti-(anti-idiotype) antibodies do not necessarily couple with the antigen. This relationship broadens the network, and an additional means of cascade damping results. The corollary that the "internal image" of the antigen carried by some anti-idiotype antibodies can serve as an antigen substitute has been confirmed with novel vaccines and the amazing mimicry of biologically active molecules, such as hormones and enzymes.

Jerne's immunological network seems to provide the fine adjustment in regulating responses. Antigen-specific helper T cells can act synergistically with idiotype-specific cells; suppression by T cells can be aided by anti-idiotypic antibody. The idiotypic governing mechanisms maintain immunological memory and keep the lymphocytes in a ready state. They also may serve as a selective influence in evolution by providing antigenic configurations that are infrequently encountered in the environment. Therefore, the dynamics of antibody formation, thanks to Jerne and the experiments instigated by his theory, have become even more complex and highly regulated than could be imagined only fifteen years ago when cooperation of lymphocyte subpopulations was first discerned. Jerne, a Leeuwenhoek of theoretical biology, had fashioned a microscope of speculations and discovered a hitherto unseen world.

For further information:

Jerne, N. K. 1960. Immunological speculations. *Annual Review of Microbiology* 14:341–358.

Jerne, N. K. 1985. The generative grammar of the immune system. *Science* 229:1057–1059.

Greene, M. I. and A. Nisonoff (editors). 1984. *The Biology of Idiotypes*. Plenum Press, New York. 507 p.

Köhler, H. 1984. The immune network revisited. In: *Idiotypy in Biology and Medicine* (H. Köhler, J. Urbain, and P-A. Cazenave, editors). Academic Press, Orlando. pp. 3–14.

Silverstein, A. M. 1986. Anti-antibodies and anti-idiotype immunoregulation, 1899–1904: the inexorable logic of Paul Ehrlich. *Cellular Immunology* 99:507–522.

Steinberg, C. M. and I. Lefkovits. 1981. *The Immune System. Festschrift in honor of Niels Kaj Jerne on the occasion of his 70th birthday. Volume 1. Past and Future.* S. Karger, Basel. 438 p.

The Paper*

. . . I think there is now a need for a novel and fundamental idea that may give a new look to immunological theory, similar to the impact that the idea of selection had on theoretical developments in the period 1950–1970. Before coming to this, I shall make a few suggestions on terminology and then start out by considering: (I) Repertoires, (II) Dualisms, and (III) Suppression.

Immunological terminology is sometimes clumsy and I now take up a proposal I made many years ago, namely to replace the term "antigenic determinant" by "epitope", and the term "antibody combining site" by "paratope". An epitope is a patch on an antigen molecule, which presents a certain relief or pattern that can be recognized with various degrees of precision by complementary patterns of paratopes located on antibody molecules. . . . Two outstanding accomplishments of the recent period are the discoveries of allotypes and idiotypes, or the finding that antibody molecules present epitopes and that these can play a functional role, as experimentally demonstrated by allotype and idiotype suppression. I draw particular attention to idiotypes which were defined by Oudin as the antigenic specificities of antibodies produced by an individual or a group of individuals in response to a given antigen. An idiotype thus is a set of epitopes displayed by the variable regions of a set of antibody molecules. Each single idiotypic epitope I shall call "idiotope". An idiotype then denotes a certain set of idiotopes. The patterns of idiotopes are determined by the same regions of antibody polypeptide chains that also determine the paratopes. In short, each Fab arm of an

---

*Jerne, N. K. 1974. Towards a network theory of the immune system. *Annales d'Immunologie* (Institute Pasteur) 125 C:373–389. [With permission.]

antibody molecule displays one paratope and a small set of idiotopes.

Let us now come to the "repertoires", and first consider the repertoire of antibody combining sites or the total number of different paratopes in the immune system. . . . The "potential" repertoire is obviously far larger than the "available" repertoire which is the number of different paratopes in the immune system of an individual at a given moment. . . . For the moment I shall simply assume that the available repertoire of paratopes in a given immune system is of the order of several millions. . . .

[E]xperiments . . . suggest that the repertoire of idiotypes is enormously large. This conclusion is supported by the findings by Nisonoff that a given idiotype is exceedingly rare in normal serum globulin. For the moment, I shall simply assume that the repertoires of paratopes and of idiotopes are both of the same order of magnitude. . . . I therefore find it reasonable to assume that, within the immune system of one given individual, any idiotope can be recognized by a set of paratopes and that any paratope can recognize a set of idiotopes. I have tried to show in an earlier paper that this recognition of antibody molecules by other antibody molecules in the same serum will result in only a negligible concentration of complexes if the production of the concentrations of reacting paratopes and idiotopes remains sufficiently small. This proviso can be satisfied by assuming sufficiently large repertoires of paratopes and idiotopes. If we accept these propositions we can conclude that, formally, the immune system is an enormous and complex network of paratopes that recognize sets of idiotopes, and of idiotopes that are recognized by sets of paratopes. I here make the additional assumption that the presence of identical paratopes on two antibody molecules does not necessarily imply that these molecules present identical idiotopes.

The second point I need to make is that the immune system displays a number of dualisms. The first of these is the occurrence of T lymphocytes and B lymphocytes with partly synergic, partly antagonistic interactions. The second dualism is the one we have just discussed, namely that antibody molecules can recognize as well as be recognized. These properties lead to the establishment of a network, and as antibody molecules occur both free and as receptor molecules on lymphocytes, this network intertwines cells and molecules. The third dualism I draw attention to is the ability of an antigen-sensitive lymphocyte to respond either positively or negatively to a recognition signal. A positive response leads to cell proliferation, cell activation and to antibody secretion, a negative response results in tolerance and suppression. . . . Thus, a lymphocyte can respond in

two ways when the paratopes of its receptor molecules recognize an epitope, or an idiotype.

What happens to a lymphocyte in the reverse situation when the idiotopes of its receptor molecules are recognized by the paratopes of free antibody molecules or by the paratopes of the receptors of another cell? Most experimental findings suggest that the lymphocyte is then repressed.

My third point is to stress the importance of suppression. I have become increasingly convinced that the essence of the immune system is the repression of its lymphocytes. Lymphocytes are suppressed by anti-allotypic antibody. As Herzenberg and Jacobson have shown, this allotype suppression is maintained by T cells that recognize the allotype of B cell receptors. The situation is similar for the suppressive effect of anti-idiotypic antibody and, by analogy, T cells recognizing the idiotopes of B cell receptors may be assumed likewise to maintain B cell suppression. Conversely, we could conclude that, normally, B cells remain functional because of the absence of sufficient numbers of specific suppressive T cells, or in other words, that B cells can suppress the emergence of recognizing T cells in certain situations. In general, this seems to lead to some dynamic equilibrium or steady state among the elements of the immune system. As tolerance induction shows that B cells and T cells can also be suppressed when the paratopes of their receptors recognize a foreign epitope or an idiotope, the number of negative, suppressive situations appears to exceed the number of positive, stimulatory situations.

Even if conceding the possibility of viewing the immune system as a formal network, one may question whether the concentrations of individual paratopes and idiotopes are sufficient to establish an internal functional network. Experiments have shown that the concentrations of epitopes needed to induce low-zone tolerance are often far lower than what most of us would estimate to be the average concentration of a single paratope or idiotope in the system. If, for example, we assume a repertoire size of five millions, both for paratopes and for idiotopes, then the average concentration in our blood of antibody molecules representing one member of a repertoire would be 10^{10} per ml, whereas low-zone tolerance has been achieved with epitope concentrations ranging from 10^6–10^{12} per ml.

We conclude that the immune system, even in the absence of antigens that do not belong to the system, must display an eigen-behavior mainly resulting from paratope-idiotope interaction within the system. By its eigen-behavior the immune system achieves a dynamic steady state as its elements interact between themselves, and as some elements decay and new ones emerge. . . . [T]he following exposition is meant only as an illustration of certain interpretative potentialities of such a theory.

Let us start with considering an immunogenic substance which presents epitope E to the immune system. This epitope is recognized (with various degrees of precision) by a set of different antibody combining sites, or paratopes. I call this set p_1 and note that these paratopes occur on antibody and receptor molecules together with certain idiotopes, so that the set p_1 of paratopes is associated with a set i_1 of idiotopes. The symbol $p_1 i_1(E)$ denotes the total set of recognizing antibody molecules and potentially responding lymphocytes with respect to epitope E (see Fig. 1). Within the network of the immune system, each paratope of the set p_1 recognizes a set of idiotopes, and the entire set p_1 recognizes an even larger set of idiotopes. This set i_2 of idiotopes is, as it were, the "internal image" of epitope E because it is recognized by the same set p_1 that recognized E. The set i_2 is associated with a set p_2 of paratopes occurring on the molecules and cell receptors of the set $p_2 i_2(E)$.

Furthermore, each idiotope of the set $p_1 i_1(E)$ is recognized by a set of paratopes, so that the entire set i_1 is recognized by an even larger set p_3 of paratopes which occur together with a set i_3 of idiotopes on antibodies and lymphocytes of the anti-idiotypic set $p_3 i_3(E)$. We come in this way to ever larger sets that recognize or are recognized by previously defined sets within the network. As a first gross approximation to a functional network we could assume that the elements (molecules and cells) of the

"internal image" set $p_2 i_2(E)$ are largely stimulatory towards the potentially responsive set $p_1 i_1(E)$ of lymphocytes, whereas the elements of the anti-idiotypic set $p_3 i_3(E)$ are largely inhibitory. In the eigen-behavior of the immune system these opposite forces result in a balanced suppression which must be overcome in order to obtain an immune response to E. . . .

The weakness of this incipient network theory lies in its lack of precision. The formal sets $p_1 i_1$, $p_2 i_2$, $p_3 i_3$, etc., refer to sets of antibody molecules that can occur both as freely circulating antibodies of all immunoglobulin classes and as functional receptors on T cells and B cells. This leaves an ambiguity in the answer to the question whether the relations between two sets is suppressive or stimulatory, or partly one and partly the other, and thus permits us to postulate interactions that suit our explanatory needs. The properties of all possible different types of interaction must therefore be clarified in order to be able to understand and eventually to manipulate the immune system. . . . Another question that needs consideration is the ontogenic development of the network in the adult immune system from a small germ-line determined, embryonic set of elements. We suspect that the initial shaping of the immune network is influenced to a large extent by the genes that cluster around the histocompatibility locus. . . . Partly because of polymorphisms in the cluster of genes at the histocompatibility locus, and partly because of a certain randomness in the ontogenic emergence of new paratopes and idiotopes, each in-

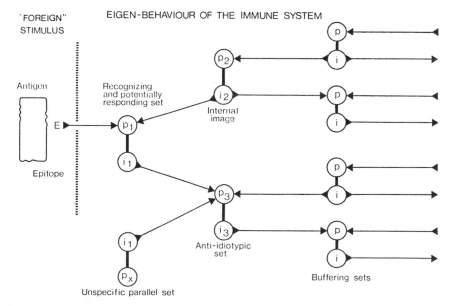

Figure 1 Eigen-behavior of the immune system.

dividual will develop a different immune network. When established, the immune network must be hard to undo later. This may be relevant to Fazekas de St. Groth's concept of the original antigenic sin and it suggests that immunological memory may be more firmly deposited in a persistent network modulation than in the persistence of a population of so-called "memory cells". . . .

In finishing, I should only like to point out that the immune system when viewed as a functional network dominated by a mainly suppressive eigen-behavior, but open to stimuli from the outside, bears a striking resemblance to the nervous system. These two systems stand out among all other organs of our body by their ability to respond adequately to an enormous variety of signals. Both systems display dichotomies and dualisms. The cells of both systems can receive as well as transmit signals. In both systems the signals can be either excitatory or inhibitory. The two systems penetrate most other tissues of our body, but they seem to be kept separate from each other by the so-called blood-brain barrier. The nervous system is a network of neurons in which the axon and the dendrites of one nerve cell form synaptic connections with sets of other nerve cells. In the human body there are about 10^{12} lymphocytes as compared to 10^{10} nerve cells. They do not need connection by fibers in order to form a network. As lymphocytes can move about freely, they can interact either by direct encounters or through the antibody molecules they release. The network resides in the ability of these elements to recognize as well as to be recognized. Like for the nervous system, the modulation of the network by foreign signals represents its adaptation to the outside world. Early imprints leave the deepest traces. Both systems thereby learn from experience and build up a memory that is sustained by reinforcement and that is deposited in persistent network modifications, which cannot be transmitted to our offspring.

These striking phenotypic analogies between the immune system and the nervous system may result from similarities in the sets of genes that govern their expression and regulation.

Part 6
Agents and Adjuncts

Too simple to distinguish right from wrong,
Inconscious agents they.   —Robert Browning

Our antagonist is our helper.   —Edmund Burke

We humans are lazy creatures. Perpetually in want of simple answers to the most complex matters of mind and the universe, we always seek first the single causative agent of phenomena—the one environmental factor, the individual cell, the key molecule. Assuming that the bactericidal or hemolytic quality of serum was related to one particular substance, early immunologists were plagued by divergent data dependent on their test systems and conditions. Bitter polemics arose on the existence and nature of the responsible factor or factors and their possible differentiation from agglutinins and other antibodies. Confusion blocked progress as the merits of hypothetical components termed alexine, complement, and cytotoxin were argued in journals and congresses. The debate was rekindled in the 1950s with the proposal of a new but similar entity called properdin. A hundred years after its first recognition, researchers shake their heads and sigh at the mention of complement, for complement is not a single substance but (with properdin) a complex, branched series of at least 20 major proteins, whose ultimate activity is dependent on the pathway, a sequence of interactions. These various proteins include both enzymes, which activate other members of the series and open target cell membranes, and structural units, which line the newly fashioned pores.

The following short series of milestones begins with two reports establishing the unique properties of complement. As we have already seen, George H. F. Nuttall in 1888 noted the occasional existence of a heat-labile bactericidal substance in defibrinated blood. The following year Hans Büchner determined that the lethal property was dependent on mineral salts, since it would disappear with dialysis against distilled water but not salt solutions. Modern investigations ascertained that calcium ions are responsible for keeping the series of complement components together for proper activity. In the classic paper presented here, Richard Pfeiffer in 1894 astonished even the ardent serologists with his demonstration of the rapid granulation and lysis of cholera vibrio in the cell-free peritoneal fluid of immunized guinea pigs. This dramatic dissolution of bacteria was the foremost weapon of the humoral school of immunity against Elie Metchnikoff's phagocyte theory. However, numerous exceptions to the phenomenon were soon found, since all Gram-positive and some Gram-negative bacteria are resistant to immune bacteriolysis.

Experimentally, the second report has nothing to do with infectious diseases; interpretively, it has everything to do with it. The hemolysis of foreign red blood cells in immune sera, first observed by Büchner, was now investigated in depth by Jules Bordet. Realizing that the reaction shared characteristics with Pfeiffer's phenomenon, Bordet set to prove that the two were in fact one. This he eventually accomplished, but more significantly he clearly separated the heat-resistant antibody or sensitizer from the lytic agent. Bordet, furthermore, discovered that this effector, which Büchner termed alexine (from the Greek for defender) and which Paul Ehrlich called complement (for obvious reasons), was nonspecific and present in normal serum as well. In the ensuing years, when researchers began to apply protein separation techniques, they isolated four components that attached sequentially to antibody and to the target cell. The idea that complement consisted solely of these four substances lasted for 32 years. In 1958, as new protein purification methods were developed, the dam began to crack, and each year thereafter would find a new component added to the cascade. In addition, complement was found to be responsible for other effects besides punching and lining holes in membranes. Various components stabilize immune complexes, and are involved in vasodilation, chemotaxis, opsonization, and viral neutralization. Among their cellular synthesizers is the macrophage, the factotum or jack-of-all-trades of immunity.

The immune response, as Metchnikoff emphasized, goes hand-in-hand with inflammation. There are many inflammatory agents of which the first and most powerful discovered was histamine (beta-iminazolylethylamine). The discovery of histamine is the third milestone. Sir Henry H. Dale and Sir Patrick P. Laidlaw observed that their isolated substance caused a wide variety of physiological effects, such as capillary dilation and smooth muscle contraction, which strongly resembled the symptoms of anaphylaxis. The often unpleasant action of histamine has at the microscopic level the benefit of infusing antibodies and complement to the offended area and easing the passage of phagocytes. Other notable inflammatory adjuncts are bradykinin, serotonin, fibrinogen, leukotrienes, and heparin. These various inflammatory agents, which are synthesized by platelets, mast cells, and basophils, affect the pulmonary and cardiovascular system, shifting lymph and blood flow, causing phagocytes to adhere to the nearby vessel, attracting them to the damaged area, and stimulating neural and endocrine centers to activate and regulate immune responses. Inflammation, like other biological activities, has its checks and balances; eosinophils, for example, secrete regulators that control the degree of mast cell degranulation and hence influence dose of mediators, which makes the difference between a healthful and a pathogenic response.

The next paper in this section concerns a nonspecific antiviral protein produced by most tissue cells including lymphocytes and macrophages. It is called interferon, and it helps prevent the spread of virus from infected cells by rendering the cells' neighbors resistant not to infection, but to viral multiplication. Interferon also recruits natural killer (NK) cells to assist in the defense, and also blocks the growth of certain cancers. Discovered by Alick Isaacs and Jean Lindenmann in 1957, interferon seemed to be a new wonder drug. It is not, but nevertheless it does have a promising future for some diseases and situations.

The numerous lymphokines and monokines (mediators secreted by monocytes and macrophages) so important in regulating the immune response are represented by a report of John R. David, who independently established along with Barry R. Bloom that the inhibition of lymphoid cell migration involves a dialyzable agent later dubbed appropriately migration inhibitory factor, or MIF, for short. Most such mediators are functionally rather than biochemically defined, and the same agent, as with complement components, may have various activities. Some one hundred lymphokine factors have been described and named. Other noteworthy agents are leukocyte chemotactic factor (LCF), macrophage chemotactic factor (MCF), lymphotoxin, lymphocyte mitogenic factor, and interleukin-2 (IL-2). IL-2, an immunoregulator formerly known as T-cell growth factor, is unique in that it and antibodies to its T-cell receptor have been applied therapeutically in immune deficiency diseases, autoimmune disorders, and adult T-cell leukemia.

Transfer factor deserves particular mention. It bears the same heterodoxy as the infectious prion, the name given to the agents of "slow virus" diseases. Both postulated agents transfer specific information to the genome of cells, although they apparently lack nucleic acid. Both are small molecular weight proteid substances. Transfer factor, discovered in 1955 by H. Sherwood Lawrence in extracts of disrupted blood leukocytes, is dialyzable and able to transfer delayed hypersensitivity to normal subjects. It has been used clinically with some apparent success in immunodeficiency, chronic fungal infections, and malignant diseases. Some slow virus diseases are elicited as degenerative encephalopathies, and genes for prion-associated protein are carried on a host cell chromosome, suggesting that the agent may act as a derepressor/inducer of the associated operon. Thirty years of research into the nature of transfer factor have been unable to discern its exact composition or mechanism. Perhaps an "internal image" of the antigen is involved, and the immunological equilibrium of Jerne's idiotypic network of T cells is similarly shifted through derepression/induction of the specific genes. Of course, transfer factor may be an artifact. It may also be that crucial enigmatic anomaly that leads to a new paradigm.

For further information:

Friedman, H. (editor). 1979. Subcellular Factors in Immunity. *Annals of the New York Academy of Sciences* 332:1–625.

Lepow, I. H. 1980. Louis Pillemer, properdin, and scientific controversy. *Journal of Immunology* 125:471–478.

Osler, A. G. 1976. *Complement. Mechanisms and Functions.* Prentice-Hall, Englewood Cliffs, NJ. 193 p.

Ratnoff, W. D. 1980. A war with the molecules: Louis Pillemer and the history of properdin. *Perspectives in Biology and Medicine* 23:638–657.

Sehgal, P. V., L. T. May, I. Tamm, and J. Vilcek. 1987. Human β_2 Interferon and B-cell differentiation factor BSF-2 are identical. *Science* 235:731–732.

Taylor-Papadimtriou, J. (editor). 1985. *Interferons. Their Impact in Biology and Medicine.* Oxford University Press, Oxford. 148 p.

Further investigations on the nature of immunity to cholera and specific bactericidal processes

1894 • Richard Pfeiffer

Comment

That serum or plasma could kill bacteria had been established. Had not Joseph Fodor, George Nuttall, Hans Büchner, and others described the effect in detail? That serum could cause bacteria to degenerate into granular clumps of debris within minutes, however, was a far different matter. Such a striking phenomenon was seen by Richard Pfeiffer (1858–1945) in the spring of 1894, when he examined the peritoneal exudate of immune guinea pigs after he had reinoculated them with cholera bacilli. Furthermore, the reaction took place without the presence of phagocytes. Pfeiffer's experiments also demonstrated the specificity of the effect and the existence of responsible chemical substances in immune serum.

Cholera, which we tend to regard as a disease of India and other tropical areas, had several episodes of pandemics reaching as far as the United States. In 1892 cholera came to Hamburg. The cholera agent is a vibrio, a comma-shaped bacterium. With the bacterium now again in Europe, research into its immunity became even more urgent.

Pfeiffer's work did not entirely vindicate the humoral theory of immunity. Pfeiffer was unable to produce bacteriolysis in immune serum alone; it required the body environment or at least "activated" peritoneal exudate. Some physical or chemical condition seemed necessary. In retrospect, his use of diluted and presumably aged serum, hence deficient in complement, may have contributed to the failure, since Jules Bordet later achieved bacteriolysis using fresh serum. However, the degree of lysis was never as extensive as within the animal. Elie Metchnikoff, who could not accept Pfeiffer's conclusions without some experimental rebuttal, showed in 1895 that excellent lysis could occur in vitro even if the serum was previously heated to inactivate the agent, provided that phagocytes were included in the test. We now know that complement reactions are sensitive to dose and to the density of antibodies on target membranes, and that macrophages, among other cells, can secrete complement.

Complement obeys a law of two. The complement cascade does not commence unless two IgG antibodies are sufficiently juxtaposed on the target for complement unit Clq to bridge them. Other examples of this principle in immunology are the signal for antibody formation, given when the two B cell receptors to antigen hapten and helper T cell are "squeezed," and the signal for mast degranulation, which occurs when two adjacent IgE Fc receptors are bridged (usually by antigen joining the membrane-bound immunoglobulins). (One unit of IgM can do the trick, but since it functions like a fusion of $2\frac{1}{2}$ IgG units, the point still holds.) If IgM resembles a ten-armed starfish, then Clq is a six-headed hydra. Each head binds to an immunoglobulin having the appropriate Fc receptor; not all subclasses have this capacity.

Then there is the matter of the test bacterium. Pfeiffer was fortunate to have first investigated cholera vibrio. Bacteriolysis is best observed with vibrios and salmonella, both Gram-negative groups with outer membranes. A Gram-positive streptococcus or Bacillus resists the activity of complement. Indeed, the inconsistency of susceptibility would prolong and confuse the debate on the nature of complement. Pfeiffer naturally assumed at first that his degenerative factor was a unique single chemical agent with a single activity like Emil von Behring's antitoxins. The subsequent description of agglutinins, precipitins, and hemolysins in immune and in some instances normal serum would exacerbate the polemic.

Pfeiffer was fortunate in other ways as well. His family's financial situation forbade his pursuit of a university medical degree, but he was admitted to a preparatory school, later the Kai-

ser Wilhelm Akademie, that led to a commission in the Prussian army medical service. Pfeiffer received his M.D. in 1880. Seven years later he was assigned to Robert Koch's laboratory at the Institute of Hygiene at the University of Berlin, where he joined other military physicians in bacteriological training and research. Pfeiffer first isolated and characterized *Haemophilus influenzae* and *Neisseria catarrhalis,* and introduced blood agar as a growth medium. He was among the few who developed a strong friendship with Koch. He became Koch's First Assistant, and when Koch's Institute for Infectious Disease was opened in 1891, Pfeiffer was appointed director of the scientific section. He also accompanied Koch on his plague expedition to India. Pfeiffer's childhood dream of a university career was fulfilled in 1899 with the appointment as a professor of hygiene and bacteriology at the University of Konigsberg and in 1901 at the University of Breslau, now Wroclaw, Poland. During World War I, he served as Director of Hygiene at the Western Front with rank of general. He retired in 1926, Carl Prausnitz taking his chair, but he remained active for ten more years. In 1928 the Royal Society of London elected him a foreign member.

For further information:

Fildes, P. 1956. Richard Friedrich Johannes Pfeiffer. 1858–1945. *Biographical Memoirs of Fellows of the Royal Society* 2:237–247.

Fine, D. P. 1981. *Complement and Infectious Diseases.* CRC Press, Boca Raton, FL. 157 p.

Mayer, M. M. 1973. The complement system. *Scientific American* 229(5):54–66.

The Paper*

In my studies with Issaeff . . . I demonstrated that the serum of animals that are actively immunized

---

*Pfeiffer, R. 1894. Weitere Untersuchungen über das Wesen der Choleraimmunität und über specifische baktericide Processe. *Zeitschrift fur Hygiene und Infektionskrankheiten* 18:1–16. [With permission of Springer-Verlag, Heidelberg.]

against cholera has a specific effect only on this vibrio, while toward other bacterial species, it behaves as normal serum. We further showed that the specific activity against the intraperitoneal cholera infection of guinea pigs is exclusively based on bactericidal processes, which are somehow caused by the serum of immunized animals. In this study I will try to analyze as far as possible the mechanism of this peculiar bactericidal activity in guinea pigs.

Another explanation for the rapid killing of the injected cholera bacteria is that chemical bactericidal substances, which originate in the body of actively immunized animals and which are transmitted through the serum during passive immunization, may play a part. . . . Therefore, it would be wise to look for such differences in the behavior of the blood of normal and immunized animals. Indeed, they were found. Normal guinea pig serum contains hardly any bactericidal attributes against virulent cholera cultures. . . . Totally different results are obtained when the cholera bacteria are transferred to the serum of immunized guinea pigs. Under these circumstances, very clear bactericidal effects are realized, which, if the amount of the inoculum is not too great, can lead to sterilization of the serum. . . .

Lazarus, Wassermann, and I found that only small amounts of serum from convalescent cholera patients, a few milligrams, can produce the strongest bactericidal effects against cholera vibrio injected into the abdominal cavity of pretreated guinea pigs. If these effects are based on the amount of preformed bactericidal substances in the serum, then the undiluted serum against Koch's comma bacteria should be a disinfectant of the first order. . . . However, the lethal strength of such highly efficient human serum is weaker in a test tube, and even fails when large amounts of cholera culture are added. The serum of immunized guinea pigs behaves similarly.

From these experimental results we can conclude that the process of passive immunization through serum can not be founded on the transmission of preformed soluble chemical bodies, and we must look for other possible explanations. Next in question is Metchnikoff's teachings on phagocytosis. According to Metchnikoff, the immunizing serum works like a specific irritation on the leukocytes, which are thereafter caused to engulf the pathogenic microorganisms and destroy them. . . . Findings were made that stand in harmony with the demands of Metchnikoff's scheme.

Nevertheless, a thorough microscopic examination of the guinea pig abdomen under the influence of immunizing serum convinced me that the phagocytes are solely an accompaniment of the dying vibrios. . . .

A guinea pig of 530 g was injected on March 28, 1894 with 1/3 loopful of cholera agar culture sterilized by chloroform vapor. The guinea pig was seven days later injected intraperitoneally with 1/2 loopful of living cholera organisms. Samples of peritoneal exudate were harvested in intervals, and examined in hanging drop and stained smear preparations. Within a hour, many of the vibrios were no longer motile, and there were many granules and degenerative forms. By microscopy, the phagocytes held large numbers of granules and comma bacilli. Within 4–5 hours the process was complete, and after symptoms of intoxication, the animal survived.

On April 12, 1894, another guinea pig was injected with a prophylactic dose of one loopful of killed cholera agents. On April 18 and 27, 1894, it was reinjected intraperitoneally with two loopfuls of organisms. . . . Immediately after the injection, all the vibrios stopped moving. After 10 minutes, many granules and swollen vibrios but almost no leukocytes were seen. After 20 minutes of the infection, all the vibrios disappeared and many granules remained. Approximately 95% of the granules were extracellular and 5% were in the protoplasm of the leukocytes. Before my eyes, the cholera vibrios were lysed free of phagocytic influence. . . .

I obtained the same results with a passively immunized guinea pig. The following experiment was especially dramatic. One loopful of a 20-hour old culture was mixed with 1 cc of a 50 to 100-fold dilution of immune serum in broth. The mixture was injected intraperitoneally into a guinea pig of 200 g. At 10-minute intervals, samples of exudate were removed by glass pipette and examined with the microscope. Almost all the vibrios had degenerated into granules within 20 minutes, and after 30 minutes the process was complete without any noticeable participation of phagocytes.

As a control, I placed a sample of the same mixture of bacteria and diluted immune serum in the incubator to learn whether the bactericidal process occurs outside the animal. Unexpectedly, the vibrios replicated rapidly. The animal body plays a major and active role. It reacts to the stimulus of the vibrios under the influence of the immune substances in serum to produce the bactericidal activity. . . .

The killing and degeneration of vibrios in the abdomen of actively or passively immunized guinea pigs are caused a priori by physical or chemical influences, since phagocytes are not essential. . . . There is no need in preforming the chemicals; they are formed and are activated the moment they are needed. . . .

Guinea pigs that were passively immunized to cholera through serum were injected with a mixture of cholera and nordhafen vibrios to determine how the animals would react. A priori the following possibilities were construed: (1) The presence of the other vibrios would block the reaction of the animal so that no bactericidal effects would occur at all, or (2) the bactericidal action would develop nonetheless. . . . If there were physical effects involved, then I could assume that both vibrio species, since they were under the same conditions, would be influenced in the same fashion. . . . The cholera bacteria were dissolved, and the nordhafen vibrios were not at all affected.

I had to consider that the unexpected results could be explained by the weak resistance of cholera bacteria, which could easily be destroyed in an animal by infuences that might have little effect on the tougher and more virulent Metchnikoff vibrios. This caused me to repeat the experiments in inverted arrangement. I immunized guinea pigs with the serum of animals that were highly active against nordhafen vibrio [*V. nordhafen,* meaning north harbor, was also known as *V. metschnikovii*]. Then I injected a mixture of both vibrio species. This time the nordhafen vibrios were killed and the cholera bacteria survived.

The results of these experiments allow only one interpretation. The immunized animal is capable to form specific bactericidal substances, which are effective only against the bacterial species that was used for immunization. These facts are certain and seem to have far-reaching significance for the theory of immunity. . . .

The specific bactericidal substances are not preformed, occur only when needed, and, I assume, are consumed immediately after dissolving the vibrios. Therefore, they do not accumulate in the exudate. Nevertheless, it is possible under certain conditions to demonstrate such activity outside the animal body. For example, I injected a large dose of cholera bacteria intraperitoneally into a guinea pig that was actively immunized against cholera. After 20 minutes of dissolution, I removed large drops of the now sterile abdominal contents. It is now possible to observe specific bactericidal effects upon reinoculation of this exudate with cholera or nordhafen vibrios in a hanging drop at incubation temperature. The cholera bacteria became motionless at once, and many transformed into granules, while the nordhafen vibrios generally retained motility. . . . The killing of the cholera bacteria was seldom complete, and survivors eventually grew again and filled the drop densely. . . .

I next determined the strength of the effect. Earlier with Issaeff's help, I intraperitoneally injected guinea pigs with certain amounts of serum 24 hours before the intraperitoneal or subcutaneous injection of cholera bacteria in order to find the smallest quantity of serum that would keep the experimental animal alive. Of course, the animal weight and given dose had to be consistent. . . . I diluted the serum in broth. For each cc of these different dilutions, 1 loopful (2 mg) of fresh, 20-hour old cholera agar culture was dispersed and immediately injected intraperitoneally into a guinea pig slightly over 200 g in weight. About 30 minutes later, I tested the peritoneal exudate and examined the behavior of the comma bacteria in hanging drop and stained preparations. . . . From the above protocol it was concluded that the tested immunizing serum was quite strong. 6 mg caused within 30 minutes a full dissolution of 1 loopful of the cholera agent. At 0.003 cc, the effect appeared less complete and more retarded; nevertheless, the guinea pig remained alive. At 0.001 cc and 0.005 cc, the specific activity was only slight, and the animal died from cholera infection, which also occurred with control guinea pigs treated with 0.2 cc of normal serum. . . .

On the agglutination and dissolution of red blood cells by the serum of animals injected with defibrinated blood

1898 • *Jules Bordet*

Comment

Irony has been pap for historians, a banal approach to analysis, but who can resist pointing out that the single most significant contribution to serology and humoral immunity came from the Pasteur Institute, from Elie Metchnikoff's own laboratory? The independent thinker was Jules Bordet (1870–1961), and his remarkable career in immunology and bacteriology earned him membership in the Royal Society in 1916, the Nobel Prize for medicine in 1919, and other honors.

With an interest in chemistry, Bordet entered the University of Brussels at age 16. In 1892 he received his M.D. along with his older brother Charles. While Charles published in 1890 his research on leukocyte chemotaxis, Jules was completing his experiments on enhancing the virulence of *Vibrio metschnikovii* by passage in immunized aimals. Having received a travel grant in 1894, Jules Bordet made arrangements to work at the Pasteur Institute under the guidance of Metchnikoff. Bordet remained in Paris until 1901, except for a visit in 1897 to the Transvaal to study rinderpest. Despite the entreaties of the Pasteur Institute staff, Bordet decided to accept the directorship of the newly organized rabies and bacteriology institute of the Belgium province of Babant. In 1903 Madame Marie Pasteur granted Bordet's request to rename it the Institut Pasteur de Bruxelles. Four years later, Bordet also became Professor of Bacteriology in the medical faculty of the Free University of Brussels. At the age of 70, Bordet resigned the directorship, his son taking over the post, but Jules Bordet continued his scientific and teaching endeavors for almost another twenty years.

Bacteriologists are familiar with Bordet's discovery of the bacillus of whooping cough (*Bordetella pertussis*), the first description of the mycoplasma of bovine pleuropneumonia, the first but unpublished observation of the spirochete of syphilis, and his study of bacteriophage lysogeny. However worthy these accomplishments may be, they follow his numerous advances in immunology: the recognition of specific agglutination in 1895; the establishment in 1899 and 1904 that foreign serum, including antibodies and complement, is antigenic, forming precipitiates in antisera; the determination in 1900 of erythrocyte stroma antigenicity and its phylogenetic relationships; the analysis in 1909 of conglutination; and the discovery of co-agglutination in 1911. Paramount is the large body of studies on complement, among which is the following milestone.

Complement reacions were confusing. Bordet proceeded cautiously, one step at a time over seven years, to ensure that the phenomenon would be thoroughly elucidated and that his developing hypothesis of independent but cooperative agents would be understood. Like everyone else, he was fascinated with Richard Pfeiffer's specific lytic phenomenon of vibrio, but Bordet was the first to see its basic similarity with the phenomenon described in Hans Büchner's report on hemolysis. Bordet found the red blood cell system an excellent means to probe the related reactions. He did not have to depend on microscopy, since the clumping of erythrocytes was easily distinguished, and the red color of hemoglobin imparted to the test solution was an obvious indicator of lysis. Furthermore, he avoided the hazards associated with pathogenic bacteria.

The fundamental questions addressed were (1) whether the lysis of vibrio and erythrocyte is due to an antigen-specific single entity with the two properties of agglutination and lysis, the latter being sensitive to heat; (2) whether two agents are involved, and if so, (3) whether one or both are antigen-specific; and (4) whether bacteriolysis and hemolysis are different manifestations of the same phenomenon, meaning that there is only one kind of alexine or complement. Bordet recognized the slim possibility of different lytic agents for each sensitizing antibody. Pfeiffer's and Bordet's own earlier studies showed that unheated normal serum even from a different species possessed the ability to restore lytic activity to heat-inactivated immune serum. The presence of two reactants was clear, and Büchner's original conception of alexine (complement) had to be modified. Bordet correctly concluded that complement is nonspecific but unable to act unless the target was already sensitized. Complement opened the now unlocked door. His paper fully established the parallel nature of bacteriolysis and hemolysis. He even duplicated the Pfeiffer phenomenon by injecting rabbit erythrocytes and heated antisera into the peritoneal cavity of normal guinea pigs. The last point of Bordet's report deserves emphasis: Neither cellular nor humoral immunity arose to ward off infectious microorganisms; the elimination of pathogens is a dividend of a general physiological function. This statement and the credit Bordet gave to Metchnikoff managed to provide support for the serological approach while not abandoning the cellular concepts of his teacher.

The coda would come in 1900, when Bordet erased any trace of doubt about complement nonspecificity by using the same complement source for both bacteriolysis and hemolysis. He would even establish that complement (now specifically identified as component C1) becomes fixed to bacteria known to resist lysis. This led to the very sensitive complement-fixation test for detecting the presence of specific antibodies in serum. Bordet and Octave Gengou's description of this technique will be presented in a later section (see Part 8/Bordet, 1901).

For further information:

Beumer, J. 1962. Jules Bordet 1870–1961. *Journal of General Microbiology* 29:1–13.

Delaunay, A. 1971. Jules Bordet et l'Institut Pasteur de Paris. *Histoire de la Medecine* 21(April):2–45.

Porter, R. R., P. J. Lachmann, and K. B. M. Reid (editors). 1984. *Biochemistry and Genetics of Complement*. Royal Society, London, 152 p.

Ruddy, S., I. Gigli, and K. F. Austen. 1972. The complement system of man. *New England Journal of Medicine* 287:489–494; 545–549; 592–596; 642–646.

The Paper*

In an article published in 1895 we called attention to the following facts:

*Bordet, J. 1898. Sur l'agglutination et la dissolution des globules rouges par le serum d'animaux injectes de sang defibrine. *Annales de l'Institute Pasteur* 12:688–695. [With permission.]

1. The serum of animals vaccinated against the cholera vibrio cause some remarkable phenomena when blended with a culture of vibrios suspended in a liquid of physiological saline or bouillon. A small dose will rapidly bring about the immobilization of microbes and their gathering into masses or clumps. If the serum is freshly extracted and added in a sufficient dose to the emulsion, the action on the microorganism is more pronounced. The clumped vibrios are soon transformed into granules identical to those which Pfeiffer has observed in the peritoneal cavity of immunized guinea pigs when he injected a culture, and that which Metchnikoff has produced in vitro by mixing an emulsion of vibrios, a little preventive serum, and peritoneal exudate containing leucocytes. This granular transformation is the visible indicator of intense bactericidal action.

2. Serum warmed to 55° or kept for some time loses the property to transform the vibrios into granules, but it maintains the capability of clumping them. This clumping always occurs with preventive serum. It therefore can be very distinct in a serum previously stripped of its bactericidal power. . . .

3. If to anti-cholera serum previously heated to the mentioned temperature, and which consequently no longer transforms the vibrios into granules, but still clumps them, one adds fresh serum from a normal animal, the bactericidal power is restored to the preventive serum, that is, its capability to produce granules. And yet heated preventive serum lends itself well to the culture of the vibrio, and normal animal serum has only slight microbiocidal activity. The two constituents of the mixture are, when isolated, only slightly bactericidal; together, however, they attack the vibrio with great energy. Normal serum gives preventive serum that which heat had removed, but it is incapable of this restoration if itself was previously exposed to a temperature of 55°. It is remarkable that the addition of a very small quantity of preventive serum, intact or heated to 55–60°, is sufficient to endow normal serum with great microbiocidal activity. We concluded from these facts that the intense vibriocidal power present in immune serum was due to the combined action on the microbe of two highly distinct substances, the first being a property of the serum of immune organisms, endowed with specificity, capable of acting even in very reduced doses, and resistant to heat,—the sera which is responsible for

the phenomenon of clumping; the second, being present in normal as well as immunized animals, destroyed at 55°, nonspecific, and having only slight activity when not associated with the first substance. . . . Without abandoning ourselves to hypotheses on the intimate mechanism of the action of the two substances, we expressed the idea that probably the specific matter, by immobilizing the microbes and causing their gathering into masses, renders them more sensitive to the influence of the bactericidal substance (alexine) distributed in the serum of normal as well as immune animals.

One can easily then comprehend why the injection into normal animals of either fresh or previously heated anti-cholera serum causes the appearance of specific vibriocidal power in their serum: The specific substance joins the alexine already present in the body of normal animals. . . .

Other facts were soon added to those mentioned. . . . We also called attention in 1895 and subsequently to the fact that generally the serum of one animal will clump the red blood cells of an animal of a different species. . . . We have known for some time, thanks to the research of Professor Büchner, that a given serum possesses, sometimes very distinctly, the property of destroying the red blood cells of an animal of a different species by diffusing their hemoglobin and rendering them transparent. . . . Büchner has showed that a temperature of 55° will destroy this lethal power for red blood cells, the same temperature that abolishes the bactericidal power of serum. . . .

It is evident that there is a striking parallel between the modifications shown by the vibrios placed in contact with cholera serum and those which red blood cells manifest under the influence of serum from a foreign species. We verified that the clumping actions more or less active in the two cases is due to material resistant to heating at 55° or even more. One also observed that the destructive influences necessitate the presence of a susceptible substance which a temperature of 55° eliminates. . . .

When one immunizes an animal against the cholera vibrio, the original clumping and destructive powers of the serum is considerably increased. On account of the parallelism that we had indicated and on account of the analogies which we observed in the action of sera on cells and microbes, a question is posed. Would it be possible by repeatedly injecting normal animals with defibrinated blood of a different species to increase the clumping and destructive powers exercised by the serum on cells identical to that injected?

Experiments gave an affirmative reply. Guinea pigs received intraperitoneally five or six successive injections of 10 cc of defibrinated rabbit blood. . . . After a time their blood was withdrawn, and the collected serum presented the following characteristics:

1. When placed in contact with defibrinated rabbit blood, it clumps the red cells with great vigor. . . .

2. These aggregated cells subsequently undergo the phenomena of rapid and intense destruction. If one mixes, for example, one part of defibrinated rabbit blood to two or three parts of active serum, the mixture becomes red, clear and limpid within two or three minutes. Microscopically, nothing more than cellular stromata is seen in the fluid, more or less deformed, very transparent, without brightness, and indistinct.

3. If this active guinea pig serum is heated to 55° for half an hour, it loses the property of destroying rabbit corpuscles, but it strongly clumps them.

4. If to a mixture of defibrinated rabbit blood and of immune serum previously heated to 55° one adds a certain quantity of normal guinea pig or rabbit serum, one can demonstrate the phenomena of destruction in their entirety. The mixture becomes clear and red within minutes. Remarkably, the experiment succeeds perfectly if to the mixture of defibrinated normal rabbit blood and heated immune serum one adds fresh serum from the same rabbit. The corpuscles of this rabbit have thus become sensitive to their own alexine under the influence of a foreign clumping substance from a guinea pig treated with injections of the defibrinated blood.

5. Although it is true that active guinea pig serum loses its destructive property by heating at 55°, it would not be entirely accurate to say that defibrinated rabbit blood mixed in such a serum remains wholly intact. There is sufficient destruction of red blood cells to give the liquid a more or less red tint, although the destruction is slow and partial. This is due to fact that defibrinated blood contains not only corpuscles but also serum containing a certain amount of alexine, and we have seen that alexine from normal rabbits acts on the red cells of the same animal when the latter have been affected by the clumping substance of active serum. However, the proportion of alexine contained in

defibrinated rabbit serum is not sufficient to destroy the enormous quantity of red cells present. . . .

6. It goes without saying that the phenomena mentioned do not occur if one uses normal guinea pig serum instead of serum from guinea pigs subjected to frequent injections of defibrinated rabbit blood. . . .

7. Active guinea pig serum does not exert any influence on defibrinated normal guinea pig blood. It furthermore has no action on pigeon red blood cells. It strongly clumps rat and mouse corpuscles, but to the same degree as with normal guinea pig serum. . . .

8. If one injects a certain quantity (2 cc, for example) of defibrinated rabbit blood into the peritoneal cavity of treated guinea pigs (successively injected with rabbit blood), the introduced red cells are rapidly destroyed. The liquid withdrawn ten minutes later from the cavity is red and limpid. . . . When the injection is made in the peritoneal cavity of normal guinea pigs, the cells are not altered in the exudate and they are finally engulfed by the macrophages.

9. If rabbit blood plus a small amount of active serum previously heated to 55° is injected into the peritoneal cavity of a normal guinea pig, the same phenomenon of cell destruction is produced.

10. Such as can be expected, the active serum, which has so vigorous an effect on rabbit red cells, is toxic for this animal. A dose of 2 cc injected into the vein of an ear is fatal. . . .

The reader will have seized, without it being necessary to insist, how close an analogy there is between the action of anti-cholera serum with that of anti-red cell serum, as sketched in this brief note. It is suitable, from the previous pages whose description so much resembles that of specific cholera serum, to replace in the text the words "defibrinated blood" with "culture of vibrios" and the term "destruction of red cells" with the expression "transformation of vibrio granules."

The analogy is still more striking if one considers that the alexine active with red blood cells is very probably identical to that which transforms the vibrio into granules. . . .

What can be concluded from the group of analogies? It may be concluded that the properties which anti-cholera serum possesses have not been created by the body for merely an anti-infectious purpose, if we may so express it, but are due simply to initiate against the vibrio some preexisting functions that may be applied, if circumstances lend themselves, to some by no means dangerous elements, such as red blood cells. We can, in fact, inject into animals not just vibrios but very different corpuscles, red blood cells, incapable of constituting a serious danger for the organism, to obtain a serum that affects these bodies exactly as the cholera serum acts on the vibrio. These properties do not arise spontaneously to defend against microbe, any more than phagocytosis, the hub of immunity, does not owe its existence to the struggle against an infectious agent. One of the most significant conclusions that is derived from the work of Metchnikoff is that immunity is a special case of intracellular digestion. . . .

The physiological action of β-iminazolylethylamine (histamine)

1911 • Sir Henry H. Dale and Sir Patrick P. Laidlaw

Comment

The discovery of histamine and its physiological effects stemmed from a pharmacological and chemical examination of ergot. Ergot is the hard mycelial sclerotium of a fungus that infects

grains, especially rye. From the Middle Ages and to as late as 1926, the consumption of such affected rye produced massive epidemics of food poisoning, whose symptoms were either gangrenous or convulsive. The fungus had long been part of folk medicine, since a herbal of 1582 noted even then its ancient use by midwives to induce childbirth. In 1808 ergot entered the mainstream medicine first to promote labor through uterine contractions, but after its hazard to the child was recognized, then to stop postpartum bleeding. Chemical analysis of the drug began in 1907 with George Barger and F. H. Carr's extraction of an alkaloid mixture, which they called ergotoxine. Barger's pharmacological colleague Henry H. Dale (1875–1968), the senior author of the following milestone, examined ergotoxine, and discovered that it was an epinephrine antagonist, affecting the nervous system. Further purification by Arthur Stoll in 1918 yielded ergotamine, which, being free of major toxic contaminants, became part of the pharmacopoeia as a hemostatic and migraine treatment.

Dale was introduced to the powers of ergot when in 1907 he attended the International Congress of Physiology in Heidelberg. There he observed a demonstration given by a gynecologist in which the dialysate from ergot initiated a contraction of the isolated uterus horn of a cat. Dale suspected that putrefaction by contaminating bacteria had a part in the effect. He believed that ergot dialysate *per se* is inactive until enzymatically or chemically processed. Since microbial biochemistry was yet an undeveloped discipline, he tested the notion through chemical manipulation. Barger and Dale in 1910 derived and isolated histamine from ergot by the chemical decarboxylation of the amino acid histidine. They knew that the substance was "histamine," but used the long organic chemical name (β-iminazolylethylamine) to prevent any legal problem that might arise from a possible infringement of trademark rights of a drug with a somewhat similar name.

Dale was a foremost pharmacologist, who was awarded knighthood in 1932 and the Nobel Prize in 1936. He was also a leading scientific administrator: director of the National Institute for Medicine Research (NIMR) between 1928 and 1942; president of the Royal Society, the British Association for the Advancement of Science, and the Royal Society of Medicine; chairman of the Scientific Advisory Committee to the British cabinet during World War II; and director of the laboratories of the Royal Institution. He began his scientific education at Cambridge University in 1894, and took his medical training at St. Bartholomew's Hospital and at University College, London. Between 1904 and 1914, Dale worked at the Wellcome Physiology Research Laboratory, becoming its director in 1906. He never had a university appointment.

Dale was assisted in the physiological analysis of histamine by Sir Patrick P. Laidlaw (1881–1940). Also a graduate of Cambridge University, in 1904, Laidlaw had earned his M.D. with academic specialty in physiology at Guy's Hospital in London. In 1909 Dale offered him a post at the Wellcome laboratory, where they collaborated for four years. Laidlaw was already examining the physiological effects of ergot when he joined Dale to focus on histamine. In 1914 Laidlaw was appointed Sir William Dunn Lecturer in Pathology at Guy's Hospital. In 1922 he became a virologist at the National Institute of Medical Research, thanks again to Dale. In 1933 Laidlaw, Sir Christopher H. Andrewes, and Wilson Smith introduced the ferret as an experimental animal for research in influenza. Laidlaw became Deputy-Director of NIMR in 1936 and Head of its Department of Pathology and Bacteriology. Fellowship in the Royal Society came in 1927; he was knighted in 1935. Dale and Laidlaw observed the similarity between the physiological effects of histamine and the symptoms of anaphylaxis. Subsequent investigations in 1927, designed to exclude bacterial influence, showed histamine to be present in a variety of tissues in appropriate levels for target organs, but its storage in mast cells, basophils, and platelets would not be known until the early 1950s. Despite their warnings that other agents can produce similar effects, histamine was long assumed to be the main instrument of inflammation. We now know that it is only one of many.

For further information:

Beaven, M. A. 1976. Histamine. *New England Journal of Medicine* 294:30–36; 320–325.

Dale, H. H. 1941. Patrick Playfair Laidlaw 1881–1940. *Obituary Notices of Fellows of the Royal Society* 3:427–447.

Feldberg, W. S. 1970. Henry Hallett Dale 1875–1968. *Biographical Memoirs of Fellows of the Royal Society* 16:77–174.

Kazimierczak, W. and B. Diamant. 1978. Mechanisms of histamine release in anaphylactic and anaphylactoid reactions. *Progress in Allergy* 24:295–365.

Noah, J. W. 1964. Anaphylactic histamine release and the Schultz-Dale reaction. In: *Immunological Methods* (J. F. Ackroyd, editor). Blackwell Scientific Publications, Oxford. pp. 285–312.

The Paper*

β-iminazolylethylamine [histamine] is the amine which is produced when carbon dioxide is split off from histidine. It was first prepared synthetically by Windaus and Vogt [1907]. Recently [1910] Ackermann obtained a large yield of the base by submitting histidine to the action of putrefactive organisms. It has been shown that several of the amines thus related to amino acids possess marked physiological activity. The activity of β-iminazolylethylamine was discovered in the course of the investigation of ergot and its extract by G. Barger and one of us, who attributed this structure to a base which they obtained, and which in minute doses produced tonic contraction of the uterus. The synthetic substance, and the base produced by splitting off carbon dioxide from histidine by bacterial action or by chemical means, were found to have an identical action. . . .

All the experiments here described were made with β-iminazolylethylamine prepared from histidine by a chemical process. . . .

No conveniently short name being yet available we shall refer to the base in this paper as β-I. The

hydrochloride was used in all our physiological experiments, and weighed without allowance for the difference in molecular weight. . . .

The frog is but slightly affected by β-I. Injections of one to ten mg into the dorsal lymph-sac caused gaping movements of the lower jaw, succeeded by depression of the central nervous system for periods increasing with the dose, and the effect lasting for about 30 min after ten mg. . . .

In rodents the effects are very different in the case of intravenous and of subcutaneous injection. In a rabbit of medium size an injection of 2 mg intravenously (ear vein) caused marked prostration, the respiration became irregular and labored and the heartbeat intermittent and feeble. These effects passed off gradually and recovery took place if no further injection were given. . . .

In large guinea pigs, weighing 800–1000 g, injection of 0.5 mg into the external saphena vein caused death in a few minutes. The immediate effect was a marked respiratory impediment, resulting in violent but largely ineffective respiratory efforts. . . . Death was clearly due to asphyxia, evidently resulting from progressive obstruction to the respiration, sufficient in its early stages to prevent the exit of the air sucked into the lungs by the violent inspiratory spasms, and later becoming complete. . . . Preliminary injection of atropine, though it did not abolish the action, had decided protective value. . . .

It may be noted, at this point, that the symptoms and post-mortem condition in the guinea pig correspond in a suggestive manner with those described by several observers as the effects of poisoning in that animal by Witte's peptone, or by serum or other protein in the sensitized guinea pig ("anaphylactic shock"). . . .

When the injection is made subcutaneously much larger doses are easily tolerated, both by the rabbit and the guinea pig. 25 mg thus administered to a rabbit caused a gradual increase in rate of both heartbeat and respiration, the effect first becoming marked about 15 minutes after the injection. Defecation, with semi-fluid feces, and micturition occurred, and during the hour succeeding the onset of the symptoms the animal showed signs of prostration, with moderately deep narcosis. The attitude was sprawling, the head sunk on the table, the ears pale and cold. Recovery then set in, and in a few hours the animal was apparently normal.

In the cat the discrepancy between the effects of intravenous and subcutaneous injections was not so marked. Intravenous injections of two, four, eight and ten mg caused immediate vomiting and purging, profuse salivation, and labored respiration, with a subsequent period of collapse and light narcosis, increasing with the dose. . . .

---

*Dale, H. H. and P. P. Laidlaw. 1911. The physiological action of β-iminazolylethylamine. *Journal of Physiology* 41:318–344.

The effect of iminazolylethylamine on the arterial blood-pressure is complex and not easily interpreted. It not only varies in different species, but shows very wide variations in individuals of the same species, especially in rabbits. These variations appear altogether out of proportion to the small differences of experimental conditions, and it is probable that individual differences of sensitiveness are also concerned. . . .

It can be seen that a rise of pulmonary pressure, amounting to about 40 mm at its maximum, follows closely on the injection [0.5 mg i.v. into a cat], its commencement preceding that of the systemic fall by about two seconds. Since the action on the heart is but slight, this large rise of pulmonary pressure can be attributed to constriction of the pulmonary arterioles. . . .

The plethysmographic results . . . show clearly that the fall of arterial pressure is mainly due to a general vasodilation, in which the arterioles of the kidney do not participate . . . There is, therefore, no escape from the conclusion that β-I has a vasodilator effect

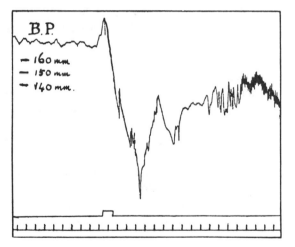

Figure 9   Rabbit. Urethane. Effect of 1 mg β-I on blood pressure.

when injected into the animal, a vasoconstrictor effect when perfused through isolated organs. In other words, the systemic arterioles respond to the drug, like most other plain muscle, by increase of tonus when isolated from the body. Their dilation in the body must, therefore, be attributed to some intermediate mechanism which does not survive excision and artificial perfusion. . . .

The action of β-iminazolylethylamine . . . appears a somewhat complicated one. It cannot be summarized with reference to any division of the autonomic system, like that of some other amines. The fundamental and characteristic feature of its action is its direct stimulant effect on plain muscle, in which it produces exaggeration of rhythm with increased tonus, or steady maximal tonus unbroken by rhythm, according to the concentration in which it is applied. The sensitiveness of plain muscle from different organs and in different species varies within wide limits. The most sensitive of all appears to be the plain muscle of the uterus: the nonpregnant uterus of some species responds to the drug in extreme dilution. The muscular coats of the bronchioles are also highly sensitive to the action, especially in rodents. The plain muscle of the intestinal wall, of the arterioles and of the spleen appears to occupy an intermediate position as regards responsiveness: that of the bladder and the iris was not perceptibly affected by the direct action of such doses as we employed. Cardiac muscle is mildly stimulated by the drug; skeletal muscles not perceptibly affected any way. . . .

Biedle and Kraus drew attention to the identity of the symptoms of anaphylactic shock with those produced by intravenous injection of "peptone", which, as we have seen are again very largely identical with those of β-I. The correspondence cannot yet be regarded as sufficient basis for theoretical speculation, and we content ourselves with recording, as a point of interest and possible significance, the fact that the immediate symptoms with which an animal responds to an injection of a normally inert protein, to which it has been sensitized, are to a large extent those of poisoning by β-iminazolylethylamine.

Interferon

1957 • Alick Isaacs and Jean Lindenmann

Comment

Interferon sounds as if it is a character in a science fiction thriller, and the therapeutic agent did in fact make an appearance in a "Flash Gordon" comic strip three years after its discovery. Despite the initial favorable and hopeful reviews in the medical literature, interferon has yet to be placed on the pharmacist's shelf.

What is interferon actually, and why has it not met expectations? The short answer is that interferon is an anti-viral agent synthesized by various host cells in response to an initial infection, and its clinical problems are side effects and an efficacy less than predicted by tissue culture and animal experiments. The long answer begins in 1937 with the work of George W. M. Findlay and F. O. MacCallum, who observed that monkeys infected with Rift Valley fever virus resisted the fatal, antigenically distinct, yellow fever virus. Reports of interference among other viruses appeared, and in 1943 Werner and Gertrude Henle discovered that ultraviolet- or heat-killed viruses are still able to interfere with secondary inoculations of live viruses. The scientific literature was soon filled with speculations on mechanisms for this transient form of viral immunity that apparently involved neither antibody nor phagocyte. The discovery and premier analysis of the agent came in 1957 with Alick Isaacs (1921–1967) and Jean Lindenmann (1924–   ).

Isaacs saw the outbreak of World War II as a medical freshman at the University of Glasgow. An outstanding student, he became a researcher in the Department of Bacteriology between 1945 and 1947, making numerous contributions to diagnostic microbiology. A traineeship next took him to the University of Sheffield, where he began investigations of influenza. In 1948 he received another fellowship, which brought him to Sir Macfarlane Burnet at the Hall Institute in Melbourne. Isaac now examined the viral interference phenomenon with Margaret Edney, hypothesizing incorrectly that it was due to competition for a key cellular constituent. He returned to England in 1951 for an appointment in the World Influenza Center Laboratory at the National Institute for Medical Research (NIMR). In 1954 he received his M.D., and in 1961 he was promoted to Head of the Division of Bacteriology and Virus Research at NIMR. Fellowship in the Royal Society came in 1966, a year before his untimely death.

Lindenmann came to NIMR in 1956 from the Institute of Hygiene at the University of Zurich on a Swiss fellowship. A research microbiologist, he shared an interest in viral interference with Isaacs, who invited him to join his laboratory. Lindenmann returned to Zurich at the end of his travel grant, but then went to the University of Bern, followed by a professorship at Florida State University. He then returned to the University of Zurich, this time at the Institute for Medical Virology.

When Isaacs and Lindenmann isolated the immune factor from the culture supernatant of chicken chorio-allantoic membranes inoculated with heat-killed influenza virus, Lindenmann offered in jest the name interferon. Everyone liked it. Fibroblast interferon, now designated IFN-β, has been joined by macrophage inferferon IFN-α, and T cell interferon IFN-γ, all differing in acid stability and other properties. Among these three families are over 20 distinct interferons. Mechanisms of their induction and function have for two decades been the major research goal, clinical application being economically and technologically prohibitive because of the difficulty of large-scale production. Still, much was learned. For instance, in some systems viruses are not even needed to elicit interferon! Synthetic double-stranded RNA, bacterial lipopolysaccharide, the plastic polyvinylsulfate, and the antibiotic kanamycin are all examples of inducers. Although the agent restricts all viruses, it is generally host-specific. This means that chicken interferon induced by influenza virus will prevent multiplication of unrelated viruses in the chicken, but will have no effect on the replication of influenza virus in the ferret. Secreted interferons do not themselves destroy viruses; rather, they serve as derepressors or initiators of two enzymes, the first leading to a blockage of viral mRNA transcription, and the second indirectly activating ribonucleases. The net result is that the viral nucleic acid can not be replicated and is soon degraded. Less than ten interferon molecules can render a cell resistant. Interferon, furthermore, activates NK (natural killer) cells and modulates the immune response by curtailing lymphocyte proliferation. Interferon may also have a more general regulatory function, with viral immunity being a fortuitous result.

By the 1950s, antibiotics had significantly lowered the mortality rate from infectious disease but the statistics of cancer were rising alarmingly. Certain cancers, including non-viral-induced tumors, are similarly affected by interferon. Isaacs, considering this exciting, medically and sociologically important application, faced the gauntlet of disbelievers. Another problem was that technology then could not surmount the great problems of mass production and purification of human interferon. The first trials using only 1 percent pure human interferon were promising, and side effects seemed minor. After a long series of setbacks, sufficient human interferon from white blood cells was harvested for larger-scale clinical studies. Kari Cantell at the Central Public Health Laboratories in Helsinki had devised a suitable method using affinity chromatography, but it was expensive. However, with the prospect of controlling cancer, funding rapidly

became available. For example, in 1978 the American Cancer Society allocated $2 million for the purchase of 40 billion units, which could treat only some 150 patients. By this time, the recombinant DNA revolution was taking effect, and budding biotechnology companies were cloning human interferon genes into bacteria for efficient production of the agent, betting that interferon would be worth the investment of research and development. The early results are mixed: interferon nosedrops do appear to help prevent rather than cure colds, but the agent is not the cancer panacea.

For further information:

Andrewes, C. H. 1967. Alick Isaacs 1921–1967. *Biographical Memoirs of Fellow of the Royal Society* 13:205–221.

Ho, M. and J. A. Armstrong. 1975. Interferon. *Annual Review of Microbiology* 29:131–161.

Isaacs, A. 1961. Interferon. *Scientific American* 204(5):51–57.

Panem, S. 1984. *The Interferon Crusade*. Brookings Institution, Washington, D.C., 109 p.

Steward, W. E. II. 1981. *The Interferon System*. Second edition. Springer-Verlag, Wien. 493 p.

The Paper*

One of the most useful situations for studying interference among animal viruses has been the interference produced by inactivated influenza viruses with the growth of live influenza virus in the chorioallantoic membrane of the chick embryo. In this system, a number of variables have been measured, e.g., the effects of varying the dose of interfering and challenge virus or the time interval between the two inoculations, the effects of different methods of virus inactivation and the use of different virus strains. As a result of studies by different workers, it is generally agreed that interference cannot be explained

*Isaacs, A. and J. Lindenmann. 1957. Virus interference. I. The interferon. *Proceedings of the Royal Society, London*. Biology. 147:258–267. [With permission of the Society.]

by blockage of cell surface receptors. Fazekas de St. Groth, Isaacs, and Edney found that interference by influenza virus inactivated at 56°C took some hours until it was fully established, but it was difficult to decide by experiments in the intact chick embryo whether this time was required for the inactivated virus to be absorbed by the cells or for some further reactions to occur. We have studied this point with pieces of chorio-allantoic membrane suspended in buffered salt solution in vitro, a method which allows observation of fluid and cells separately and manipulations which are not possible in the chick embryo. As a result, a number of new features of the interference reaction have emerged. . . .

The Melbourne strain of influenza virus A was used as freshly harvested allantoic fluid. It was mixed with 2% sodium citrate solution in normal saline and borate buffer, pH 8.5, in the ratio 6 parts virus, 2 parts citrate-saline and 1 part borate buffer, and heated at 56°C for 1 hr. This treatment abolished the infectivity and enzymic activity of the virus while retaining its interfering activity. . . . The heated virus is referred to as heated MEL. . . .

An interference experiment was carried out in the following way: Six pieces of membrane were placed in $6 \times 5/8$ inch test-tubes, and to each was added 1 ml of test material. Six other tubes were similarly incubated with 1 ml buffer. In each case 100 units of penicillin were added per ml fluid. The tubes were stoppered and placed in a roller drum at 37°C (8 rev/hr). After 24 hr incubation the membranes were removed, washed in two changes of buffer and put in fresh tubes along with 1 ml buffer in which MEL virus at a final dilution of 10^{-3} was incorporated. . . . The tubes were placed in the roller drum for a further 48 hr at 37°C after which the fluids were titrated individually for their haemagglutinin content. . . .

In preliminary experiments it was found that interference could be induced in pieces of chorio-allantoic membrane in the following way. Heat-inactivated MEL virus was added to the suspending fluid along with a piece of membrane, and this was then incubated in the roller drum for 24 hr at 37°C; controls were incubated in buffer. The membranes were then washed, placed in fresh tubes with live MEL viruses diluted 10^{-3} in 1 ml buffer, and incubated for a further 40 to 48 hr at 37°C. Previous treatment of the membranes with heated MEL in this way caused pronounced interference with the growth of live MEL. In this system, 200 to 400 agglutinating doses of heated MEL almost completely suppressed haemagglutinin production by live virus. . . .

It was soon found that the time interval between the application of interfering and challenge viruses

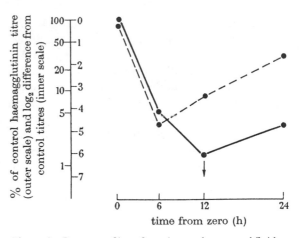

Figure 1   Presence of interferon in membranes and fluids; solid line—fluids, dashed line—membrane extracts.

had an influence on the degree of interference. In order to see what was the importance of the time interval, the following experiment was carried out. Pieces of membrane were mixed with a small dose of heated MEL virus in order to produce slight interference, and at varying time intervals, groups of membranes were removed, washed thoroughly in buffer, resuspended in buffer and further incubated either at 2 or 37°C. The total incubation time was 24 hr and this was divided between a primary incubation period in contact with heated MEL at 37°C and a secondary incubation period of the washed membranes at 2 or 37°C. After the secondary incubation, the membranes were again washed and challenged with MEL virus. . . . The results show that a primary period of 15 min contact between heated MEL and the membrane was sufficient to establish nearly as much interference as a primary period of 24 hr at 37°C, provided the secondary incubation was carried out at 37°C. The finding suggests that the heated MEL virus is rapidly adsorbed to the cells, and thereafter that it does not act as an inert blocking agent. The fact that after 4 hr primary incubation there is a slight difference in interference, depending on whether secondary incubation is carried out at 2 or 37°C, implies that some active metabolic process in the membrane requiring at least 4 hr incubation at 37°C is necessary before interference is fully established. . . .

Incidental observations had pointed to some instability of the interfering activity of heated MEL during incubation at 37°C. . . . [T]he interfering activity of heated MEL virus was reduced about tenfold by incubating it for 24 hr at 37°C before adding the membranes. . . .

When an attempt was made to measure the amount of unabsorbed heated MEL virus after varying times of contact with chorio-allantoic membrane, a difficulty was soon encountered. Apparent rapid "disappearance" of the haemagglutinin was found to be caused by combination of the virus with an inhibitor of agglutination released by the membrane into the surrounding fluid. This could be shown by incubating pieces of membrane with buffer at 37°C in the roller drum, when after 2 hr sufficient inhibitor of agglutination was released by the membrane into the surrounding fluid to block agglutination by an equal volume of heated MEL virus with an agglutinin titer of 100. . . .

An experiment was carried out to see what effect this membrane inhibitor might have on the interfering activity of heated MEL. A sample of inhibitor was prepared by incubating normal membranes in buffer. Heated MEL virus was then tested for its interfering activity diluted in this membrane extract or in buffer as a control; also, interfering activity was tested by adding the membranes to these reagents at once, or after the two preparations of heated MEL had been incubated for 4 hr at 37°C. . . . [T]he membrane extract had a pronounced inhibitory effect on the interfering activity of heated MEL. Also, the degree of instability of the interfering activity of heated MEL during 4 hr incubation at 37°C was not affected by the presence or absence of membrane inhibitor.

These experiments have indicated that the interfering virus is rapidly taken up by the cells, although interference in the cells takes some time to be established. One would expect, too, that in these experiments little interfering activity would remain in the fluid after 24 hr contact between heated MEL and the membrane, since any unabsorbed virus would lose interfering potency as a result of inactivation at 37°C and combination with inhibitor. It was surprising, therefore, to find that after 24 hr incubation considerable interfering activity remained in the surrounding fluid. . . .

In an effort to explain the results of the last experiment the possibility was considered that fresh interfering activity was produced by the membrane. This possibility was confirmed by the following experiment. Heated MEL virus was incubated with pieces of membrane for 2 hr at 37°C. The membranes were then thoroughly washed and incubated in fresh buffer at 37°C. It was found that after some hours' incubation at 37°C fresh interfering activity could be detected in the incubating fluid. . . . [T]he newly released interfering agent is a non-haemagglutinating macro-molecular particle which has many different properties from those of heated influenza virus. To distinguish it from the heated influenza virus we have called the newly released interfering agent "interferon." It was also found that the mem-

branes which were liberating "interferon" showed a diminished production of MEL virus on challenge, i.e. establishment of interference was accompanied by liberation of interferon.

We next studied the appearance of interferon in the membranes and its liberation into the surrounding medium at different time-intervals after inoculating heated MEL virus. . . .

Pieces of chorio-allantoid membrane were mixed with a large dose of heated MEL (4000 agglutinating doses/membrane piece) and incubated in the roller drum for 3 hr at 37°C. The membranes were then removed, washed thoroughly in buffer, resuspended in fresh test-tubes with 1 ml of buffer/membrane piece and reincubated at 37°C. The end of this time was taken as zero hour and at various time intervals thereafter groups of tubes were removed, and the fluids and membranes tested separately for interferon activity. . . . The fluids and membrane extracts tested at 0 hr showed no interfering activity, although the membranes had absorbed large amounts of heated MEL virus, and would themselves probably have been resistant to challenge as shown by control experiments. At 6 hr there was a high degree of interferon activity in the membrane extracts and slightly less in the fluids. The greatest interfering activity in the fluids was found at 12 hr. . . . At 24 hour there was little remaining activity in the membrane extracts and most of the interferon had been liberated into the medium. . . .

In another experiment, the differential release of interferons into the fluid was studied. Heated MEL and membranes were kept 2 hr in contact at 37°C and the membranes were then washed and incubated in buffer. At two-hourly intervals thereafter the membranes were removed, washed and incubated in fresh buffer; all the manipulations were carried out with warm reagents and at 37°C. . . .

The maximal liberation of interferon occurred between the second and sixth hours. The yield of interferon was much smaller at each interval, largely due to the fact that the total yield was divided among so many samples. . . .

The amount of interferon produced depends on the amount of heated MEL used. . . . [I]nterferon production is also dependent on the possession of interfering activity by the heated MEL. It is based on the fact that MEL virus heated for 1 hr at 56°C had strong interfering activity, whereas the same virus heated for 1 hr at 60°C had no significant interfering activity. . . .

The results obtained have not made it clear whether interferon is part of the heated MEL virus which is liberated by the membrane, or whether it is newly synthesized in the membrane. In either event it was interesting to test the possibility that interferon might be able to replicate in series. In order to test this, advantage was taken of the fact that interferon exerts its activity if it is left in contact with the membranes for 4 hr at 37°C, and the membranes are then washed and incubated in buffer for a further 20 hr at 37°C before challenge. Under these conditions no new interferon activity could be detected in ground membranes or in the medium after a single passage or after two serial passages. Controls showed that the interferon grown in eggs or tissue cultures did not produce live virus. . . .

The present results suggest . . . that interference shows some of the characters we might expect of an abortive attempt at a single cycle of virus multiplication. A second finding which supports this idea (in addition to the fact that interference requires some metabolic activity on the part of the membrane) is that the interfering action of heated MEL is inactivated during incubation at 37°C to approximately the same extent as is the infectivity of unheated virus. But the best support for the idea arises if we consider the interferon provisionally as an abortive product of virus multiplication. . . .

Mediation of delayed hypersensitivity by cell-free substances

1966 • John R. David

Comment

Science has often chronicled bitter rivalries and polemics centered on priority of discovery, but such vanities would not affect the independent investigators John R. David and Barry R. Bloom. They were on intersecting research paths using the same technical advance to produce related data. They also simultaneously reached the same conclusion: immune lymphoid cells stimulated by their corresponding antigen secrete a substance that inhibits the migration of macrophages, a characteristic of delayed hypersensitivity. Although the work of David is next featured as representative, both researchers share the honor of discovery.

John David, born in England in 1930, received his Bachelor of Arts from the University of Chicago in 1951, and continued there for B.S. and M.D. diplomas four years later. He interrupted his clinical training at Massachusetts General Hospital with studies at the National Institute of Arthritis and Metabolic Diseases between 1957 and 1959 and the following year in England at the Rheumatism Research Unit. In 1964 he joined the medical faculty of New York University, but transferred to Harvard Medical School, where he became Professor of Medicine and Tropical Public Health.

His competitor Barry Bloom, younger by seven years, graduated from Amherst College in 1958. After earning the Ph.D. in immunology at Rockefeller University in 1963 under the guidance of Merrill Chase, Bloom spent a year as a fellow at the Wright-Fleming Institute in London. The Albert Einstein College of Medicine has been his academic home; he advanced to Professor of Cell Biology, Microbiology, and Immunology in 1973 and chairman in 1980.

What sparked their famous investigations was the development of a remarkably simple and literally graphic in vitro method to demonstrate cellular immunity. In 1961 Mariam George and John H. Vaughn at the University of Rochester were examining the thirty-year old observations of Arnold Rice Rich and Margaret Reed Lewis on fragments of spleens and separated white blood cells of guinea pigs that were immunized against the tubercle bacillus. Upon culturing, cells would migrate from the fragments, spreading along the vessel wall. However, when tubercle antigen was introduced, the phenomenon would not occur; the wandering cells remained localized. Sera from immunized animals mixed with normal, nonactivated cells in the presence or absence of tuberculin had no inhibiting effect. George and Vaughn withdrew peritoneal exudate cells from guinea pigs using capillary tubes. They next centrifuged the tubes and broke them at the interphase of cells and fluid. When placed in culture medium without antigen for 18 to 20 hours, cells left the capillary, extending out as a fan. When antigen was present, only a confined bulbous concentration would be seen. The extent of inhibition was measured by calculating—using photographs—the proportional difference in cellular area between unstimulated controls and stimulated test preparations.

David began his study on advice of Lewis Thomas, who had visited Vaughan and obtained the still unpublished manuscript. When David and his associates confirmed the results with a modified technique, they urged George and Vaughn to submit the original work to a journal. At a meeting of the Federation of American Societies of Experimental Biology, where he presented his data, David met Bloom for breakfast and imparted to him some of the technical arts of the method. Both recognized that inhibition of migration could be correlated with delayed hypersensitivity. Whether the effect was strictly cellular or mediated by a soluble factor was the immediate question to be answered. David had his solution by January 1966, but decided not to report it at a winter immunology conference until he had performed further supportive experiments. Several months later at another FASEB meeting, Bloom presented his own results. David later remarked that he "never held back anything like that since."

After determining that a secreted factor was indeed involved, both researchers began to characterize the agent, which they called migration inhibitory factor (MIF). David found MIF unable to pass through a dialyzing membrane, indicating a molecular weight of over 10,000 daltons. He further concluded that the agent was not preformed, since treatment of splenic cells with the antibiotic puromycin, an inhibitor of protein synthesis, would block any retardation of cellular movement. Bloom and his associates, by separating the cellular populations, clearly established that lymphocytes produced the factor and that macrophages were its target. They noted inhibition using antigen-sensitized lymphocytes and normal macrophages. When antigen was introduced and maintained, the factor could be detected within 4 to 6 hours and as long as 4 days afterward.

Later research countered the doctrine that stimulation by a specific antigen was necessary for the effect. Lymphocytes that were activated by mitogens, such as concanavalin A and purified protein derivative of tuberculin (PPD), could synthesize and release the factor, and such agents have been used as positive controls. Remarkably, MIF is not species specific despite some chemical differences: human MIF is a protein resistant to neuraminidase, while guinea pig MIF is a glycoprotein susceptible to that enzyme, yet human or mouse MIF can act on guinea pig macrophages. MIF seems to affect glycolipid sites on macrophage membranes, causing stickiness and permitting cohesion and clumping of the cells.

Here then was the first indication that soluble factors regulate immunity and serve in intercellular communication. While macrophages seem to process large particulate antigens for presentation to lymphocytes, and helper T cells and B cells also interact directly, migration inhibition is action at a distance. Dividing clones of lymphocytes, responding to the presence of antigen, signal macrophages to stop their amoeboid wanderings. Soon a host of other molecule mediators, dubbed lymphokines by D. C. Dumonde, were discovered. Among them is macrophage chemotactic factor, which directs the phagocytes to the area of its greatest concentration. The macrophage in turn secretes mediators that influence both T and B cells. David and Bloom laid the first strands of a chemical and cellular immunological network. Their friendly rivalry developed into a true friendship, and both have served on a WHO committee on the immunology of tuberculosis.

For further information:

Bloom, B.R. 1971. In vitro approaches to the mechanism of cell-mediated immune reactions. *Advances in Immunology* 13:101–208.

Melnick, H. D. 1971. Inhibition of macrophage migration and the mediation of cellular immunity: a review. *Annals of Allergy* 29:195–208.

The Paper*

It has long been thought that delayed hypersensitivity is mediated by cells or cell-associated substances. In an attempt to investigate the mechanism of delayed hypersensitivity, in vitro studies using the inhibition of cell migration by specific antigen as an assay have been carried out. In this in vitro system, it has been shown that peritoneal exudate cells taken from guinea pigs exhibiting delayed hypersensitivity and placed in capillary tubes are inhibited from migration by specific antigen. Moreover, when mixed populations of normal and sensitive cells were prepared, it was observed that if as few as 2.5 per cent of the cells in a population were from a sensitive animal, the whole population (97.5% normal cells) would be inhibited by antigen.

The results of recent experiments suggest that the lymphocyte is the specifically sensitive cell in this system. . . . It is of note that such sensitive lymphoid cells, when assayed alone in culture, are not themselves inhibited from migrating by antigen.

Experiments were initiated in an attempt to determine the manner by which these sensitive lymphoid cells achieved their effect. These results, where reported, demonstrate that, following incubation of sensitive lymphoid cells with specific antigen for 24 hr, a nondialyzable substance is detected in the cell-free supernatants which inhibits the migration of normal peritoneal cells.

The antigens used were ovalbumin and o-chlorobenzoyl chloride conjugated to bovine gamma globulin (OCBC-BGG). . . .

Twelve to twenty-one days after sensitization axillary, inguinal and popliteal lymph nodes were obtained aseptically from guinea pigs. . . . The nodes were diced into tissue culture medium. . . . The suspension was allowed to stand for 4 min so that the tissue fragments settled by gravity. The supernatant was then removed to a fresh tube. After three such settlings the cell suspensions were essentially free of tissue fragments. The preparations contained 90–95% lymphocytes by Wright's stain and phase microscopy. Suspensions were adjusted to a final concentration of 1.8×10^7 cells per ml. Aliquots of these suspensions were made to contain ovalbumin, or OCBC-BGG 100 μg/ml. Suspensions not containing antigen were also prepared. In each experiment, suspensions were incubated in specific antigen and an unrelated antigen. . . .

Peritoneal cells from normal guinea pigs were induced by oil and collected. . . . Capillary tubes were filled with this suspension, sealed with wax, and centrifuged. The tubes were cut, and the portion containing the packed cells was placed in Macaness type chambers, two tubes per chamber. In each experiment at least two to three chambers were prepared for each media to be tested. The media include supernate from sensitive lymphoid cells incubated with (1) specific antigen, (2) unrelated antigen, (3) without antigen; tissue culture media containing (4) specific antigen, (5) unrelated antigen, and (6) without antigen. The concentration of antigen was 100 μg/ml. It should be noted that where OCBC-BGG was the sensitizing or specific antigen, OCBC-BGG was the unrelated. Chambers were incubated for 24 hr, and the area of migration was measured by planimetry. . . . In calculating the data from these experiments, the following formula was used:

$$\frac{\text{Average area of migration in supernatant with antigen}}{\text{Average area of migration in media with the same antigen}} \times 100 = \%\ \text{migration}$$

Cell-free supernatants from sensitive lymph node cells incubated 24 hr with specific antigen produced inhibition of migration of normal peritoneal exudate cells. In contrast, supernatants from the same cells incubated with an unrelated antigen, or incubated without antigen, had no effect.

In 14 experiments the average migration of normal peritoneal exudate cells in supernatants prepared with specific antigen was 52 per cent as compared to migration in control media containing the same antigen. The average migration on normal cells

---

*David, J. R. 1966. Delayed hypersensitivity in vitro: its mediation by cell-free substances formed by lymphoid cell-antigen interaction. *Proceedings of the National Academy of Sciences (USA)* 56:72–77. [By permission.]

in supernatants prepared with unrelated antigen was 97 per cent. In eight additional experiments, the total area of migration was not significantly inhibited; however, there was marked clumping of cells migrating in supernatants prepared with specific antigen, which was reminiscent of the effects of antigen on sensitive cells when added after 24 hr of incubation in normal media. This clumping may be a qualitative expression of the same phenomenon as inhibition of migration and a function of the amount of active material present. If the specific supernatant is diluted 1:5 or 1:10, the effect is abolished.

The possibility that sensitive lymphoid cells incubated without antigen produced cell-free substances which would subsequently interact with antigen and inhibit the migration of normal peritoneal exudate cells was investigated. Lymphoid cells from guinea pigs with delayed hypersensitivity to OCBC-BGG were incubated without antigen, with OCBC-BGG, and with ovalbumin. After 24 hr the cells were removed by centrifugation and the supernatants passed through Millipore filters. OCBC-BGG was added to half of the supernatant from the group of sensitive cells incubated without antigen. In three experiments, normal peritoneal exudate cells migrated normally in the supernatants to which the specific antigen had been added *after* 24 hr. The average migration was 106 per cent. In contrast, the same cells were inhibited by the supernatant which had been prepared by adding OCBC-BGG before the start of incubation, migrating an average of only 51 per cent. Supernatant obtained from cells incubated for 24 hr with ovalbumin, an unrelated antigen, had no effect; the average migration in these chambers was 101 per cent. . . .

[T]he dialyzed and nondialyzed supernatants prepared with specific antigen were equally effective in inhibiting the migration of normal cells. . . .

In three experiments, supernatants prepared with specific antigen were divided into two aliquots, and one portion heated to 56°C for 30 min. It was found that normal peritoneal cells were still inhibited by the heated supernatants.

In two experiments, sensitive lymphoid cells were exposed to 5 μg/ml puromycin during 24 hr of incubation with specific antigen; control sensitive cells were incubated in specific antigen alone. After 24 hr the cells were removed by centrifugation and the supernatants dialyzed over 24 hr to remove puromycin. The supernatants were assayed for their effect on normal cell migration. The results showed that exposure to puromycin during incubation abolished the ability of supernatants prepared with specific antigen to inhibit normal cell migration; cells migrated normally in these supernatants, averaging 100 per cent. On the other hand, supernatants prepared with specific antigen, but not exposed to puromycin, inhibited the migration of normal cells. The average migration was 54 per cent in one experiment, and marked clumping was observed in the other.

The data presented here indicate that sensitive lymphoid cells during incubation with specific antigen elaborate a soluble substance into the media which inhibits the migration of normal peritoneal exudate cells. This material is not detected in supernatants from lymph node cells incubated with an unrelated antigen, or incubated without antigen, thus suggesting that the production or release of this material is the result of a specific immunologic reaction.

The most attractive interpretation of these findings is that specifically sensitive lymphocytes are stimulated to form inhibitory substances by antigen. Another interpretation could be that the substances are normally produced when the cells are incubated without antigen; but in the presence of antigen, complexes are formed which inhibit the migration of normal cells. Evidence against this interpretation is the finding that the supernatants are ineffective when antigen is added after 24 hr of incubation without antigen. It is not known whether the material stimulated by antigen inhibits the migration of normal peritoneal cells of itself or whether the continued presence of antigen is necessary. . . .

The results of experiments with puromycin provide additional evidence that the lymphocytes are actively synthesizing material(s) in response to antigen. In this group of experiments, it was found that the presence of puromycin during the incubation of sensitive lymphoid cells with antigen resulted in supernatants which had no effect on normal cells. The results are in agreement with earlier studies where puromycin was shown to prevent the inhibition of migration of sensitive peritoneal cells by antigen and this effect correlated with inhibition of protein synthesis by puromycin. . . .

It should be noted that cells destroyed [by puromycin] did not release substances into the media which inhibited the migration of normal cells. This result provides further evidence against the existence of preformed inhibitory materials.

Previous attempts to detect cell-free substances which would inhibit the migration of normal cells from sensitive peritoneal exudate cells (approximately 20% lymphocytes) have been unsuccessful. These experiments were repeated with sensitive lymph node cells (approximately 95% lymphocytes). . . . A possible explanation for failures to produce this effect with sensitive peritoneal cells may be that the material produced by the lymphocytes in the sensitive peritoneal populations is immediately taken up by the surrounding macrophages and little

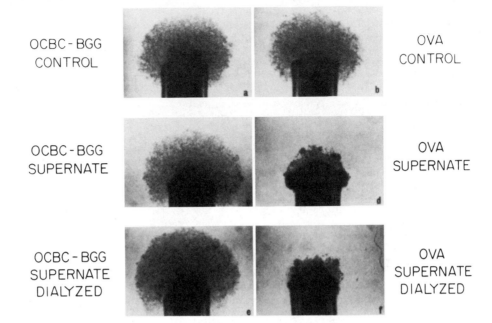

Figure 1 Effect of supernatants from ovalbumin-sensitive lymph node cells incubated with specific and unrelated antigens on the migration of normal peritoneal exudate cells. (*a*) Normal peritoneal cells in media containing OCBC-BGG. (*b*) Normal cells migrating in media containing ovalbumin. (*c*) Normal cells migrating in supernatant from ovalbumin-sensitive lymph node cells incubated with OCBC-BGG. (*d*) Normal cells inhibited by supernatants from ovalbumin-sensitive lymph node cells incubated with ovalbumin. (*e*) Same as (*c*) except that supernatant was dialyzed for 24 hr. (*f*) Same as (*d*) except that supernatant was dialyzed for 24 hr. Peritoneal cells in all photographs came from the same pool.

diffuses out into the media. In contrast, the material appears readily to diffuse away from populations containing a majority of lymphocytes.

Recently, an abstract by Bloom and Bennett has appeared describing experiments using lymphocytes from peritoneal exudates obtained from animals sensitive to PPD [purified protein derivative of tuberculin]. Supernatants of these cells incubated with PPD inhibited the migration of normal peritoneal cells, whereas sensitive lymphocytes incubated without antigen or normal cells incubated with PPD had no effect.

The data available suggest an explanation of the phenomenon of inhibition of peritoneal cell migration by specific antigen. The first event may be the reaction of specifically sensitive lymphocytes in the population of antigen. This interaction results in the production of substances that, either alone or in combination with antigen, affect the remaining nonsensitive cells, presumably macrophages, to inhibit the migration of the whole population.

It is of interest that mixed populations containing 20 percent sensitive peritoneal cells and 80 per cent normal peritoneal cells are inhibited by antigen; in contrast, other populations containing 20 per cent of the same sensitive peritoneal cells and 80 per cent normal spleen cells are not inhibited by specific antigen. Furthermore, sensitive lymphoid cells themselves are not inhibited by specific antigen. These findings suggest that two cell types are important in these reactions, sensitive lymphocytes and cells from the peritoneal exudate, presumably macrophages, which need not be sensitive. . . .

Part 7
Immunogenetics

Am not I consanguineous? Am I not of her blood? —William Shakespeare, *Twelfth Night*

Perpetual in perpetual change,
The unknown passing through the strange. —John Masefield

How appropriate it is to begin this section with investigations of the blood. The science of heredity, whose roots reach back to the domestication of animals and the breeding of livestock, once regarded blood as the purveyor and symbol of life, of individuality and of familial relationships. We speak of bloodlines, blood brothers, and talents being in the blood. Immunology, however, has treated blood as merely another physiological tissue, whose cells and fluids help provide resistance to environmental intruders and maintain the integrity of self. Blood cells in Hans Büchner and Jules Bordet's studies on immune hemolysis were merely tools of inquiry, since they served as test systems for antibodies and complement. Short of the recognition of antigenic differences between species and the minor individual variation in antibody production and susceptibility to pathogens, heredity simply was not considered important. Then came Paul Ehrlich and Karl Landsteiner, who discovered that red blood cells of individuals can differ antigenically. Soon familial and racial traits in blood types were discovered. Blood remained a tool, but now it was a touchstone of genetics, which is a study of biological creation, change, and development.

Three milestones cover this foundation. The leader is Landsteiner's elegant, definitive report on blood groups. By simply mixing serum and erythrocytes from different persons and comparing their pattern of reactions, he could classify blood into three groups. The occurrence of agglutination indicated the existence of natural or preexisting antibodies against foreign blood groups. Those with group A blood cells had antibodies to group B cells; those with group B blood cells reacted with group A cells; and the serum of group C people agglutinated erythrocytes of both group A and B people. Today group C is known as group O. The fourth group, AB, was discovered a year later, and these rare individuals lack both isotypic agglutinating antibodies. Landsteiner's work led to a reduction in the risk of blood transfusions, which had previously and unpredictably resulted in toxic shock. At the same time, it provided both a scientific explanation and a method for determining transfusion compatibility. The life-saving procedure of blood transfusion, first described in the seventeenth century but rarely attempted, soon became routine. The legal profession also was quick to take advantage of this new tool of biological identification, such as in determining the species of an unknown blood stain or in helping solve the questioned parentage of a child.

The first four blood groups to be discovered did not distinguish individuals, but with the addition of the minor erythrocyte antigens, individualistic sets emerged. Fortunately, these minor blood groups rarely are a problem in transfusion. However, blood incompatibility in the special yet common circumstance of the Rh antigen can be fatal, and is the theme of the next report by Philip Levine and his colleagues. It concerns how one self accepts or rejects another self within its territory, specifically how an Rh negative mother becomes sensitized to and subsequently kills an Rh positive fetus developing within her. The disease is erythroblastosis fetalis, and the milestone established its immunological origin. Levine's team knew that, like ABO blood groups, the Rh antigen was inherited by Mendelian processes, but the underlying genetic mechanisms were unknown.

M. Robert Irwin is the geneticist who first attempted to determine the genetic control of antigenicity through traditional techniques, such as genetic cross matings. He also introduced the term immunogenetics to describe the union of the two sciences. His report analyzing blood antigens in species of birds and their hybrids opened the doors of chromosome mapping and comparison of alleles, and ushered in studies on the origin and expression of characteristic antigens. On investigating this antigenic correlation of species, he discovered the creation of a hybrid-specific antigen and the interaction of genes.

Irwin, as a geneticist, focuses on immunology as a tool. Other immunogeneticists have been immunologists who applied methods of genetics to advantage. The next four milestones describe the clinical problem of tissue transplantation. Although analogous to blood transfusion, the immune mechanisms are different, being mainly T cell- rather than B cell-mediated. The paper of Peter A. Gorer, besides being a pioneer work on the subject, nicely ties together the previous reports with this next set of papers, since he first determined the blood groups of mouse strains to obtain immunological markers of genetic individuality. He investigated the variable resistance of individuals to tumors, and discovered that one strain that was especially susceptible to injected tumor cells possessed a certain blood antigen, which was later found on other normal and cancerous cells. It was the first histocompatibility antigen, H-2, and its controlling genes soon described the major histocompatibility complex of mice.

Sir Peter Medawar, under the emergency of World War II, examined transplantation of normal tissues in burn patients and then in rabbits. He established that the rejection of grafts is an immunological rather than a physiological phenomenon. Indeed, he observed in the same animals enhanced and faster rejection responses with the second application of tissue from the original donor but again a primary response with tissue from a different source. Medawar likened the secondary response to tissue hypersensitivity, such as the Arthus reaction, and thereby indicated the presence of individually unique tissue antigens.

Rupert E. Billingham, Leslie Brent, and Medawar next found that animals not only can acquire immunity to foreign tissues, but that they can also acquire tolerance, so that allogeneic (of the same species) and even xenogeneic (of different species) grafts can be accepted. Their article relates back to the immunology of reproduction, for tolerance was achieved by the preliminary introduction of tissues into the yet immunologically incompetent fetus. Thus, foreign histocompatibility antigens became self-antigens. The role of genes in determining immunity was no longer simple, and a significant somatic effect now had to be considered.

The last paper of this set, introduced here because it is related, is by N. Avrion Mitchison, who demonstrated that immunity to foreign tissues can be transferred to normal animals by the injection of cells from lymph nodes that drained the graft site. In his system, as with Landsteiner and Chase's observations on delayed hypersensitivity, normal animals could not acquire tissue immunity through serum factors, although antibodies do contribute in some instances to graft and tumor rejection.

Histocompatibility antigens are again directly considered in the report by Jean Dausset. He found that human leukocytes themselves also possess unique antigens. Persons who received multiple transfusions and women who went through many pregnancies possessed antibodies that agglutinated certain leukocytes. Dausset described the first human histocompatibility antigen, known today as HLA-A2. Such an immunological component of individuality is a class I antigen of the major histocompatibility complex.

Immune response (Ir) antigens and genes have been a focus of Baruj Benacerraf. These substances belong to the regulatory class of histocompatibility antigens. In his report featured here, Benacerraf noted that synthetic antigens of polypeptide carriers conjugated to haptens were not recognized by all strains of guinea pigs. Different antigens would initiate antibody formation and delayed hypersensitivity reactions in different strains of animals, and the carrier was the responsible portion. Much later the helper T cell receptor was found to be carrier-specific; the receptor of its B cell partner is hapten-specific. The regulatory T cell receptor also engaged the Ir or class II histocompatibility antigen.

The last milestone in this section is the discovery of immunoglobulin idiotypes. The work of Henry G. Kunkel, who shares this honor with Jacques Oudin, is featured. Kunkel and his students immunized rabbits with isolated human antibodies to different antigens, and observed that the rabbit antisera could differentiate them. The rabbit antibodies were also person-specific. The question of immunoglobulin genetics was hence brought forward, since their data showed that lymphocyte clones synthesize antigenically unique immunoglobulins. This implied either that genetic codes existed for hundreds of millions of different immunoglobulins, or that the immunoglobulin genes have an extraordinarily high rate of somatic mutation. It soon became apparent that both notions were partly correct.

Immunogenetics, which is almost automatically equated with immunoglobulins and the major histocompatibility complex, also pertains to the multitude of other immunological functions and agents, such as lymphokines, macrophage enzymes, interferons, and complement proteins. Immunogenetics is a perfect match of disciplines: genetics, which concerns the development of self and its relationship with other selves, and immunology, which is said to distinguish self from nonself. The field is rooted in DNA, chance, shape, and process: DNA, the genetic code and blueprint of the organism; chance, the seemingly random effects leading to genetic mutation and recombination and to altered somatic expression; shape, the patterns of molecules and molecular interactions; and process, the cause of structure or form and the expression of the genetic code. Where then is self? From a less lofty and more practical position, immunogenetics explores the creation and development of the immune system through hereditary units and, reciprocally, examines these genes through the development of the immune system. The immunological engineer prefers the tangible aspects; the immunological philosopher, the abstract; but should we not be like students of Zen, who are at home in both, penetrating the interrelationships?

For further information:

Dorf, M. E. (editor). 1981. *The Role of the Major Histocompatibility Complex in Immunobiology.* Garland STPM Press, New York. 406 p.

Paul, W. E. (editor). 1984. *Immunogenetics.* Raven Press, New York. 211 p.

Hildemann, W. H., E. A. Clark, and R. L. Raison (editors). 1981. *Comprehensive Immunogenetics.* Elsevier, New York. 368 p.

Fudenberg, H. H., J. R. L. Pink, A-C. Wang, and G. B. Ferrara. 1984. *Basic Immunogenetics.* Third edition. Oxford University Press, New York. 302 p.

On the phenomenon of agglutination in normal human blood

1901 • Karl Landsteiner

Comment

Karl Landsteiner's Nobel Prize of 1930 stems from the following paper he had written 30 years earlier. In it he established the existence of human blood groups, and at the outset, he could hardly believe his own results. The existence of these hemagglutinins countered contemporary notions about immunity. First, the antibodies were present in normal, healthy individuals. Second, the antibodies were naturally produced without apparent stimulation. Third, the target antigen was the healthy intact red blood cell, not a microorganism, toxin, or denatured host constituent. Fourth, individuals could be classified into four groups depending on the blood group antigens present. If in accepting the nonteleological Darwinian approach he did not ask the question Why?, the question How? remained, taking on greater significance.

Landsteiner did not actually discover these isoantibodies (alloantibodies). Previous researchers, who described the agglutination of human erythrocytes by patient sera, had misinterpreted their findings. It was commonly believed that agglutination was symptomatic of an underlying infectious disease, since agglutination itself was described several years before as a diagnostic tool for identifying or monitoring typhoid fever. Furthermore, while the capability of producing antibodies against blood cells of different species, as observed by Jules Bordet among others, challenged the defensive purpose of immunity, its importance was dulled by its artificiality. The first person to recognize the genetic relationship of isoantibodies was Paul Ehrlich.

Ehrlich had no problem in accepting natural antibodies, since they were even predicted by his side-chain theory of antibody formation. For him, antibodies were not defensive, although they could by chance provide protection. Ehrlich and his assistant Julius Morgenroth had immunized nine goats with the blood of each other animal. The number of different hemagglutinins varied with each animal. Despite repeated injections, some animals were unable to produce any antibodies, and none had antibodies against its own cells. Ehrlich concluded that the results reflected normal physiological variation among individuals.

Joseph Halban, a gynecologist in Vienna, agreed with Ehrlich, emphasing that erythrocytes as well as antibody-producing cells differ in receptors. He also speculated on the origin of isoagglutinins. Suggested possibilities included the mutual immunization of mother and child; the absorption of products from indigenous intestinal bacteria; the normal denaturation of host tissue; and antigenic by-products of metabolism. As will be discussed shortly, Halban guessed well.

Landsteiner began his definitive report by first cross-testing the serum and erythrocytes from volunteers in his laboratory, including himself. He next interacted the blood of women who had just given birth, and finally examined their sera against blood cells from the various placenta. He built his experiments around the results of others, but Landsteiner went further in his checkerboard analysis, allowing him to recognize consistent clusters of reactivity, which he conveniently termed A, B, and C (now O). Landsteiner himself was type O. In 1902 his associates and students Alfred von Decastello-Rechtwehr and Andriano Sturli (one of Landsteiner's Group A subjects) discovered individuals whose cells carried both antigens, their serum having neither agglutinin. This group was designated eight years afterward as AB. Also at this time, through absorption studies with anti-A sera, a subset of group A was found among 20 percent of this population. Group A could thus be divided into A_1 and A_2.

Landsteiner immediately saw the important medical and forensic applications of such classification. In 1903 he published a report on its potential use in forensic practice, comparing fresh blood with samples dried on linen, glass, and wood. The tests were recorded by an independent reader, and although the dried material gave weaker agglutination, the accuracy was excellent. These studies also gave physical anthropologists a new tool, and racial and regional differences in distribution frequency were soon recognized. Beginning in the 1920s, blood grouping was required before transfusions of blood, which helped reduce the risk of traumatic hemolysis.

The Mendelian inheritance of blood group antigens was suggested in 1908, verified in 1910, and analyzed mathematically in 1924. The paramount question, however, was why preformed antibodies to the other isotypic antigens were present at all in blood? Halban was on the right track. The blood cell antigens A and B are found in many foods and are almost ubiquitous in the environment; antibody induction begins at birth in those so predisposed, and is maintained by the constant infusion and ingestion of antigenic substances. Consisting of oligosaccharide chains of up to 60 residues of mainly galactose and N-acetyl-glucosamine, the blood group antigens are found in the cell walls of microorganisms colonizing the intestine, upper respiratory tract, and other host tissues. In humans, these antigens exist as free oligosaccharides in urine, colostrum, and milk; as glycoproteins in saliva, vaginal and seminal fluids, and mucus secretions of goblet cells and glands of the respiratory, genito-urinary, and gastrointestinal tracts; and as membrane-bound glycolipids on erythrocytes and cells of the liver, spleen, kidney, and stomach. The A and B antigens are truly of blood, sweat, and tears. Despite their multiple locations, their absence from blood cells, as in type O individuals, seems to make no difference. Attempts to correlate certain diseases with blood type have failed. These markers could have a yet obscure evolutionary function.

For further information:

Farr, A. D. 1979. Blood group serology—the first four decades (1900–1939). *Medical History* 23:215–226.

Mazumdar, P. M. H. 1975. The purpose of immunity: Landsteiner's interpretation of the human isoantibodies. *Journal of the History of Biology* 8:115–133.

Race, R. R. and R. Sanger. 1954. *Blood Groups in Man.* Second edition. Charles C Thomas, Springfield, IL. 400 p. [and subsequent editions].

Rose, N. R., H. Friedman, and J. L. Fahey. 1986. *Manual of Clinical Laboratory Immunology.* Third edition. American Society for Microbiology, Washington, D.C., 1002 p.

The Paper*

I have recently observed and stated that the serum of normal people is capable of clumping erythrocytes of other healthy individuals. At the time, I had the impression that in certain illnesses the clumping attribute of serum is more obvious with foreign blood cells, and I assumed this is in connection with the lytic capacity of pathological serums to normal cells . . . since the agglutination and dissolving capacity often, but not always, occur in tandem. . . . [An] essential difference between my observations and Maragliano's is that in his case the serum acted also on the cells from the same individual, and his reaction only succeeds with blood from ill patients. My own observations showed quite amazing differences between the serum and cells of different healthy people. . . .

The agglutination of human blood by human serum is called isoagglutination by Ehrlich and Mor-

---

*Landsteiner, K. 1901. Ueber Agglutinationserscheinungen normalen menschlichen Blutes. *Wiener Klinische Wochenenschrift* 14:1132–1134.

genroth. These two researchers described some investigations based on my reports in which they were able to produce isolysin and isoagglutinin through injection of blood from the same species, i.e., sera that react with cells of the same species. Because of the variable proportions in the single experiment, this very detailed study does not provide clear evidence to confirm predetermined blood differences within a single animal species. . . .

Many researchers are examining the behavior of isoagglutination in people. The judgment of their studies is that this reaction is specific for a certain illness. Other studies noted the intensity and frequency of the reaction particularly in ill cases. . . . These results contradict my data.

The tables from my recent experiments are easy to understand. About the same quantity of serum and a 5% blood suspension were mixed in 0.6% salt solution and observed either in a hanging drop or in a test tube. [Table I concerns the blood of six apparently healthy men; Table II, of the blood of six apparently healthy women in labor (puerpera); and Table III, of the blood of five puerpera and six umbilical cords. The + means agglutination.]. . . . In a study of 10 or more normal persons (with 42 combinations of the same kind) the proportions were similar.

The experiments confirm my previous statements. All 22 examined sera from healthy adults gave a reaction. The result would obviously have been different had I not used different blood cells for the test.

Halban, Ascoli and lately Eisenberg have already called attention to the differing resistance of blood cells to the reaction. Resistance is also shown in the tables. Furthermore, there was a peculiar regularity in the behavior of the 22 examined blood samples. Notwithstanding a few occurrences of sera from fetal placental blood that did not cause agglutination, Halban, too, found that fetal blood agglutinated less often. Most of the sera could be divided into three groups:

In a few cases (Group A), the sera reacted with cells of another group (B) but not on the cells of group A, while the A cells and serum B were influenced in the same manner. In the third group (C), the serum agglutinated the cells of A and B, while the C cells were not influenced by the sera from A and B.

As commonly expressed, it can be said that in these cases at least two different kinds of agglutinins exist, one kind in A, the other in B, both together in C. The cells are naturally regarded as insensitive to the agglutinins that are situated in the same serum.

It can not be denied that the statement on the existence of different agglutinins in the examined cases sounds awkward, even though similar conditions have been observed in the experiments on isolysin by Ehrlich and Morgenroth, and it would be much more satisfying to find another interpretation through further research. Naturally, these regularities should also be examined in pathological cases.

The origin of agglutinins led Eisenberg back to the idea of resorption of the components of erythrocytes. . . . I have not succeeded in instilling the capacity of autoagglutination in animals by injections of their own dissolved blood cells. . . . The origin of naturally occurring hemagglutinins and bacterial agglutinins should be explained separately.

My experiments also show that the different sera in regard to the agglutination do not act identically. If one can accept the capacity for agglutination as a kind of autoimmunity through resorption of cellular components, one must therefore assume individual differences in order for different sera to react. In fact, even fetal blood cells behave differently. Differences occur in sera or cells. Agglutination within species can be understood with the same ease or difficulty as that with sera from foreign species. Nevertheless, this explanation can not be excluded. . . . It is hard to avoid it, and one would have to look at the physiological decomposition of the body tissue as a source of efficient serum stuff. . . .

The described agglutination can also be performed with serum that is dried and readily dissolved. I even succeeded using the solution of a blood drop that had been stored for 14 days dried onto

Table I   Experiments with blood from six male subjects

Source of serum	Source of blood cells					
	Dr. St.	Dr. Plecn.	Dr. Sturl.	Dr. Erdh.	Zar.	Landst.
Dr. St.	−	+	+	+	+	−
Dr. Plecn.	−	−	+	+	−	−
Dr. Sturl.	−	+	−	−	+	−
Dr. Erdh.	−	+	−	−	+	−
Zar.	−	−	+	+	−	−
Landst.	−	+	+	+	+	−

Table II   Experiments with blood from six pregnant females

Source of serum	Source of blood cells					
	Seil.	Linsm.	Lust.	Mittelb.	Tomsch.	Graupn.
Seil.	−	−	+	−	−	+
Linsm.	+	−	+	+	+	+
Lust.	+	−	−	+	+	−
Mittelb.	−		+	−	−	+
Tomsch.	−	−	+	−	−	+
Graupn.	+	−	−	+	+	−

Table III   Experiments with blood from five females and blood from six umbilical cords

Source of serum	Source of blood cells					
	Trautm.	Linsm.	Seil.	Freib.	Graupn.	Mittelb.
Lust.	+	+	−	−	−	+
Tomsch.	−	−	+	−	−	−
Mittelb.	−	−	+	−	−	−
Seil.	−	−	+	−	−	−
Linsm.	+	+	+	−	−	+

cloth. It is possible that the reaction in some cases may be suitable for forensic use to help identify or, better, recognize the nonidentity of blood. If rapid fluctuations of the agglutinin attributes appear, which is possible, it could prevent this procedure. On the other hand, the six sera of Table I showed the same behavior in a second test as that of nine days earlier.

Finally, it should be mentioned that the stated observations allow an explanation for the differing consequences of therapeutic human blood transfusions.

The role of iso-immunization in the pathogenesis of erythroblastosis fetalis

1941 • Philip Levine, Lyman Burnham, E. M. Katzin, and Peter Vogel

Comment

How does a fetus survive in its genetically and immunologically different mother? This challenging question has yet to be fully solved; however, a variety of mechanisms seem to act together to form a normally effective anatomical and process barrier. The embryo, possessing foreign paternal antigens, becomes surrounded by the trophoblast, a wall formed by the massive fusion of trophoblastic cells that are deficient in Class II major histocompatibility antigens. Protection may be aided by locally synthesized immunosuppressants and an antigen-masking layer of hyaluronic and sialic acid-rich mucoproteins and mucopolysaccharides. The mother herself may become tolerant through low-dose exposure. Maternal and fetal blood circulation are not fused but are juxtaposed within the placenta. Only very small numbers of blood cells manage to cross over, but—and here is the rub—IgG passes freely.

The presence of maternal antibodies in the fetus provides the neonate with broad passive immunity against the onslaught of worldly toxic and microbial hazards. The shield lasts approximately six months, during which the child's immunological system matures. Occasionally, however, maternal antibodies can attack fetal antigens on erythrocytes, killing the developing child. This is the concern of the next paper, which establishes the immunogenetic basis of Rh incompatibility.

Blood groups numbered only four until 1927, when Karl Landsteiner and Philip Levine (1900–1987), continuing cross-absorption studies of rabbit antisera to human blood, discovered three minor antigens, M, N, and P. By this time, Landsteiner had begun a quest to "fingerprint" individuals by their blood type, and today immunohematologists work with some 200 different antigens organized in 20 blood groups. The ABO group is the most important because of the high concentration of the particular antigen on erythrocyte membranes. The other major human antigenic group is the Rh group. At least 35 different Rh antigens exist, some found in 100 percent of humans. The classic Rh antigen is called Rhl, D, or Rh_0, depending on nomenclature system; it is carried by 85 percent of Caucasians. This is the antigen referred to when stating that an individual is Rh positive or Rh negative.

Levine, born in Russia, came to the United States in 1908. After service during World War I, he attended New York City College, and in 1923 he earned the M.D. at Cornell University. He continued there another two years for his M.A. Levine also had his research skills shaped at the Rockefeller Institute, where between 1925 and 1932 he was Assistant and then Associate. Failing to gain further promotion, his next stop was the faculty of the University of Wisconsin Medical School. However, it was a short stay. Beginning in 1935, he worked in bacteriology and serology at the Beth Israel Hospital in Newark, New Jersey, and completed his career at the Ortho Research Foundation, where in 1944 he became Director of the Department of Immunohematology.

The first Rh antigen, a red herring, was discovered by Landsteiner and Alexander S. Wiener in 1940. Wiener, who at this time was head of the blood-transfusion departments of Brooklyn Jewish Hospital and Adelphi Hospital in New York, had for three years collaborated with Landsteiner on several serological studies. They had injected rabbits with the blood of rhesus monkeys, and after appropriate absorptions with human blood cells, an antiserum was obtained that still agglutinated the erythrocytes of some humans. They designated the new antigen "Rh," for rhesus. However, the response was actually a cross-reaction of the two primate systems. Cells of many Rh-negative humans still reacted weakly with this absorbed antiserum. The human equivalent was first described a year earlier by Levine and Rufus Stetson, who found the agglutinin in the blood of a woman whose fetus was dead for six weeks prior to delivery. In publishing this report, Levine broke his previous agreement with Landsteiner that he would not independently seek new blood groups, a project Landsteiner had reserved for himself. The rhesus antigen of monkey erythrocytes, on Levine's suggestion, had been redesignated LW in honor of its discoverers to prevent further confusion—and to mark the end of a bitter polemic with Wiener on priority of discovery. Human Rh, thus, is a misnomer too ingrained in clinical science and public knowledge to be remedied.

In 1940 Wiener and H. Raymond Peters published a report linking Rh incompatibility with transfusion reactions. Thus, basic and clinical researchers were approaching a common element. The milestone of Levine and colleagues put the matter in sharp focus, showing that the paternal Rh-positive antigens of the fetus could induce an Rh-negative mother to produce anti-fetal antibodies. Usually the antigen is introduced in sufficient dose only after the trauma of the first childbirth. Each succeeding pregnancy leads to further antigenic stimulation, thus increasing the risk. Rh hemolytic disease, of which erythroblastosis fetalis is one clinical manifestation, is in practice a complex process. For instance, maternal Rh-negative serum usually does not agglutinate Rh-positive cells. The concentration of Rh antigen is too low for effective cross-linking, and the antibodies must be detected by the Coombs test, which involves bridging with secondary (anti-immunoglobulin) antibody. What then causes the destruction of fetal blood cells? It seems that the antibodies act as opsonins for macrophage engulfment and mediated lysis of the red cells. Affected newborns die shortly after birth from bilirubin neurotoxicity. It might seem that even the first type A or B fetus should likewise be at risk with a type O mother, but hemolytic disease is somehow less common and so weak that the rare affected newborn child can be effectively treated.

Prophylaxis is through the immunological strategy of antibody-mediated suppression. The observation that stronger ABO incompatibility reduced the incidence of Rh disease led to the hypothesis that fetal blood cells were intercepted and rapidly removed from maternal circulation before Rh sensitization could occur. This in turn provided the regimen of injecting the Rh-negative mother with anti-Rh antibodies within three days of each delivery. The key to successful treatment is beginning with the first pregnancy.

For further information:

Beer, A. E. and R. E. Billingham. 1976. *The Immunobiology of Mammalian Reproduction.* Prentice-Hall, Englewood Cliffs, NJ. 240 p.

Levine, P. 1984. The discovery of Rh hemolytic disease. *Vox Sanguis* 47:187–190.

Potter, E. L. 1947. *Rh. Its relation to congenital hemolytic disease and to intragroup transfusion reactions.* Year Book Publishers, Chicago. 344 p.

Zimmerman, D. R. 1973. *Rh. The Intimate History of a Disease and Its Conquest.* Macmillan Publishing Co., New York. 371 p.

___

The Paper*

Studies on the cause of intra-group transfusion accidents associated with pregnancy have established the importance of the concept of iso-immunization of the mother by blood factors in the fetus transmitted from the father. More recently it was found that the same theory of iso-immunization may serve as the basis for a theory on the pathogenesis of erythroblastosis fetalis, the well-described familial hemolytic disease of the newborn.

The data to be presented indicate that erythroblastosis fetalis results from (1) iso-immunization of the mother by dominant hereditary blood factors in the fetus, as evidenced by the production of immune intragroup agglutinins and (2) the subsequent passage of these maternal agglutinins through the placenta and their continuous action on the susceptible fetal blood. In the great majority of the cases the blood factor involved has been shown to be either identical with or related to the Rh (Rhesus) agglutinogen first described by Landsteiner and Wiener with the aid of rabbit sera prepared by injection of Rhesus blood. In other words, the rabbit anti-Rhesus immune sera and the sera of pregnant women suffering from intra-group transfusion accidents gave almost identical agglutination reactions on all human blood tests. Accordingly, a pregnant woman whose blood does not contain the Rh factor (Rh−, occurring in about 15 per cent of the general population) if married to an Rh+ husband (85 per cent in the random population), may produce anti-Rh agglutinins as a result of immunization with the Rh fetal blood. Should these agglutinins penetrate the placenta in suitable concentration they may serve as the source of the intrauterine hemolysis of fetal blood, the characteristic feature of erythroblastosis fetalis.

The term iso-immunization denotes immunization within the same species, i.e., the individual being immunized and source of the antigenic (immunizing) stimulus belong to the same species. It is obvious

___

*Levine, P., L. Burnham, E. M. Katzin, and P. Vogel. 1941. The role of iso-immunization in the pathogenesis of erythroblastosis fetalis. *American Journal of Obstetrics and Gynecology* 42:925–937. [With permission of C. V. Mosby Company.]

that patients receiving repeated blood transfusions may be subjected to iso-immunization. A prerequisite condition is an antigenic difference in the blood of recipient and donor. In each instance, this difference is expressed by the presence of a particular blood factor in the donor and its absence in the recipient. . . .

Iso-immunization in pregnancy as the cause of the production of atypical agglutinins responsible for an intra-group transfusion accident was suggested by Levine and Stetson in 1939. In this case the patient (Group O), who harbored a dead fetus for two months, was transfused with her husband's blood (Group O) after the delivery of a macerated fetus. This transfusion was followed by an immediate severe reaction resulting in jaundice, anuria, and ultimate recovery. . . . In 1940 . . . it could be shown that the patient was Rh− and her husband Rh+. . . .

[O]ne of us (L. B.) observed a patient who suffered from a severe transfusion accident following the delivery of an infant in whom a diagnosis of erythroblastosis fetalis was established. The obstetric history in this case (R. C.) and in still another case (J. L.) not transfused, were so striking as to suggest a theoretical basis for the pathogenesis of erythroblastosis fetalis. One of these mothers (R. C.) had three pregnancies, the first and third of which resulted in infants with erythroblastosis fetalis and the second pregnancy terminated in a macerated fetus. In the other case (J. L.), there had been 10 pregnancies, the first of which resulted in a normal infant; there were 3 spontaneous abortions and the remaining 6 pregnancies resulted in infants who survived one to three days. In at least 3 of these neonatal deaths there was sufficient evidence to support a diagnosis of erythroblastosis fetalis. This woman's blood was tested in the eighth month of her eleventh pregnancy. Since atypical agglutinins were already present, it was anticipated that the baby to be born would be affected. Actually, the infant suffered from anemia of the newborn, one of the several manifestations of erythroblastosis fetalis.

The two cases mentioned were among the seven patients with 37 pregnancies which formed the basis for the preliminary observation that the pathogenesis of erythroblastosis fetalis depends on iso-immunization of the mother by the fetus. . . .

In 6 of the 7 women in whose blood atypical agglutinins were demonstrated, there were indications that the specificity of the antibodies corresponded to the anti-Rh. . . . If iso-immunization with the Rh factor plays a significant role in the pathogenesis of this disease, one should expect to find (1) a high incidence of Rh-reactions in this group of selected mothers and (2) a high incident of anti-Rh agglutinins in their sera.

Whenever possible, the bloods of the fathers and the affected children were also tested, for, if the iso-immunization theory is correct, then 100 per cent of the fathers and the affected children in the series of Rh− mothers should be Rh+. . . .

This study is based chiefly on blood tests of 153 mothers who delivered one or more infants suffering from one of three clinical forms of erythroblastosis fetalis. . . .

One or more drops of anti-Rh serum are mixed in small test tubes (75 × 10 mm) with 2 drops of a washed 1 per cent to 2 per cent cell suspension. . . . The tubes are shaken and incubated in a water-bath at 37°C for one hour, at the end of which period . . . all tubes are centrifuged at low speed (500 rpm) for one minute. After replacing the tubes in the rack, the sedimented cells are resuspended by gently shaking and readings are recorded. . . . Bloods showing no agglutination are Rh−.

Two drops of the serum to be tested are added to each of 10 small test tubes and each tube receives two drops of washed cell suspension of ten different Group O bloods. As a rule, at least one Rh− blood is included. The tests are incubated at 37°C for one hour, and readings are made after centrifuging the tests and resuspension of the sediments as indicated above. . . .

The findings in [Table IV] strongly indicate the iso-immunization of the Rh− mother by the Rh factor in fetal blood. The final proof for such iso-immunization can be supplied only by the demonstration of anti-Rh agglutinins in the mother's blood. Obviously, the likelihood of finding such agglutinins will be greater if the mother's blood is tested soon after the delivery of an infant suffering from erythroblastosis fetalis. This is borne out by the findings presented in Table V.

The failure to detect anti-Rh agglutinins in many cases tested shortly after the delivery of an affected infant does not exclude their presence at some previous period during the course of their pregnancy. . . .

The findings presented establish the significant role of iso-immunization of the mother by blood factors in the fetus in the pathogenesis of erythroblastosis fetalis. Of prime importance is the Rh factor in fetal blood which is transmitted as a dominant mendelian gene from the father. . . . It is the continuous intra-uterine action of anti-Rh agglutinins with the Rh positive fetal blood over a period varying from weeks to months which causes a progressive hemolysis of fetal blood. . . .

One of the most striking features of erythroblastosis fetalis is the wide variety of clinical syndromes it embraces, such as, the extremely fatal form of fetal hydrops and the mild, frequently unrecognizable

Table IV. Incidence of Rh+ and Rh− in Husbands and Affected Infants of the 141 Rh− Mothers

	NUMBER TESTED	Rh+	Rh−	EXPECTANCY OF Rh− IN RANDOM POPULATION
Husbands	89	89	0	13 (89 × 15%)
Affected infants	76	76	0	11 (76 × 15%)

The findings in this table are based on tests with serum M. F. which gives an incidence of 15% Rh− reactions.

Table V. Incidence of Anti-Rh Agglutinins in 141 Rh− Mothers

INTERVAL AFTER LAST DELIVERY OF AN AFFECTED INFANT	AGGLUTININS PRESENT	AGGLUTININS NOT FOUND
2 months post partum	33	37
2 months to 1 year past partum	5	15
1 year or longer post partum	2	39
During next pregnancy	2	5
No data	0	3
Total	42	99

anemia of the newborn. These clinical forms are probably the result of varying degrees and duration of iso-immunization during the course of the pregnancy. . . . [I]t is conceivable that the prolonged action of immune iso-agglutinins on the susceptible fetal blood may induce more severe damage than the action of agglutinins produced very late in the course of a pregnancy.

The clinical observation has been made that some infants may be born apparently free from the condition, but in the course of a few days, severe anemia and jaundice make their appearance. It is difficult to correlate this fact with the iso-immunization theory since the infant after birth should be free from any further action by the maternal agglutinins. . . .

The hereditary nature of erythroblastosis fetalis, hitherto unknown, can now be stated in terms of the iso-immunization theory. In some families, every pregnancy but perhaps the first, terminates in either an abortion, a still-birth, or an infant with erythroblastosis fetalis; while in other families, only one of several pregnancies results in an affected infant. Since the Rh factor is inherited as a simple mendelian dominant, it is obvious from a genetic standpoint, that this striking difference in familial incident of this disease is determined by the homozygosity or heterozygosity of the father's blood. . . . [T]he first born is frequently but not always spared because more than one pregnancy with an Rh+ fetus may be required before a sufficient degree of iso-immunization is attained. . . .

Immunogenetic studies of species and of species hybrids in doves

1936 • M. Robert Irwin and Leon J. Cole

Comment

Ernest W. Lindstrom, a plant geneticist, had some good advice for his new graduate student M. Robert Irwin (1897–1987): Get some training in bacteriology, immunology, and biochemistry as well as traditional genetics. In the 1920s this was a fairly avant-garde idea, since genetics was steeped in classical zoology and botany with emphasis in cytology. Irwin complied with the suggestion. Thus, when he left Iowa State College, after earning his Bachelor's in 1920 and the Ph.D. in 1928, he had an extraordinarily broad scientific background, extending from agricultural breeding to the serological techniques for diagnosing infectious diseases. While at Harvard University as a National Research Council Fellow, he was amused but pained to find the famous microbiologist Hans Zinsser struggling to comprehend the genetic principles of blood group inheritance. Most immunologists and physicians lacked training in genetics; geneticists were not particularly interested in the medical sciences.

In 1929 Irwin came to the Rockefeller Institute for Medical Research, which was the place to be at this time for those who wanted to work at the frontier of medical science. He was fortunate to find a place in the laboratory of Leslie T. Weber, who was sympathetic to the concept that heredity influences natural resistance to disease. Weber had helped to organize a mouse colony and to develop model epidemics of mice with *Salmonella typhimurium* and *Klebsiella pneumoniae* to refute the view of William W. C. Topley of the London School of Hygiene and Tropical Medicine. Topley had suggested that during epidemics sickness among nonimmunized individuals was merely a result of population density, pathogen virulence, and chance. Weber was quick to tap Irwin's expertise in genetics in order to produce inbred strains of mice with differing resistance to the test bacterium. Soon two diverse colonies were obtained; in one, on average, 95 percent of the mice were susceptible to the bacterial infection. In the other, only 15 percent of the mice could be infected. When members of both colonies were mixed in the model epidemic, they reacted as if in their isolated units, vindicating the importance of genetics in infectious disease. Subsequent studies established that the two susceptibilities were pathogen-specific.

Irwin in 1930 joined the faculty of the Department of Genetics at the University of Wis-

consin. His first projects concerned infections that caused abortion in rabbits and cattle, but an idea he had put aside at the Rockefeller Institute now had an opportunity to be developed. He had learned about the antigenicity of carbohydrates from the research of Michael Heidelberger and Oswald Avery. This was important to genetics, since proteins were then obscure in structure and composition, but polysaccharide chemistry was much better understood. The comparative simplicity of sugars meant that they had the potential to serve as known molecular and immunological markers of genetic alterations. Furthermore, serum proteins of similar species were poorly differentiated by standard serological methods. At first he considered the pollen of maize as a test material, but recalling the success of Karl Landsteiner in differentiating the erythrocytes of horses, donkeys, and their hybrid, the mule, Irwin decided to make use of the colonies of pigeons and doves within the department to search for antigenic differences in their blood. Rabbits injected with the red cells provided the antisera, which could be characterized by cross-absorptions and comparative hemagglutination.

The bird colonies had been bred by Leon J. Cole (1877–1948), the chairman of the Department of Genetics and co-author of the following milestone. Cole, who had his training at the University of Michigan and Harvard University, was a traditional geneticist. His first post was in 1906 as chief of the Division of Animal Breeding and Pathology at the Rhode Island Experimental Station. In 1910 Cole came to the University of Wisconsin College of Agriculture, and in 1918 he founded the Department. He also held in 1923 a concurrent appointment as Chief of the Animal Husbandry Division of the Bureau of Animal Industry, United States Department of Agriculture.

Irwin was able to formally link immunology and classic genetics through a laboratory blood rite. Indeed, he coined the term "immunogenetics" over the previous candidate "serological genetics," because of the familiar precedent of Svante Arrhenius's "immunochemistry." The testing of cross-species hybrids and backcrosses eventually allowed studies of antigen linkage and chromosome mapping, investigations of alleles and phenotypic effects of heterozygosity, and mechanisms of evolution from an immunological perspective. Irwin described "unit antigens" which met both genetic and immunological criteria in frequency of expression. The presented paper noted that the hybrids did not contain the antigenic complement of both parents, but data from a later, more extensive study did show that some hybrid birds could fully carry both sets of antigens. The existence of a unique "hybrid substance" was the key finding of the report, besides establishing the genetic relationship of antigenicity. A report in 1944 determined that the hybrid substance was antigenic even in the parent animals. The origin of such antigens was afterward shown to arise from the interaction of parental alleles and also from the interaction of genes on different chromosomes, both between and within species.

For further information:

Irwin, M. R. 1974. Comments on the early history of immunogenetics. *Animal Blood Groups and Biochemical Genetics* 5:65–84.

Irwin, M. R. 1976. The beginnings of immunogenetics. *Immunogenetics* 3:1–13.

Jacob, F. 1973. *The Logic of Life. A History of Heredity* (B. E. Spillmann, translator). Pantheon Books, New York. 348 p.

Johansson, I. 1961. Leon Jacob Cole 1877–1948. *Genetics* 46:1–4.

The Paper*

Representatives of the domesticated Ring dove (*Streptopelia risoria*), an Asiatic species (*Spilopelia chi-*

---

*Irwin, M. R. and L. J. Cole. 1936. Immunogenetic studies of species and of species hybrids in doves, and the separation of species-specific substances in the backcross. *Journal of Experimental Zoology* 73:85–108. [With permission of Alan R. Liss, publisher.]

nensis) commonly called Pearlneck, and of F_1 (hybrids) from male Pearlnecks × Ring dove females have served as donors of [red blood] corpuscles for injections and agglutinations. In this paper, the terms F_1 or hybrid will designate the species hybrid. . . .

Antisera were prepared by injecting rabbits with washed erythrocytes from representatives of each species and of the F_1. The agglutinations were performed by adding to 0.1 cc of the immune serum in varying dilutions (by halves) 1 drop of a 2.5% saline suspension of washed red blood cells. For the absorptions, the immune serum was diluted according to its titer and mixed with a proportionate amount (generally one-half) of washed cells. The mixture was agitated gently at intervals, and allowed to stand at room temperature from 1 to 2 hours. The process was repeated until absorption was complete at the original dilution. . . .

The differentiation of species, of the F_1's from their parents, and of the individuals of the backcross generation from one another and from the F_1 parents, is based on agglutinations of the corpuscles following absorption of agglutinins from the immune serum. . . .

The direct agglutination tests for each serum fail to differentiate the cells. However, when anti-Pearlneck serum is exhausted by the cells of Ring doves, with no trace of agglutinin for Ring dove cells at the serum dilution used for the absorptions, the agglutinins remaining cause clumping of the cells of both Pearlneck and the F_1 at one-half the dilution for the direct agglutinations. This constant difference occurred without exception for each of several different anti-Pearlneck sera employed, and for all the many tests of each of these absorbed sera.

If anti-Pearlneck serum is absorbed by cells of the F_1, the agglutinins for Ring dove cells are removed at the same time, the exhausted fluid in these tests producing agglutination only with Pearlneck cells at a low titer. Absorption by Pearlneck cells removed all agglutinins for the three types of cells. . . .

The erythrocytes of the Pearlnecks have antigenic components in common with Ring doves (the agglutinins for the common substances are those absorbed) as well as components specific for themselves—"species-specific" Pearlneck substances not shared by Ring doves.

In like manner, the cells of Ring doves, in addition to the constituents shared with Pearlnecks, also possess substances specific for themselves. . . . There is some indication that these specific Ring dove substances are quantitatively less than those of Pearlneck for itself, as suggested by the greater drop in the titer of Ring dove serum absorbed by Pearlneck cells than is found in the reciprocal test.

The F_1 cells lack a small part of the total complement of both Pearlneck and Ring dove cells, since

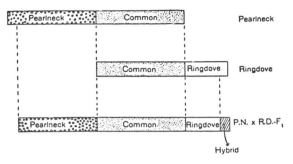

Figure 1 Diagrammatic representation of the antigenic components of the corpuscles of dove species and their hybrids.

each anti-parental serum absorbed by hybrid cells still retains agglutinins for the parental cells of the anti-serum employed. . . .

A very significant finding is that some agglutinins remain in anti-F_1 serum for F_1 cells after exhaustion with both Pearlneck and Ring dove cells. Therefore, the cells of this hybrid contain a substance or substances not found in either parent. This is a new, or "hybrid" substance. . . . The cells of all the F_1 progeny tested (sixteen) were alike in containing this new substance. . . .

A diagrammatic representation of the antigenic components of the corpuscles of these species and of the hybrids is shown in Figure 1. . . .

With a technic for determining specific antigenic characters of a species and their presence in the F_1, it is possible by an examination of the cells of the offspring of a backcross, in this case to Ring dove, to determine whether or not the species-specific substances (Pearlneck) are divisible and heritable. . . .

Complete exhaustion at the first dilution of the agglutinins for Ring dove cells and for those of each backcrossed hybrid . . . allows the general conclusion that the individual differences displayed are due to a separation of different component specific Pearlneck substances. . . .

The production in the cells of the hybrid of a substance, or substances, not found in the cells of either parental species is the first instance recorded of its particular kind. Hence the distribution of this character in the cells of the backcross generation is of special importance, since thereby its unity or complexity, and, possibly, the specific genetic factors involved from at least one species parent may be determined.

There is some indication from the distribution that quantitative differences of the substance exist; certainly its absence in the cells of several of the birds tested is beyond question. . . .

If these biochemical components of the cells are the result of the action of genes, a segregation of the characters specific for the Pearlneck is to be expected in offspring from backcrosses of the F_1 to Ring doves. . . . The most critical genetical evidence that these data afford is that absorption of anti-Pearlneck serum by F_1 cells removes completely the agglutinins for the cells of the backcross progeny, a finding easily explained on genetic grounds, but otherwise not at all understandable. . . .

Between ten and twenty different biochemical constituents imply at least as many genes, which in this experiment are not alleles, are required to explain the segregation of the Pearlneck substances in the first backcross generation. . . .

Our studies show that the antigenic characters specific for Pearlneck, not shared by Ring dove, are multiple, requiring many genes (not alleles) to account for their presence. Assuming that the substances common to the two species are also numerous, it becomes evident that the number of cellular components within the species is indeed very great. Obviously, these substances can be detected within a species only if the causative genes, for any or all, have alleles with different effects. . . .

The specific "hybrid" substance of the F_1 offers evidence that a different biochemical character of the cells may be produced by the interaction of two or more genes than is produced in conjunction with their normal alleles. It is logical to assume that this new substance is the result of interaction of genes which within each species produced only species-specific effects. . . .

The genetic and antigenic basis of tumor transplantation

1937 • Peter A. Gorer

Comment

Teleological immunology has retreated to a new, hardened line of defense at the major histocompatibility complex (MHC). Apparently, certain molecules exist solely as reference markers of self. They have been organized into two classes. Class I antigens are carried on virtually every cell, especially lymphocytes and macrophages, although even here they compose less than 1 percent of membrane proteins. They are exceedingly low in concentration in embryonic cells, and may be absent from trophoblasts. They are recognized with incompatible transplants, serving as the tocsin for cytotoxic T_8 lymphocytes. MHC Class I antigens consist of two chains, with the heavy chain being anchored to the membrane and coded by genes on chromosome 6 of humans. Its light chain, noncovalently bound partner, coded on human chromosome 15, is the intriguing β_2-microglobulin, whose origin is shared by immunoglobulins and neuronal cell Thy-1 glycoprotein. Class II MHC antigens are expressed on fewer cell types, mainly the immunological cells. Consisting of two glycoprotein chains, they are associated with regulation of the immune response, requiring to be recognized by T_4 cells simultaneously with a foreign antigen, such as a viral glycoprotein, before the process can be advanced. Histocompatibility antigens are generally coded on at least four clustered loci of a single chromosome.

How extraordinary! The mathematical form of individuality is recognized by the sequences of chromosomal nucleic acid. But what about twins? Surely, they are individuals. Somatic random factors, such as messenger transcription and peptide recombination during anti-body synthesis, could provide structural uniqueness. The mental recognition of the individual is through a synergistic combination, or gestalt, of image, behavior, and other comparative memory patterns. But what is thought? What immediately concerns us is that at the functional molecular level, through the recognition agency of a particular subset of T lymphocytes and the psychoneuroendocrinoimmunological network (see Part 9), individuality is the configuration of a molecule on the surface of mature somatic cells encoded in a narrow region of DNA. However, all forms of self are patterns impossibly frozen in time-space and founded on the gossamer of nonlocal acting particle-wave behavior patterns of matter-mind. Thus, while we all are cognizant of life, of individuality, of concrete matter and abstract mind, any definition will ultimately fail. Recalling Lao Tzu: The Tao that can be fixed is not truly the Tao—nameless, it is the source of heaven and earth; named, it is the mother of all things.

The remainder of the milestones in this section, concerning the development of our knowledge of histocompatibility and its relation to genetics, begins with the work of Peter A. Gorer (1907–1961). Gorer entered Guy's Hospital, London, in 1924 as a dental student, switching to medicine three months later with emphasis in physiology. Having received his medical degree in 1932, he went to University College, London, to study genetics under J. B. S. Haldane. Two years later, for its better facilities, he transferred to the Lister Institute. Like M. Robert Irwin, Gorer examined in mice the inherited variation in resistance to bacterial infections. The highly resistant and susceptible strains were so far apart that immunization could not bring them on par. The genetic regulation of infectious disease led to the genetic analysis of tumor immunity. World War II took him back to Guy's Hospital as a hematologist with more practical matters to be accomplished than basic research. Gorer spent 1946 at the Roscoe B. Jackson Memorial Laboratory at Bar Harbor, Maine, as a fellow of the National Institutes of Health in order to further his research on the genetics of transplantation. He continued his investigations at Guy's, but before he could secure a faculty appointment, he was struck down by cancer.

Gorer chose mice for his genetic studies because they were already being used for tumor studies and pure inbred strains were available. Mouse blood groups being unknown, on a lark he tested his own blood against the erythrocytes of several mouse strains. He was pleasantly surprised to find good agglutination with mouse strain A, a weak response with strain CBA, and no effect with strain C57. Next he cross-bred the strains and produced antisera in rabbits. Three antigens were distinguished: antigen I in cells of A and CBA; antigen II plentiful in A, sparse in CBA, and absent in C57; and antigen III in all three strains. Later, on the suggestion of George D. Snell, antigen II became Histocompatibility-2 (H-2). Gorer confirmed Mendelian inheritance and the genetic control of tumor susceptibility previously observed by the Bar Harbor group. His new finding, however, was the correlation of resistance to tumor transplantation to the absence of a particular blood group antigen. He offered tumor studies an immunological perspective, and provided the first linked marker of histocompatibility.

Further research located antigen II on various other normal and tumor cells. Also, C57 mice, which lacked the antigen, were able to produce antibodies to it. He found no reason to link the resistance of C57 mice to A strain tumors with antibody formation, although in 1942 an experiment demonstrated that animals could not acquire strain A leukemia when inoculated with cells mixed with antisera. Gorer's research made no waves. Surgeons who attempted transplantation were little interested in genetics, and most tumor researchers could not yet appreciate the necessity of using inbred, homozygous animal strains. However, the situation soon changed with the war, when transplantation of tissues to the wounded became crucial. Gorer outlined the genetic problem, and provided the first techniques for its analysis. He replaced the terms "homologous" and "isologous" with the more precise "allogeneic" and syngeneic." He firmly planted immunogenetics in the ground of immunology. Gorer was honored with fellowship in the Royal Society in 1960, a year before his tragic death.

For further information:

Cunningham, B. A. 1977. The structure and function of histocompatibility antigens. *Scientific American* 237(4):96–107.

Klein, J. 1975. *Biology of the Mouse Histocompatibility-2 Complex. Principles of immunogenetics applied to a single system.* Springer-Verlag, New York. 620 p.

Medawar, P. B. 1961. Peter Alfred Gorer 1907–1961. *Biographical Memoirs of Fellows of the Royal Society* 7:95–109.

Snell, G. D. 1981. Studies in histocompatibility. *Science* 213:172–178.

The Paper*

Several of the earlier workers on tumor transplantation suggested that heredity might play a part in determining the fate of transplants. The pioneer researches along these lines were made by Loeb (1909) and by Tyzzer (1909). . . .

In order to make a thorough genetic analysis it is necessary to secure stocks of the utmost degree of genetic purity by continued brother-sister matings. Stocks obtained after twenty to thirty generations of

*Gorer, P. A. 1937. The genetic and antigenic basis of tumor transplantation. *Journal of Pathology and Bacteriology* 44:691–697. [With permission of the Pathological Society of Great Britain and Ireland.]

such matings may legitimately be described as pure lines. . . .

If a tumor arises in a member of a pure line it will usually grow in 100 per cent of cases when transferred to other members of the same pure line; with few exceptions such tumors are highly specific and will not grow in animals of different genetic constitution. If two pure lines are crossed, one susceptible and the other resistant, the first generation hybrids (F_1) are all susceptible; similarly the progeny produced by backcrossing the F_1 to the susceptible pure line are also all susceptible. The number of susceptible individuals in the backcross to the resistant line and in the F_2 generation varies with the tumor used; in some cases 50 per cent of the former and 75 per cent of the latter generations may be susceptible, whilst in other cases the number is much less. The interpretation of the observed results is that susceptibility is determined by dominant genes, the number of genes required varying with the tumor used; in some cases only one gene is required whilst in other cases 10 or more are needed.

The study of blood groups in man and animals has shown that antigenic differences are determined by dominant genes and the suggestion has been put forward that the genes determining susceptibility to tumor transplantation might be identical with those determining antigenic differences. A study by Haddow (1934) along these lines using a fowl sarcoma gave a negative result. Since pure lines of fowls cannot be obtained, it was thought worth while to perform a similar experiment with pure lines of mice.

Two pure lines of mice were used, viz. a line of blacks and line of albinos. . . . The albinos have been shown to possess an antigen (described as antigen II) in their erythrocytes, detectable with sera from immunized rabbits, which is lacking in those of the blacks; its presence is determined by a single dominant gene).

The following crosses were made:

Black by albino = F_1 generation
F_1 by albino = A backcross
F_1 by black = B backcross
F_1 by F_1 = F_2 generation

The tumor arose in an albino female about 12 months old, and macroscopically it appeared to be a typical mammary carcinoma. . . . For the first transfer it was successfully inoculated . . . into 12 albinos and failed to grow in 12 blacks. . . . [T]he tumor (now in its seventeenth transfer) appears to be a pure spindle-cell sarcoma and has shown remarkably constant behavior in successive transfers. Growth is somewhat more rapid when trocar and cannula are used instead of the saline emulsion and the former technique has been employed for genetic analysis. . . .

[Transplantation in pure lines, the F_1 hybrid, and the A backcross gave typical dominant gene results as described above.]

Tables II and III deal with transplantation in F_2 and B backcross mice. In them we get segregation of the genes required for tumor transplantation and of the gene determining the presence of antigen II. In the F_2 generation 70 animals were tested for the antigen, of which 52 were positive and 18 negative. Five animals were lost or died prior to inoculation and Table II shows the result of inoculating the remaining 65 animals, inoculation being into both flanks. The figures in parenthesis are the numbers expected on the hypothesis that two genes are needed, one of which is identical with the gene for antigen II. It will be seen that the agreement is excellent.

The B backcross generation affords a more sensitive test of the above hypothesis, since only one half should possess antigen II and one half of these should grow the tumor. Of 84 animals tested for

TABLE II.

Results of inoculation of F_2 generation (progeny of F_1 by F_1).

Antigenic type of mouse.	Result of inoculation.		
	+	−	Total.
With antigen II . . .	35 (36·56)	13 (12·19)	48 (48·75)
Without antigen II . .	0	17 (16·25)	17 (16·25)
	35 (36·56)	30 (28·44)	65

Figures in brackets = number expected if there are 2 dominant genes influencing the growth of the tumour, one of which determines the presence of antigen II.

TABLE III.

Results of inoculation of B backcross (progeny of F_1 hybrid by black).

Antigenic type of mouse.	Result of inoculation.		
	+	−	Total.
With antigen II . . .	17 (19·5)	17 (19·5)	34 (39)
Without antigen II . .	0	44 (39)	44 (39)
	17 (19·5)	61 (58·5)	78

Figures in brackets as in table II.

antigen II 37 were positive and 47 negative (the deviation from expectation is not significant) and 78 were available for inoculation. The results are shown in Table III. It will be seen that the observed values agree with those expected (figures in parentheses). Actually in the experiment with this cross 56 per cent lacked antigen II so the experiment was slightly biased in favor of disclosing any susceptible animals that lacked the antigen. . . .

If the animals with atypical growth are classified as negative, the agreement with a two factor ratio is less satisfactory and one cannot exclude the hypothesis that though two genes will allow growth for a limited period, three genes are needed for a typical progressive growth. However, this does not influence the chief point at issue, namely that antigen II must be present in the tissues of the host, otherwise the tumor will regress.

It is possible to obtain more direct evidence on the importance of antigenic differences by an ex-amination of the sera of animals in which the tumor has regressed. Ten blacks were bled between 14 and 17 days after inoculation, at which time the tumors had either disappeared completely or were obviously regressing rapidly. When such sera were tested against the cells of blacks and albinos at 37°C, those of the latter were specifically agglutinated. The titer of the sera varied from about 1:5 to 1:100. . . . Rabbit sera containing antibody II behave in this way but . . . at present it is impossible to say more than that iso-agglutinins are formed when the tumor regresses. . . .

The nature of the immunity reactions that follow transplantation of a tumor has been subject to dispute. It is important to decide whether the reactions are directed against malignant tissues per se or are elicited by antigenic differences between the tissues of the host and those of the animal in which the tumor arose. Experiments with genetically purified stocks give evidence in favor of the latter hypothesis.

The behaviour and fate of skin autografts and skin homografts in rabbits

1944 • Peter B. Medawar

Comment

Sir Peter B. Medawar (1915–1987) was not an immunogeneticist. He was a zoologist by training, a physiologist by bent, and a clinical im-munologist by circumstance of war. His work, nonetheless, clearly engaged the problem of immunological individuality, and focused on the practical aspects of histocompatibility and its associated antigens and genes. He demonstrated that the physiological rejection of foreign normal tissue has an immunological basis.

Medawar in 1935 passed his Bachelor's examinations with first honors from Magdalen College at Oxford University. His first scientific work, by way of scholarships and a favorable introduction by his tutor, was in Sir Howard W. Florey's Department of Pathology, where he gained some valuable experience in the conduct of research while developing tissue cultures. The tyro also happily found that sulfadiazine and penicillin were not toxic for wounds. In 1938 he became a Demonstrator in Zoology at Oxford, worked on a mathematical analysis of scalar growth, and considered the merits of a doctorate. After compiling a small body of research and passing the examination committee, Medawar decided at the end not to formally petition for the degree, regarding it of "no useful purpose and cost." At that time in England, the doctorate was not always necessary for advancement, and the Old Boy Network provided Medawar his positions.

One day during the Battle of Britain, a twin-engine bomber crashed close to Medawar's home. An airman was wrested from the wreckage with third-degree burns over 60 percent of his body. Once such a condition was tantamount to a death sentence, but the war with its thousands of burn casualties provided the impetus for emergency experimentation. Transfusions and antimicrobial agents were already reducing mortality. Medawar was obliged to assist on the case. Skin grafting was known for centuries, but successful treatment was restricted to the use of the patient's own skin or that of a twin. Even then, the amount of involved tissue was relatively minor. Medawar obtained remnants of plastic surgical operations from another institution. After failing to grow skin cells in culture with the aim of seeding trypsin-dispersed epidermal cells on the patient's body, Medawar tried microtome-sliced sheets of the patient's dermis. These, too, could not be integrated. Eventually the treatment

method of P. Gabarro, whereby postage-stamp-size grafts from the patient are distributed over the wound, managed to save the warrior's life.

Frustrated by the inability to render effective aid or minimally to understand the process of tissue rejection, Medawar wrote a memorandum to the War Wounds Committee of the Medical Research Council. He urged them to fund some facility to conduct research on homografts. A member of the committee asked whether Medawar himself was interested in obtaining the grant, and receiving an affirmative reply, arranged for him to visit the Burns Unit of the Glasgow Royal Infirmary under Leonard Colebrook. The collaborative homograft studies on patients were published in 1943. Back in Oxford, Medawar carefully explored the phenomenon in rabbits. This definitive investigation is the next milestone. As expected, homografts were at first incorporated and fused with the animal's skin and then shed. Histological sections showed that lymphocytes and macrophages attacked the graft after the blood supply was reestablished through linkage of host and graft capillaries. Medawar discovered that a second application of the graft from the same donor caused an accelerated rejection, while a new graft from another donor behaved much like the original. He concluded that transplantation is controlled by an unknown immune mechanism, with rejection superficially resembling the Arthus reaction.

As we know today, the timing and vigor of rejection is related to the degree of differences between histocompatibility antigens of donor and recipient. Some primary tissues will not survive even a week; others may endure for months. Another determinant is the carry-over of donor lymphocytes, which, by selective movement into patient immunological centers, hasten the antibody and cellular immune responses. Thanks to the matching of major histocompatibility antigens, at times with the temporary aid of immunosuppressants, the replacement of kidneys has become an almost routine practice, and transplantation of other organs, including the heart, is no longer creating headlines.

Medawar was soon an elected Fellow (an administrative staff member and tutor) of Magdalen College and in 1947 he took the professorship of zoology at the University of Birmingham. In 1949 Medawar was elected to the Royal Society. Two years later, he accepted an offer as Professor of Zoology at University College, London. His research on tolerance, which will be discussed in the next comment, brought a share in the Nobel Prize of 1960, and the floodgates of honors were opened. Eschewing the regular academic doctorate, Medawar now assented to the bevy of honorary degrees. In 1962 he filled the vacancy of Director of the National Institute of Medical Research. All was going exceedingly well until 1969, when he suffered a stroke from which he, like Louis Pasteur, never fully recovered while fortunately maintaining strong mental abilities. The Medical Research Council, realizing that Medawar could no longer handle the administrative chores, relieved him of the burden, and offered a research post at the Clinical Research Center, where he remained until retirement.

For further information:

Billingham, R. and W. Silvers. 1971. *The Immunobiology of Transplantation.* Prentice-Hall, Englewood Cliffs, NJ. 209 p.

Hixson, J. 1976. *The Patchwork Mouse.* Anchor Press/Doubleday, Garden City, NY. 228 p.

Medawar, P. 1986. *Memoir of a Thinking Radish. An Autobiography.* Oxford University Press, Oxford. 209 p.

Wolstenholme, G. E. W. and M. P. Cameron (editors). 1962. *Ciba Foundation Symposium on Transplantation.* J. & A. Churchill, London. 426 p.

The Paper*

The "natural" process of wound healing is always necessary, but not always sufficient, to secure an efficient functional repair of damaged tissue. The repair of injuries involving an extensive loss of skin has long been recognized to be a surgical problem; one for which, in the majority of cases, the operation of skin grafting is a fully adequate solution. . . .

Skin from another human being will not serve as a permanent graft: neither in the human subject, nor, it will be shown, in the rabbit, is there any evidence that normal cellular tissue can survive transplantation between individuals of ordinary genetic diversity. The possibility of using skin homografts in clinical practice has been almost, if not quite, universally discredited.

Although the "homograft problem," as that which relates to the grafting incompatibility of tissues may be called, has well-recognized and more or less direct implication for surgery, genetics, serology, and taxonomic zoology, no systematic attempt has been made to solve it. There is an urgent need for a straightforward description of the behaviour of homografts, and of how their behaviour varies with the quantity of tissue that is grafted and with the recipient's previous record of graftings from the same donor source. Skin is the tissue of choice, because it can be made to provide a quantitative measure of the time of survival of foreign tissue under a variety of different conditions, and because like nerve and bone (but unlike glandular tissue) it can be grafted "isotopically"—into an anatomically natural environment. The pinch or discrete graft has proved to be superior to the continuous sheet graft for the following reasons: (a) it is technically the easiest to work with; (b) it can be cut to a fairly uniform size, and so makes possible a regulation of the dosage of grafts that an animal receives; (c) it grows by lateral spread of epithelium around its margin, and the extent of this outgrowth provides a useful quantitative measure of the efficiency of grafts of various types; and (d) single members of a uniform population of pinch grafts may be removed at regular intervals for histological examination, with the object of constructing a serial record of their behaviour and ultimate fate.

The rabbit was chosen as experimental animal, more for its size and ease of supply than for any intrinsic merit. Its serological peculiarities do, how-

*Medawar, P. B. 1944. The behaviour and fate of skin autografts and skin homografts in rabbits. *Journal of Anatomy* 78:176–199. [With permission of Cambridge University Press.]

ever, throw some light on the homograft problem. . . .

The grafts are cut from the very closely clipped skin of the outer aspect of the thigh. (Although the trauma caused by shaving is ultimately repaired, it complicates the interpretation of histological specimens; and if the donor area is shaved some days before operation, the traumatic thickening of the epidermis destroys one of the most valuable measures of the extent of cellular activity in the grafts. . . .)

The average diameter of the grafts, measured along the major axis of the oval after fixation in full extension, was found to be 8.5 ± 0.3 mm standard sampling error. The epithelial area of the "large" graft is thus reasonably uniform; its thickness is the principal variable.

The small graft used in a number of experiments on the significance of graft dosage . . . ranged between 2 and 3 mm. "Large" and "small" grafts are hereafter used as technical terms. . . .

The grafts are transplanted within half an hour of removal to a rectangular raw area on the lateral thoracic wall striped down to, but not including, the vascular fascial planes immediately overlying the panniculus carnosus. . . .

The epidermal layer on top of the graft is the "graft roof," and that part of the raw area on which the graft is planted is distinguished from the rest by being called the "graft bed." The tissue between the grafts and overlying the panniculus carnosus is called the "outlying tissue"; the term "raw area," which describes its surface before, in due course, epithelium covers it, would clearly be misleading. Epithelium of new formation is "spread epithelium," and is differentiated into inner and outer rings and margin. . . .

The autograft operation is one in which eight large pinch grafts are transplanted. . . . The behaviour of autografts has been reconstructed from the serial record provided by six animals, from each of which a biopsy specimen was removed every 4th day from the 4th to the 24th days inclusive. . . .

The evidence presented above is consistent with a hypothesis first put upon a more than speculative foundation by Gibson (1942) and Gibson & Medawar (1943), namely, that the mechanism by means of which foreign skin is eliminated belongs in broad outline to the category of *actively acquired immune reactions*. The accelerated retrogression of 2nd-set homografts, here demonstrated on a scale which makes due allowance for the degree to which genetic variance governs the intensity of the homograft reaction, argues the existence of a systemic immune state. . . .

The rabbit is known to be peculiarly susceptible to *anaphylactic inflammation* (the Arthus reaction), a phenomenon usually attributed to the meeting of antigen with antibody within the tissues. The inflammation which accompanies the homograft reaction in rabbits is very probably of the anaphylactic type. Yet, though all the ingredients of the inflammatory process are present—vacular and lymphatic proliferation, oedema, and the mobilization and deployment of mesenchyme cells of every type—the reaction is nevertheless atypical; for the lymphocyte takes the place of the polymorph in the "classic picture." At no stage in the homograft reaction has the polymorph been found to plan an appreciable part. . . .

In many other ways the immune reaction is "atypical," i.e., does not conform to the clear-cut pattern defined by, for example, the bacterial antigens. . . . There should certainly be no attempt to *force* the homograft reaction into the stereotyped serological mold. . . .

The whereabouts of the antibody is equally conjectural. Its free circulation in the blood stream may be doubted. . . .

SUMMARY

1. An investigation into the behaviour and fate of skin autografts and skin homografts in rabbits is described.

2. A technique of operation and of post-operative dressing has been employed, by means of which pinch grafts transplanted from the outer aspect of the thigh to the lateral wall of the thorax may be made to undergo full primary healing in 100% of cases.

3. The evolution of autografts falls into [a period of primary union and vascularization, characterized by migratory and amoeboid activities of cells of all types;] a period of generalized hyperplasia, in which all the cellular elements of the grafts participate; and a period of partially retrograde differentiation during which the grafts return towards the condition of normal skin.

4. Homografts undergo normal primary healing in a latent period during which they provoke no specific reaction from their recipients. At some time thereafter, they are invariably destroyed.

5. The evolution of homografts in high graft dosage (0.36–0.44 g skin per rabbit) embraces the period of generalized hyperplasia of autografts, but does not usually extend into the period of differentiation. New hairs do not mature and pierce the graft roof.

6. The phenomena of acute inflammation are superimposed upon the otherwise autograft-

like behaviour of high-dosage homografts in the period of hyperplasia.

7. The inflammatory process includes vascular and lymphatic proliferation; a massive invasion of the grafts by lymphocytes and monocytes of native origin through the walls of the vessels within them; edema of such severity that the graft bed may be distended by tracts of free fibrinous matter; and a general mobilization of mesenchyme cells.

8. Inflammation reaches its peak, and passes into necrosis, with the stagnation and obliteration of the vascular system of the graft and the death of every cellular element within it. Homografts are then invaded anew by capillary vessels from the graft bed; lymphocytes and monocytes passing through their walls establish a secondary population of native cells within them.

9. The intensity of the inflammation and its rate of development vary inversely with the time of survival of foreign skin epithelium.

10. Disengagement and breakdown of the foreign epithelium begins in that which has spread from the graft, and extends thereafter to epithelium of the graft center, to the accompaniment of a variety of non-specific pathological changes in the cells. The entire process of breakdown is complete within a compass of 4 days from start to finish.

11. The median survival time of homografts is defined as that at which the foreign epithelium borne by 50% of the experimental animals has just broken down.

12. The median survival time of homografts in high graft dosage is 10.4 ± 1.1 days.

13. The survival time of homograft epithelium varies inversely with the dosage of foreign skin which an experimental animal receives.

14. The median survival time of homografts in initial dosage of 0.0006–0.006 g foreign skin per rabbit is 15.0 ± 0.9 days. The evolution of these lower-dosage grafts extends into the period of differentiation characteristic of autograft evolution. Newly formed hairs mature and pierce the graft roof.

15. The median survival time of homografts transplanted to a freshly prepared raw area

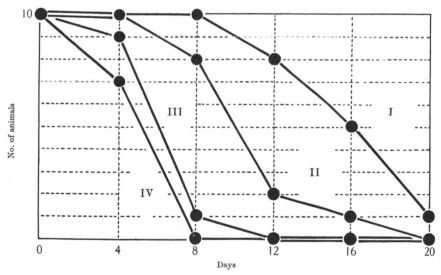

Figure 4 The survival of homograft epithelium as a function of time. Each point defines the number of animals, out of ten for each type of experiment represented, which still bear surviving foreign epithelium at the stated times. I, lower-dosage graft bearers: computed from fifty pairs of animals in five independent groups of ten; II, high-dosage graft bearers: computed from ten pairs of animals, from each of which a graft sample was removed at 4-day intervals from the 4th to the 20th day; III, standard 2nd-set graft bearers: computed from ten pairs of animals, from each of which a graft sample was removed at the 4th and at the 8th day; IV, local 2nd-set graft bearers: computed from ten pairs of animals from each of which a graft sample was removed at the 4th day. Curves III and IV are extrapolated to zero survival at the 12th and 8th days respectively without error. Curve I cannot be extended in this manner to the 24th day, since the 4-day groups of data are here independent.

of the opposite thoracic wall 16 days after a rabbit has received a 1st set of homografts in high dosage from the same donor is 6.0 ± 0.6 days. The evolution of such "2nd-set" homografts does not extend into the period of generalized hyperplasia. Inflammation is precocious in time of onset.

16. The accelerated retrogression of 2nd-set homografts has been demonstrated by a wholly independent test: one in which the survival of homograft epithelium is confirmed or refuted by transplanting a graft back to its donor after a varying period of residence on its original recipient as a 1st-set or 2nd-set homograft.

17. The accelerated retrogression of 2nd-set homografts does not necessarily extend with equal vigor to 2nd-set grafts derived from a donor source other than which provided the 1st set.

18. The breakdown of 2nd-set grafts which are transplanted to the position formerly occupied by grafts of the 1st set is far advanced, but not necessarily complete, within 4 days of transplantation. The local immune state adds little to the systemic.

19. Analysis has been made of the sampling errors of a variety of numerical estimates of survival time, intensity of inflammation, extent of hyperplasia, and degree of differentiation.

The differences between high-dosage and lower-dosage grafts on one hand, and between 1st-set and 2nd-set grafts on the other, are in each such respect greater than those for which the changes of random sampling provide a sufficient explanation.

20. The reaction elicited by homografts is sharply and precisely specific to foreign as opposed to native skin.

21. The mechanism by which foreign skin is eliminated belongs to the general category of actively acquired immune reactions.

22. The inflammatory process which accompanies it has in all likelihood the character of a local anaphylaxis.

Actively acquired tolerance of foreign cells

1953 • Rupert E. Billingham, Leslie Brent, and Peter B. Medawar

Comment

Reading the milestone paper that follows, the reader may get the impression that Sir Peter B. Medawar and his colleagues Rupert E. Billingham (1921–   ) and Leslie Brent (1925–   ), setting out to find a means by which homografts might be accepted permanently, conceived the ontological approach of introducing foreign tissue to a yet immunologically immature fetus, thus rendering it tolerant to the given foreign antigens as an adult. Assuredly, such a goal was ever present in their minds, but like many discoveries in science, the novel method was unplanned and unanticipated.

Medawar had attended the International Congress of Genetics held in Stockholm in 1948, where he met the Head of the Animal Breeding Research Organization of the Agricultural Research Council in Edinburgh. The animal geneticist, whose experiments on the influence of environment on behavior required the use of twins, asked if Medawar knew any method that could distinguish a fraternal from an identical twin in cattle. Naturally Medawar suggested, with the full confidence instilled by several years of repetitive experimentation, that the exchange of skin transplants could readily provide the solution, and offered to arrange a demonstration. Several months afterward, Medawar and Billingham obligingly drove to the experimental farm where sets of twins were held ready for the trial. Some fraternal twins were obvious, since they were of different sex. Surprisingly, the transplants of all animals, fraternal and identical twins, were accepted. Stunned and somewhat embarrassed, the researchers repeated the experiment, but obtained the same result. Why should fraternal twins of cattle react differently from those of humans or rabbits?

The following year Medawar picked up a copy of Macfarlane Burnet and Frank Fenner's book—excerpted earlier in Part 5/Burnet, 1949—*The Production of Antibodies,* which cited the work of Ray D. Owen, who had observed the same phenomenon with erythrocytes. Born on a dairy farm in 1915, Owen was a student of Leon J. Cole at the University of Wisconsin with whom he studied the developmental genetics of pigeons. After receiving his Ph.D. in 1941, he became a postdoctoral fellow of M. Robert Irwin, this time focusing on the blood groups of cattle. In 1945 Owen reported in the above influential paper cited by Burnet and Fenner that examined fraternal twins, a male Guernsey and a female Hereford, had the same blood type for the simple reason that they shared blood cells. Common placental circulation had allowed the exchange. Some mechanism in utero permitted mutual tolerance. Medawar had further demonstrated that the tolerance extended to tissues. Owen in 1946 came to California Institute of Technology as a research fellow. The next year, he was a professor turning to the immunogenetics of laboratory animals.

Some biographical notes on Billingham and Brent are also in order: After service in the Royal Navy, Billingham became Medawar's first graduate student at Oxford. He accepted Medawar's invitation to join him at the University of Birmingham, where he secured the post of Lecturer in Zoology while completing his doctoral thesis. Brent was a graduate student at Birmingham. In 1951, the troika transplanted themselves to University College, Billingham as Research Associate and Brent, in 1954, as Lecturer. When Medawar left for the National Institute of Medical Research in 1962, he was accompanied by Brent alone; Billingham, now a Fellow of the Royal Society, had in 1957 become a professor of zoology at the Wistar Institute of the University of Pennsylvania. In 1965 he switched to the medical faculty as a professor of medical genetics. Billingham's last move was in 1971 to the Southwestern Medical School of the University of Texas Health Science Center at Dallas, where he became Professor of Cell Biology. Meanwhile, Brent served as a professor of zoology at Southampton University between 1965 and 1969, and since then has held the position of Professor of Immunology at St. Mary's Hospital Medical School.

The paper by Medawar, Billingham, and Brent appeared at approximately the same time as Milan Hasek's report. Unintentionally duplicating the phenomenon described by Owen, Hasek had connected the circulatory systems of two chicken embryos in their respective egg, a condition known as parabiosis. He found the hatched chicks to be chimeras (containing somatic cells of two genetic types) tolerant of each other's blood and skin grafts. The approach of the British team, however, was more versatile. A more interesting variation was their introduction of lymph node cells from normal immunized adults: The grafts on tolerant animals were soon shed, demonstrating that the antigenicity of the grafts remained and that it was the animal's immune response that had been effectively switched off or blocked. This result also tended to discount the possibility that suppressor T cells were responsible for tolerance. Another key finding was that the resulting degree of tolerance varied among the animals, which was probably related in part to the technically difficult experimental design. Today, such experiments are performed on neonates rather than fetuses, and to avoid graft-versus-host reactions, the F_1 hybrid serves as the donor and one of the parent strains as the recipient.

Tolerance, or specific immunological unresponsiveness, has no single mechanism of induction. The exceedingly complex interaction of cellular and soluble immunological components is vulnerable—so to speak—at the many different points mentioned in the previous sections. Most likely any form of tolerance stems from a combination or perhaps synergy of several mechanisms. Certain processes, nevertheless, may dominate. The tolerance described by Medawar's team is that which normally makes the organism immunologically blind to itself. Rather than T cell suppression and antibody interference, which can provide tolerance in adults, clonal inactivation seems to be primarily responsible. However, tolerance is rarely complete. Some clones with less avid receptors may remain competent. The breaking of tolerance noted in the report was probably through antibody cross-reactivity and stimulation of T cells to the different minor histocompatibility antigens of the related grafts. Despite all the advances in immunology, the basic process of self-tolerance remains cloudy.

For further information:

Auerbach, R. and S. Clark. 1975. Immunological tolerance: transmission from mother to offspring. *Science* 189:811–813.

Hildemann, W. H. and J. Frelinger. 1981. Biographical preface. In: *Frontiers in Immunogenetics. Proceedings of a symposium in honor of Professor Ray D. Owen* (William H. Hildemann, editor). Elsevier/North-Holland, New York. pp. vii–xiii.

Landy, M. and W. Braun (editors). 1969. *Immunological Tolerance. A reassessment of mechanisms of the immune response.* Academic Press, New York. 352 p.

Lewin, R. 1981. Lamarck will not lie down. *Science* 213:316–321.

Strayer, D. S., H. Cosenza, W. M. F. Lee, D. A. Rowley, and H. Kohler. 1974. Neonatal tolerance induced by antibody against antigen-specific receptor. *Science* 186:640–643.

The Paper*

The experiments to be described in this article provide a solution—at present only a "laboratory" solution—of the problem of how to make tissue homografts immunologically acceptable to hosts which would normally react against them. The principle underlying the experiments may be expressed in the following terms: that mammals and birds never develop, or develop to only a limited degree, the power to react immunologically against foreign homologous tissue cells to which they have been exposed sufficiently early in fetal life. If, for example, a fetal mouse of one inbred strain (say, CBA) is inoculated *in utero* with a suspension of living cells from an adult mouse of another strain (say, A), then when it grows up, the CBA mouse will be found to be partly or completely tolerant of skin grafts transplanted from any mouse belonging to the strain of the original donor.

This phenomenon is the exact inverse of "actively acquired immunity", and we therefore propose to describe it as "actively acquired tolerance". The distinction between the two phenomena may be made evident in the following way. If a normal adult CBA mouse is inoculated with living cells or grafted with skin from an A-line donor, the grafted tissue is destroyed within twelve days. The effect of this first presentation of foreign tissue in adult life is to confer "immunity", that is, to increase the host's resistance to grafts which may be transplanted on some later occasion from the same donor or from some other member of the donor's strain. But if the first presentation of foreign cells takes place in fetal life, it has just the opposite effect: resistance to a graft transplanted on some later occasion, so far from being heightened, is abolished or at least reduced. Over some period of its early life, therefore, the pattern of the host's response to foreign tissue cells is turned completely upside down. In mice, it will be seen, this inversion takes place in the neighborhood of birth, for there is a certain "null" period thereabouts when the inoculation of foreign tissue confers neither tolerance nor heightened resistance—when, in fact, a "test graft" transplanted in adult life to ascertain the host's degree of immunity is found to survive for the same length of time as if the host had received no treatment at all.

The literature of experimental embryology is rich in evidence that embryos are fully tolerant of grafts

*Billingham, R. E., L. Brent, and P. B. Medawar. 1953. 'Actively acquired tolerance' of foreign cells. *Nature* 172:603–606. [By permission, copyright 1953 Macmillan Journals Limited.]

of foreign tissues. It is less well known (though no less firmly established) that embryonic cells transplanted into embryos of different genetic constitutions may survive into adult life, although their host would almost certainly have rejected them if transplantation had been delayed until after birth. . . . An exactly comparable phenomenon has been described by Owen, who found that the majority of dizygotic cattle twins are born with, and long retain, red blood cells of dizygotic origin: each calf contains a proportion of red cells belonging genetically to itself, mixed with red cells belonging to the zygote lineage of its twin. There is no reason to doubt that this is because the cattle twins, being synchorial, exchange blood in fetal life through the anastomoses of their placental vessels. . . . [W]e have found that the majority of cattle twins at birth and for long after are fully tolerant of grafts of each other's skin. Being freshly transplanted, these grafts can have no opportunity to "adapt themselves antigenically to foreign hosts, but they survived nevertheless.

The experiments of Cannon and Longmire have a direct bearing on the phenomenon of actively acquired tolerance. About 5–10 per cent of skin grafts exchanged between pairs of newly hatched chicks of different breeds are tolerated and survive into adult life; but the percentage of successes falls rapidly as the age at which the chicks are operated increased, and reaches zero by the end of the second week. . . .

A single experiment will be described in moderate detail: the recipients were mice of CBA strain, the donors of A strain. The data for transplantations between normal mice of these strains are as follows. The median survival time of A-line skin grafts transplanted to normal CBA adults (regardless of differences of sex, or of age within the interval 6 weeks–6 months) is 11.0 ± 0.3 days. In reacting against such a graft, the host enters a state of heightened resistance; a second graft transplanted up to sixty days after the transplantation of the first survives for less than six days, and immunity is still strong, though it has weakened perceptibly, after four months.

In the experiment to be described (Exp. 73), a CBA female in the 15th–16th day of pregnancy by a CBA male was anesthetized with "Nembutal", and its body wall exposed by a median ventral incision of the skin. The skin was mobilized but not reflected, and particular care was taken not to damage the mammary vessels. By manipulation of the abdomen with damped gauzes, six fetuses were brought into view through the body wall. Each was injected intraembryonically with 0.01 ml of a suspension of adult tissue cells through a very fine hypodermic needle passing successively through the body wall, uterine wall, and fetal membranes. . . . After injection of the fetuses, the skin was closed with interrupted sutures.

Five healthy and normal-looking young were born four days later; of the sixth fetus there was no trace. Eight weeks after their birth, when the lightest weighed 21 g, each member of the litter was "challenged" with a skin graft from an adult A-line donor. The first inspection of the grafts was carried out eleven days later, that is, at the median survival age of A-line skin grafts transplanted to normal CBA hosts. The grafts on two of the five mice were in an advanced stage of breakdown; the grafts on the other three . . . resembled autografts in every respect except their donor-specific albinism. Each of these three grafts became perfectly incorporated into its host's skin and grew a white hair pelt of normal density and stoutness. Fifty days later, one of the three mice received a second A-line graft from a new donor, and this graft also settled down without the least symptom of an immunological reaction.

The graft on one of the three animals underwent a long-drawn-out "spontaneous" involution, beginning before the 75th day after transplantation. . . . The other two mice were made the subjects of an experiment designed to show that acquired tolerance is due to a failure of the host's immunological response and not to an antigenic adaptation of the grafted cells. When the two grafts were of 77 and 101 days standing, respectively, and still in immaculate condition, their hosts were inoculated intraperitoneally with chopped fragments of lymph nodes from normal CBA mice which had been actively immunized against A-line skin. The grafts began to deteriorate 2–3 days later. . . . It follows that tolerant hosts are fully capable of giving effect to a state of immunity which has been elicited by proxy, and that the tolerated grafts have not lost their ability to respond to it. . . .

The results of Exp. 73 demonstrate the great (but not necessarily indefinite) prolongation of the life of homografts made possible by a preemptive exposure of their hosts to foreign homologous cells. Beyond this, they demonstrate (a) that this prolongation of life is not due to an antigenic transformation of the grafts, nor to a competitive absorption of antibodies by, for example, cells of the fetal inoculum which had survived into adult life; and (b) that acquired tolerance is either not transferred to, or is too weak or too ephemeral to make itself evident in, the offspring. . . .

The more important results obtained from the investigation of other litters may be summarized as follows. (1) The conferment of tolerance is not of an all-or-nothing character; every degree is represented, down to that which gives the test-grafts only a few days of grace beyond the median survival time of their controls. (2) The conferment of tolerance is immunologically specific. Thus a CBA mouse made tolerant of A-line tissue, or vice versa, retains the ability to react with unmodified vigor against skin from a donor belonging to a third strain, AU. But it has so far been our experience that the transplantation of (say) AU skin to a CBA mouse that is tolerant of A-line cells will elicit a reaction which, in addition to destroying the AU graft, causes an A-line graft already in residence to go through a severe immunological crisis. Although we have evidence of a sharing of tissue antigens between strains A and AU, this phenomenon is difficult to interpret, for the antigens common to strain A and AU are merely a sub-group of those to which the CBA host is manifestly unresponsive. It may therefore turn out that the continued well-being of a tissue homograft upon a tolerant host depends upon the quiescence of the antibody-forming system, and that if this is awakened by tissue antigens other than those which the host is tolerant, antibodies directed against its, until then, tolerated graft may be formed as well. (3) A wide histological variety of tissue cells is capable of conferring tolerance to homografts of skin. It is by no means obligatory that skin cells, or even epithelial cells, should be among them. (4) We have inoculated ninety-six newborn mice with adult or fetal tissue cell suspensions to decide whether tolerance can be conferred by exposure to foreign cells at this relatively advanced stage of development. The majority received a single inoculation of cells as soon as possible after birth; a small subgroup of these was injected with 0.05 mg cortisone acetate on the same occasion and several more times during the first week of life in an attempt to delay the maturation of the antibody-forming system. The remainder of the newborn mice received repeated injections of foreign tissue cells in increasing quantities over the period of a month from birth. In all, only nine mice (about 10 per cent) showed an increase of tolerance when tested with a skin graft from the donor strain, and six of these were members of a single litter of eight which had received a single inoculation of cells, without cortisone, immediately after birth. It is of particular interest that when challenged with skin grafts in adult life the great majority of inoculated newborn mice showed neither tolerance nor enhanced resistance. Newborn mice are, in general, too old for a tissue inoculum to confer tolerance, and too young for it to confer immunity; the epoch of birth represents a null period during which the net outcome of exposure to foreign cells is to leave its subjects in a state of unaltered reactivity. (5) Grafts removed from hosts which have tolerated them, and then transplanted to normal mice of the host's strain, survive 2–3 days longer than freshly transplanted homografts of normal skin. Such homografts cannot, however, be compared directly with homografts of normal skin, because a high proportion of the corium of each will probably have been replaced by cells and cellular derivatives of host origin.

[This section was followed by an account of some preliminary experiments with Rhode Island Red and White Leghorn chickens, which gave similar but less distinct results mainly because of heterogeneity in the breeds.]

It is one of the predictions of Burnet and Fenner's theory of immunity that the exposure of animals to antigens before the developmet of the faculty of immunological response should lead to tolerance rather than to heightened resistance. The homograft immunity system is particularly well suited to the appraisal of such a hypothesis, because the antigens are at once powerful, innocuous and persistent. . . . It must be emphasized, however, that our experiments do not yet bear upon the fundamental problem of whether the production of antibodies represents an *inherited* derangement of protein synthesis, that is, a transformation which can persist through repeated cell divisions after the disappearance of the antigen originally responsible for it. It would be a highly significant fact if a transient exposure to antigen in fetal life could confer a permanent or very long-lasting tolerance; but in our present experiments there is no reason to doubt that at least some of the cells of the fetal inoculum survived as long as the tolerant state which they were responsible for creating. At all events, any complete theory of antibody formation must be competent to explain two sets of facts: that although embryos do not make antibodies, they respond to antigens in a manner that prejudices their ability to do so in later life; and that acquired tolerance is highly specific, for antibody-forming cells can be prevented from responding to one antigen without impairing their capacity to respond to any other. . . .

Passive transfer of transplantation immunity

1953 • N. Avrion Mitchison

Comment

N. Avrion Mitchison came naturally to the following study on transplantation. He had been, after all, a graduate student of Peter Medawar at Magdalen College, Oxford. Tutor and student were also members there of the Theoretical Biology Club, which included such luminaries and scholars as J. H. Woodger, Francis Huxley, Karl Popper, and Joseph Needham. Mitchison completed the research while a Fellow at the University Museum and Department of Zoology and Comparative Anatomy, just before leaving for the University of Edinburgh. In 1962 Mitchison and Medawar were together again when both received appointments to the National Institute for Medical Research, Medawar as its Director and Mitchison to head the Division of Experimental Biology.

The phenomenon of transplantation immunity and its genetic relationship had been described, but what was its mechanism? Since Sir Peter Medawar's initial report, it was suspected to be a special case of allergic cellular immunity, but evidence was ambiguous. Antibodies and serum factors still dominated immunological thought, and some experiments indicated that the key role belonged to antibodies. This confusion is understandable, since foreign tissues can elicit both cellular and humoral responses, depending on circumstances. However, the T cell-mediated reactions to histocompatibility antigens, particularly the involvement of cytotoxic T cells, were experimentally the crucial element. For example, athymic mice (typically neonates whose thymus was surgically removed) have no difficulty accepting any graft, even from a different species, as demonstrated by Jacques F. A. P. Miller. The B cells of such mice remain functional, albeit somewhat dormant. The addition of normal T

cells to these animals will initiate graft rejection, and if the T cells come from immune donors, the rejection manifests an accelerated, secondary response.

Mitchison's work was an extension of Merrill W. Chase's demonstration eight years earlier that tuberculin or delayed hypersensitivity can be passively transferred by immune cells but not by antiserum. However, in contrast with Chase's finding, peritoneal exudates were not effective. While strongly resembling tuberculin sensitivity in some respects, the tissue phenomenon was obviously more complicated. Mitchison elegantly provided the first evidence that transplantation immunity, the ability to maintain immunological individuality, is effected by regional lymph node cells. Strikingly, the cells from the parallel node, on the side of the body opposite to the site tumor inoculation, were ineffective. With a different experimental design, Medawar afterwards found that peripheral blood lymphocytes also could transfer immunity. Mitchison helped dispel the long-held view that antibodies were the wherewithal of immunity. Nevertheless, in some instances with a given graft site, a particular tissue type, and a degree of antigenic deviation, antibody formation may indeed be a significant contributor to graft rejection.

Hyperacute organ transplant rejection, first observed with kidney transplants, results when preexisting antibody—synthesized by a previous infection, transfusion, or transplant—immediately attaches to the blood vessels of the transplant and activates the complement cascade. The resulting cellular damage and platelet formation of fibrin clots starve the tissue and produce necrosis. This variation of rejection is aptly called hyperacute, since the first signs of this process can be detected during the surgical operation! Natural killer cells also can contribute by homing in on the Fc portion of the tissue-attached antibodies. Insidious and delayed rejection may also occur with the deposition of immune complexes on the glomerular basement membranes.

Almost paradoxically, antibodies may also prolong the survival of incompatible grafts. The mechanism of tissue immunity is, of course, linked with the mechanisms of tolerance, as Medawar's team was concurrently exploring. In this particular process, known as enhancement, antibodies neutralize the antigenic tissue fragments—which always arise during surgery—before they reach the helper T cell. The fragments themselves can act as an intercepting screen for cytotoxic T cells. The passive introduction of such antibodies is the strategy of prophylaxis in Rh-negative mothers. An alternate mechanism calls for antibodies to alter or occlude the antigens on the graft to prevent recognition by helper or cytotoxic T cells. Thus, Mitchison's failure to provide immunity or secondary type rejection in normal mice by passive introduction of antisera may in part reflect this opposite action. Later Mitchison demonstrated that the same antigen could induce immunity or tolerance depending on dosage.

Transplantation, therefore, has no unique immune mechanism. Rejection is largely a delayed hypersensitivity reaction that involves to a varying extent cytotoxic T cells, NK cells, macrophages, complement, and antibody. The target antigen, however, is steadfastly the isotypic class I histocompatibility molecule. When Mitchison's paper was published in 1953, most of these agents were unknown. The formal disciplines of genetics, hematology, immunology, and surgical medicine were growing toward each other, and experiments in transplantation, tolerance, and cellular immunity interweaved, such that a discovery in one branch of immunology was rapidly felt in another. A unified conception, however, was still nowhere in sight. Researchers seemed to stumble over each other in the dark of ignorance. A small candle was lit two months after Mitchison's report appeared: The same journal published the double-helix model of DNA.

For further information:

Feldman, J. D. 1972. Immunological enhancement: a study of blocking antibodies. *Advances in Immunology* 15:167–214.

Levey, R. H. 1971. Immunological tolerance and enhancement: a common mechanism. *Transplantation Proceedings* 3(1):41–48.

Strom, T. B., N. L. Tilney, C. B. Carpenter, and G. J. Busch. 1975. Identity and cytotoxic capacity of cells infiltrating renal allografts. *New England Journal of Medicine* 292:1257–1263.

Turk, J. L. 1975. *Delayed Hypersensitivity.* Second edition. North-Holland Publishing Company, Amsterdam. pp. 112–128.

The Paper*

Passive transfer of transplantation immunity has never been successfully achieved in a simple way. Previous demonstrations of passive transfer have either employed special techniques giving results which are difficult to interpret, or else the nature of the immunity has been in doubt. Here is reported a simple procedure for passively transferring transplantation immunity to a tumor.

The tumor used was lymphosarcoma 6C3HED, described by Gardner, Dougherty and Williams. Mice of Strong's CBA line are uniformly susceptible to the tumor, and mice of Strong's C57 line, and the Ai line inbred in this laboratory, are uniformly nonsusceptible. The survival of grafts of the tumor in nonsusceptible mice has been measured by allowing grafts of the tumor to lie in these mice, and then regrafting them into susceptible mice, where growth of the tumor indicates that the tumor had survived in the nonsusceptible host. In this way the median survival time of the tumor in Ai mice was found to be 9.9 ± 0.8 days. If the Ai mice had been previously immunized by inoculation with the tumor, the me-

---

*Mitchison, N. A. 1953. Passive transfer of transplantation immunity. *Nature* 171:267–268. [By permission, copyright 1953 Macmillan Journals Limited.]

dian survival time was then 2.1 ± 0.3 days. In order to demonstrate passive transfer of transplantation immunity, tissues were transferred from immunized nonsusceptible mice into nonsusceptible mice from the same line, and the proportion of test grafts of the tumor which survived after eight days in these hosts was measured. Approximately 70 per cent of the grafts survived this time in untreated nonsusceptible mice, and after successful transfer of immunity this proportion was reduced.

Subcutaneous inoculations of serum and peritoneal exudate from immune mice both proved ineffective in transferring immunity, in experiments with Ai mice. However, evidence was obtained for transfer of immunity by intraperitoneal transplantation of "immune" lymph nodes, and further investigations of this method of transfer were carried out in C57 mice. Lymph nodes from immune mice were found to be highly effective in transferring immunity.

The method of transfer could be shown to be genuinely passive, and not merely a transfer with the lymph nodes of tumor cells or possibly of isoantigenic particles. Immune lymph-node mince was in-

oculated into CBA mice, but invariably failed to give rise to tumors. Furthermore, the duration of their immunity was estimated by leaving intervals between inoculation of immune lymph nodes and test tumor grafts. The immunity appeared to remain firm for four days, weaken after ten days, and disappear after twenty days. Lymph nodes taken from nonsusceptible mice ten days after inoculation with the tumor were effective in transferring immunity, but after twenty days this power was lost. At this time all the tumor cells had been killed, and the nodes, which after ten days hypertrophy to approximately double their normal weight, have almost returned to normal. Only local lymph nodes were effective in transferring immunity; the corresponding nodes from the opposite side to the site of tumor inoculation were not effective. Neither spleen nor muscle from immunized mice was found to be effective.

This investigation . . . shows that transplantation immunity shares with immunity to simple organic compounds and immunity to tuberculin the property of being transferred with greater facility by cells than by serum.

Alloantibodies to leucocytes

1958 • Jean Dausset

Comment

With the present milestone, we leave transplantation to return to the mainstream of immunogenetics, although successful transplantation of tissues and organs is the most important application of the field. Immunogenetics began with the investigation of antigens on red blood cells and their relationship to transfusion reactions, but no attention was given to the white blood cells that were also transferred. Could a patient react against them also? The pioneer of this inquiry is Jean Dausset (1916–   ), whose researches established a human equivalent for Peter A. Gorer's mouse histocompatibility system.

Blood was the hallmark of Dausset's early medical training with the Free French forces

in World War II in the North Africa campaign and the liberation of France. The occasional transfusion reactions were bitter, curious phenomena that etched his consciousness. With the battle of France won, but a war still to end, he entered the University of Paris to continue the program for his M.D. It was awarded in 1945. He completed additional medical studies in 1948 at Harvard University. When he observed in 1951 that transfusion reactions occurred after patients were given diphtheria and tetanus antitoxins, which later were found to contain blood group antigen A, Dausset was intrigued. Purely clinical pursuits gave way to research.

In 1952 he discovered that the serum of patients with autoimmune hemolytic anemias and other blood disorders contained antibodies that agglutinated allogeneic leukocytes and platelets. This led to a further study of normal subjects who received multiple transfusions. He determined that the increased opportunity for exposure to allogeneic leukocytes could initiate the formation of agglutinins. Other researchers observed leukocyte agglutination with sera from women who had repeated pregnancies, which provide similar contact with foreign antigens. At first Dausset searched for and found ABO blood group antigens, but they were inadequate to explain the result of serological absorptions. His work of 1958 is the next milestone, since it introduces the first human histocompatibility antigen, MAC, named after the initials of three donors whose leukocytes did not agglutinate the test sera. This antigen is now known as HLA-A2.

Through the 1960s, work on histocompatibility genetics was a jumble of obscure nomenclature, uncertain alleleic products, supposed genetic loci, nonstandard methods, and confused interpretations. The anarchy slowly came to an end in the course of a still continuing series of workshops launched by Bernard Amos in 1964 whereby the investigators shared their reagents of antisera and antigens and tried to reach a consensus. In 1965, Dausset with Pavol and Dagmar Ivanyi in Czechoslovakia reported that ten leukocyte antigens were controlled by a single genetic system, then termed Hu-1, with several loci, including the genes for now recognized HLA-A and HLA-B antigens. The concept of the human major histocompatibility complex was born.

From 8 to 40 alleles are associated with each of the 6 genetic loci, a condition known as polymorphism. The unique and antigenic molecular configuration of these antigens is not merely a change in the chromosome base pair or a substitution of an amino acid. Class I antigens encompass HLA-A, HLA-B, and HLA-C loci; class II antigens are coded at DC, DR, and SB loci. Class III genes code for complement factors 2 and 4 and properdin Factor B. Located on the short arm of chromosome 6,

the histocompatibility complex is one of the most thoroughly examined regions of the genetic complement of humans.

Biologists have sought an explanation for the origin and purpose of the major histocompatibility complex, particularly for the class I antigens. Are they merely, as Dausset put it, the identity card of the organism, with antigens presumably serving as the digits of a social security number? Or, to use a more precise analogy, are they but multilingual signposts marking territories, which are recognized as friendly or dangerous by the monoglot cellular constabulary responsible for immunological surveillance? As with the blood group isoantigens, population studies have been useful in determining anthropological patterns, and comparisons with the mouse H-2 system and those of other animals are aiding in evolutionary studies. "Hybrid vigor" is too simple an answer for its function. The variation among individuals certainly helps to preserve the species from the threat of infectious diseases or a hazardous mutation or recombinant; however, this is only a fortuitous emergent result, which is maintained through selection. For example, only a single form of class I histocompatibility antigen is found among Syrian hamsters, whose solitary desert life limits if not precludes epizootics. Graft rejection among these animals, when it does occur, is due to differences in their class II antigens. From correlative epidemiological studies another pattern has appeared. Predisposition to certain diseases has been linked to particular allelic products. The best example is HLA-B27 and ankylosing spondylitis; some 90 percent of patients with this rare affliction carry the antigen. Other strong associations are with multiple sclerosis, dermatitis herpetiformis, Addison's disease, and acute anterior uveitis. A variety of mechanisms have been proposed for these associations from tolerance-producing mimicry of infectious agents to receptors for viruses or toxins, from proximal linkage with unrelated functional genes to the altering of the efficacy of cytotoxic T cells. The evidence is still too skeletal for any fair judgment of worth.

Dausset, who has speculated that class I antigens have domains with various functions like their probable immunoglobulin cousins, has spent most of his career in the Faculty of Medicine of the University of Paris, rising to professor of immunohematology in 1968. In 1977 he transferred to experimental medicine at Saint Louis Hospital of the College de France in Paris. Concurrently, he was Director of the Immunogenetics Unit on Human Transplantation of the Institut National de Recherche Santé et Medicale and Co-Director of the Oncology and Immunohematology Laboratory of the Centre National de Recherche Scientifique. He retired in 1984. His chief honors are the rank of Commander, Legion of Honor, awarded in 1969, and the Nobel Prize in 1980, which he shared with George D. Snell and Baruj Benacerraf.

For further information:

Darden, A. G. and J. W. Streilein. 1986. Can a mammalian species with monomorphic class I MHC molecules succeed? In: *Paradoxes in Immunology* (G. W. Hoffman, J. G. Levy, and G. T. Nepom, editors). CRC Press, Boca Raton, FL. pp. 9–26.

Dausset, J. 1981. The major histocompatibility complex in man. Past, present, and future concepts. *Science* 213:1469–1474.

Festenstein, H. and P. Demant. 1978. HLA and H-2. *Basic Immunogenetics, Biology and Clinical Relevance.* Edward Arnold, London. 212 p.

Sasazuki, T., H. O. McDevitt, and F. C. Grumet. 1977. The association between genes in the major histocompatibility complex and disease susceptibility. *Annual Review of Medicine* 28:425–452.

Snell, G. D., J. Dausset, and S. Nathenson. 1976. *Histocompatibility.* Academic Press, New York. 401 p.

The Paper*

The relatively slow progress in the immunology of leucocytes is not due to the rarity of antibodies—on the contrary they are very frequently found in the blood of polytransfusion diseases—but mainly to the difficulties which are encountered in procuring leucocyte antigens in sufficient quantity and purity. In spite of these obstacles, a certain number of new facts have been acquired:

I. Natural isoantibodies are detected to antigens common to those of erythrocytes. Numerous studies . . . have ascertained that natural antibodies of the ABO system are capable of agglutinating leucocytes from donors belonging to the corresponding groups. Agglutination assays show that leucocytes A_2 are less strongly agglutinated than leucocytes A_1.

Absorption tests further show that leucocytes A_2 absorb a lesser quantity of antibodies than leucocytes A_1. . . . It does not seem that it is a question of simple absorption of soluble antigens A and B, because these assays had been made with leucocytes washed 5 times and the same degree of absorption has been observed with leucocytes from subjects whose plasma was rich or poor in soluble antigen. . . .

II. Do natural anti-leucocyte isoantibodies exist directed against groups of antigens independent of those of erythrocytes? . . . We have never found agglutination between normal serum and normal compatible leucocytes.

III. Immune isoantibodies seem to be much more important. These are observed extremely frequently. They appear nearly systematically in polytransfusion diseases between the 15th and 30th transfusion. . . .

Our personal experience is currently 168 cases of leuco-agglutinins. The most important are those of pancytopenia, but it is known that these patients had for the most part received a very great number of transfusions; the other cases are distributed among the other diseases of blood which necessitated transfusions. However, I direct attention to 3 groups of patients who had not received transfusions: the disseminated lupus erythromatoses, patients having received anti-tetanus serotherapy, and the agranulocytoses to pyramidon [aminopyrine] to which are added some rare cases of idiopathic agranulocytoses. In all the other cases, at least in the vast majority, the existence of anti-leucocyte antibodies can be attributed to prior transfusions.

The serological characteristics of immune leuco-agglutinins are known. These have an optimal tem-

*Dausset, J. 1958. Iso-leuco-anticorps. *Acta Haematologica* (Basel) 20:156–166. [With permission of S. Karger AG, Basel.]

perature of 37°C. These are of complete type, initiating agglutination in saline. They are present among the gamma globulins and according to Miescher, in the beta-two region. To detect them, it often requires heating serum some minutes at 56°C, which destroys a thermolabile system inhibitor.

We are especially interested in their specificity.

1. They are isoantibodies; indeed they always remain inactive toward the patient's own leucocytes, although they agglutinate more or less a large assortment of iso-leucocytes. This single fact is sufficient to demonstrate that important antigenic differences, of which exist leucocytic groups, occur among human leucocytes.

2. These isoantibodies remain inactive to red blood cells, and inversely anti-erythrocyte isoantibodies are inactive toward leucocytes. This allows the assertion that leucocytic groups are independent of erythrocytic groups.

3. Antigens that produce sensitization, and which are without doubt surface antigens, are multiple as evidenced by the progressive sensitization to an increasing number of antigens in proportion to the number of repeated transfusions. Likewise, desensitization occurs in stages.

Another proof for the multiplicity of leucocytic antigens can be found in the percentage of groups of iso-leucocytes agglutinated by leuco-agglutinins. The percentage varies from 100% to 33%.

In attempting to clarify the problem, we have for the past two years tested our leuco-agglutinins against a panel of 20 collections of normal leucocytes.... This long study did not provide all the clarity that we had hoped. It was observed that leucocytic antigens must be extremely numerous and complex, because... there were only two groups of leucocytes that had reacted identically with the 27 studied sera.... There were only two sera ... that had reacted absolutely identically with the 20 assortments of leucocytes. This seems to indicate that the anti-

bodies that are found in current practice are a mixture.

Nevertheless, we have attempted with the aid of 7 sera to sketch a primary system of leucocytic groups. These 7 sera were inactive to 3 collections of leucocytes, and were active toward 11 others. It could be thought that the 3 negative leucocyte groups did not possess a responsible antigen for the formation of a principal antibody. The 11 positive assortments possessed this or another antigen against which certain patients had produced a secondary antibody. Five other groups, which gave discordances, did not possess it but carried one or several other antigens.

If we accept this hypothesis, the antigen in question, which we have called MAC, would be present in about 60% of individuals. It is noteworthy that the antibodies of these 7 patients were inactive not only to their own leucocytes but also to the leucocytes of 6 other patients, demonstrating that all lacked at least the same antigen. From the data of this study it is evident that on leucocytes there does not seem to exist an antigen clearly more antigenic than others, as for example is the case of the Rh antigen on erythrocytes. Nevertheless, the MAC antigen could serve in a preliminary classification.

We had thought that the mixture of antibodies observed in practice was due to the fact that the patients had been transfused with multiple assortments of leucocytes. Thus to obtain relatively singular antibody, we regularly transfused patients with the blood of the same donor. Three groups of 2 individuals had received 12 such transfusions. Leucoagglutinins appeared in 4 of the 6 recipients. In these 4 instances, active leuco-agglutinins to donor leucocytes were found by the 7th transfusion. These leuco-agglutinins had been tested against the leucocytes of our panel. Antibodies arose with continued transfusions, agglutination becoming stronger for certain collections of leucocytes. Certain groups remained unagglutinated....

By another means we have compared the antigens of leucocytes from transfused patients with their donors. In this instance their leucocytes had been tested against 13 leuco-agglutinins....

The antigenic composition of human leucocytes are of extreme complexity, but these antigens reflect

Table IV   Progressive sensitization against leucocytes after multiple transfusions.

	Leucocyte No.									
	1	2	3	4	5	6	7	8	9	10
After 1 transfusion	−	−	−	−	−	−	−	−	−	−
After 31 transfusions	−	−	+	+	−	−	−	+	−	−
After 50 transfusions	+	−	+	+	−	−	+	+	+	−
After 162 transfusions	+ +	−	+ +	+ +	+ +	+ +	+ +	+ +	+ +	−

Table XI Agglutination of leucocytes of twins by sera [edited].

	Sera possessing leuco-agglutinins
Monozygotic twins	
Twin A1	− ± − + − + + − + + + + − + + + ± + + + − − −
Twin A2	− ± − + − + + − + + + + − + + + ± + + + − − −
Twin B1	+ ± − − + + ± − + + + + − + + + + + + + +
Twin B2	+ ± − − + + ± − + + + + − + + + + + + + +
Twin C1	+ + + + + + − + + + + − − + + + + +
Twin C2	+ + + + + + − + + + + − − + + + + +
Dizygotic twins	
Twin D1	+ + − + + + + − + + + − − − + + − − + + + − . −
Twin D2	+ − + + − + + − − + + + + + + + + + + + + + −

the genetic constituency of each individual as shown by our study of monozygote twins. The leucocytes of 6 monozygote twins and of 2 dizygote twins were tested with leucocyte-agglutinating sera. It was observed that reactions were absolutely identical for each pair of monozygote twins but dissimilar in the dizygote pair. . . .

What are the practical consequences of these studies? And firstly should one even consider transfusions of leucocyte antigens? . . .

Concerning at the outset the survival of transfused leucocytes, it is known that leucocytes, compatible or not, disappear very quickly from the circulation. The choice would thus not afford any apparent benefit. But we do not know anything about the survival of leucocytes outside the circulation and it is possible that the total duration of life is longer for leucocytes not attacked by antibodies. . . .

However, the choice of nonagglutinated leucocytes can be of great interest in attempting to avoid the immediate or delayed appearance of transfusion shocks. The conflict between incompatible leucocytes and leucocyte antibodies seems responsible for certain unexpected transfusion shocks following multiple transfusions. . . .

To avoid these shocks it is then necessary to inject only blood deficient in leucocytes. . . .

Lastly . . . the study of leucocytic antigens could have great importance for tissue grafts and especially bone marrow. . . .

Studies on artificial antigens

1963 • Bernard B. Levine, Antonio Ojeda, and Baruj Benacerraf

Comment

Immunity is a process of a vast network, which includes various interacting cell types, but if one cell category has to be ranked above all, it would be the T cell. The macrophage was the first king of immunology. Then the antibody-forming B cell ruled. Now it is the thymus-derived lymphocyte. The change of command, a result of ten decades of research, also reflects phylogenic evolution. The phagocyte is by far the most primitive immunological agent; the inhibitory chemical-synthesizing cell appeared in higher invertebrates, true specific immunoglobulins arising with the vertebrates; and the thymus developed fully in the advanced vertebrates. The presence of histocompatibility antigens—emphasis on *antigens*—concomitant with T cells offers a deeper understanding of the function of the allogeneic markers: Both class I and class II molecules are regulatory partners to T cell receptors, class I for effector T_C cells, and class II for affector T_H and T_S cells.

Previous milestones have been concerned with class I genes. In 1973 serological and recombinant genetic studies established the existence of class II histocompatibility genes, but ten years earlier Baruj Benacerraf (1920–) and his associates had discovered the same genes in a different functional guise. Benaceraff was born in Venezuela, and spent his later youth in France, attending the University of Paris. In 1940 he left wartime France for the United States, where two years later at Columbia University he received his B.S. His next stop was the Medical College of Virginia, which in 1945 awarded him the M.D. After his military service and upon the advice of Rene Dubos and Jules Freund, Benacerraf went back to Columbia University in 1947 as an unpaid research fellow to learn the scientific arts of immunochemistry from Elvin Kabat at the College of Physicians and Surgeons. In 1949 he returned to France as Senior Researcher at the Centre National de Recherche Scientifique. Seven years afterward he was back in New York, this time as a professor of pathology at the New York University School of Medicine. In 1968, Benacerraf became Chief of the Laboratory of Immunology at the National Institute of Allergy and Infectious Disease, but two years later he accepted the appointment as Professor of Comparative Pathology and Chairman of the Department of Pathology of Harvard University Medical School, where he at last planted roots. To the above responsibilities, he added President of the Sidney Farber Cancer Institute. As noted before, he shared the Nobel Prize in 1980.

Benacerraf came to immunogenetics through the anomaly of an experiment. Collaborating with Gerald M. Edelman in attempts to determine the molecular structure of antibody, he was hampered by the normal heterogeneity of immunoglobulins made against complex and multi-epitopic antigens. To break the impasse, Benacerraf thought that a simple synthetic antigen composed of a peptide polymer carrier, such as poly-L-lysine, conjugated to a hapten, such as dinitrophenol, would yield a restricted assortment of immunoglobulins, perhaps of a single molecular composition, i.e., monoclonal antibodies. He injected some outbred guinea pigs (of mixed genetic ancestry) with the antigen in hopeful anticipation. The results were not what he had expected. Furthermore, while some animals responded with antibodies, others seemed to ignore the antigen. Striking differences occurred when he next tested two inbred strains of guinea pigs: strain 2 responded, but strain 13 failed to produce antibody. When linear, random co-polymers of glutamic acid and tyrosine were used as a carrier in place of poly-L-lysine, the opposite result was found: strain 2 guinea pigs did not respond, but specific antibodies were isolated from strain 13 animals. Benacerraf realized that something here was of great significance. History had recorded similar failures among individual animals, but he had the advantage of a unique antigenic tool and the new knowledge of immunogenetics. He also had the curiosity and will to find out why.

Benacerraf developed the concept of Ir (immune response) genes. Individuals with this gene would be able to recognize certain carriers and thereby synthesize antibodies or manifest delayed-type hypersensitivity to the target hapten. Soon thereafter, Hugh O. McDevitt and Michael Sela discovered similar genes in mice within a new locus, "I." Benacerraf and McDevitt would later communicate their findings daily, allowing rapid verification in the other's animal system. Benacerraf next observed that the guinea pig Ir genes are part of the animal's major histocompatibility complex, and with David H. Katz he ascertained that T and B cells must be Ir-compatible to mount an immune response to a T-cell dependent antigen. Another team expanded the interaction to T cells and macrophages/dendritic cells. After Jan Klein and Donald C. Shreffler independently discovered the Ia (I associated) antigen, the two constituent chains were found to be coded on subregions of the Ir/class II loci.

Benacerraf's pioneering discovery is reported in the next milestone. The research was not immediately appreciated and its publication elicited only a few reprint requests. When Benacerraf and McDevitt later presented their findings at a meeting of the Federation of American Societies for Experimental Biology (FASEB), the symposium was sparsely attended, and McDevitt complained to his colleague that their work was not understood. Benacerraf, who was a businessman and investor as well as a scientist, replied that they were actually fortunate to have the field to themselves without the pressure of competition, and that their position was like someone who had bought stock in IBM when it was only $5 a share.

One of Niels K. Jerne's theories called for T cells differentiating in the thymus to be selected for their recognition of indigenous histocompatibility antigens followed by mutation. From this, Benacerraf speculated that T cells have a low-affinity receptor for self-histocompatibility antigens but a high affinity for slight variants, which would allow especial recognition of malignant, virus-infected, and denatured host cells. This attribute would also permit strong recognition of allogeneic antigens. He also proposed that xenogeneic histocompatibility antigens would be immunologically weak. Lo! It was indeed demonstrated that T cells to such antigens from other species are highly cross-reactive with allogeneic antigens; that T cells against allogeneic antigens cross-react with modified, hapten-conjugated syngeneic cells; and that T cells to virus-infected syngeneic cells cross-react with allogeneic antigens.

The T cell receptor is at the heart of the histocompatibility system. Its ability to recognize the combination of Ia/class II molecules on B cells and macrophages and the carrier of the hapten determines whether the individual will or will not be a good responder. Since this receptor appears to be singular and encompasses both carrier and histocompatibility antigen, which may be considered a superantigen, the absent Ia would thus result in a poor fit of the soluble antigen, and no B-cell signal will be triggered. In the case of cytotoxic T cells, the receptor may directly recognize the foreign histocompatibility antigen or the host antigen and an adjacent aberrant or nonself membrane antigen. Thus, class I molecules are more than territorial flags of self; they are the necessary components of internal immunological fine-tuning.

For further information:

Bach, F. H. and J. J. van Rood. 1976. The major histocompatibility complex—genetics and biology. *New England Journal of Medicine* 295:806–812; 872–878; 927–936.

Benacerraf, B. 1981. Role of MHC gene products in immune regulation. *Science* 212:1229–1238.

Benacerraf, B. 1985. Reminiscences. *Immunological Reviews* 84:7–27.

von Boehmer, H., W. Haas, and N. K. Jerne. 1978. Major histocompatibility complex-linked immune-responsiveness is acquired by lymphocytes of low-responder mice differentiating in thymus of high-responder mice. *Proceedings of the National Academy of Science USA* 75:2439–2442.

The Paper*

Previous studies on the genetic transmission of the capacity for an immune response have shown that there is a statistically significant relation between the abilities of parents and of offspring to respond to a given antigen. Mendelian genetic patterns were not observed, however, possibly because of the structural complexity of the immunizing antigens em-

*Levine, B. B., A. Ojeda, and B. Benacerraf. 1963. Studies on artificial antigens. III. The genetic control of the immune response to hapten-poly-L-lysine conjugates in guinea pigs. *Journal of Experimental Medicine* 118:953–957. [By copyright permission of The Rockefeller University Press.]

TABLE III

Antigenicity of Hapten-PLL Conjugates in Inbred Guinea Pigs

Guinea pig strain	No. of pigs immunized	Guinea pigs becoming hypersensitive,* immunizing conjugates	
		BPO$_{24}$-PLL$_{316}$	DNP$_{20}$-PLL$_{316}$
		per cent	*per cent*
Random-bred albino Hartley	40	10 to 40	10 to 40
Strain 2	40	100	100
Strain 13	11	0	0

* Animals becoming hypersensitive (responders) showed both Arthus and delayed allergic skin reactions and their sera contained detectible antihapten antibodies by PCA or ring precipitin test. Non-responders showed negative skin reactions, and their sera were negative for antihapten antibodies by PCA and by ring precipitin test.

ployed. Poly-L-α-amino acids and hapten conjugates of synthetic polypeptides are antigens of comparative structural simplicity. Such materials are accordingly suitable for studies of the genetic transmission of the capacity for immune responses.

In previous reports, it has been shown that only 10 to 40 per cent of random-bred Hartley guinea pigs have the capacity to respond immunologically to 2,4-dinitrophenyl (DNP) conjugates of poly-L-lysine (PLL), whereas 100 per cent of these guinea pigs can respond to DNP conjugates of homologous or foreign proteins. Only those guinea pigs capable of responding immunologically to DNP-PLL could respond also to PLL conjugates of 3 other immunogenic haptens. These findings suggest that the capacity of an individual guinea pig to become hypersensitive to hapten-PLL conjugates depends on its ability to properly metabolize the PLL carrier.

In the present work, breeding experiments were carried out in order to study the genetic transmission in guinea pigs of the capacity to become immunized by hapten-PLL conjugates. The results obtained indicate that this trait is transmitted genetically as a unigenic Mendelian dominant. . . .

DNP-PLL conjugates and benzylpenicilloyl-PLL conjugates (BPO-PLL) were prepared, purified, and analyzed. . . . The following preparations were used: DNP$_{20}$-PLL$_{316}$, DNP$_{24}$-PLL$_{316}$, and BPO$_{24}$-PLL$_{316}$ (the subscripts refer to average numbers of haptenic groups per molecule of conjugate). . . .

82 per cent of the offspring of 8 breeding pairs of responder parents showed an immune response to DNP$_{24}$-PLL$_{316}$. Responders showed both Arthus and delayed allergic skin reactions to the immunizing conjugates, and their sera contained both skin-sensitizing and hemolytic antibodies specific for the DNP haptenic group. None of 26 offspring of 9 breeding pairs of non-responder parents showed a demonstrable immune response. The animals showed negative skin reactions, and antihapten antibodies could not be demonstrated in their sera [by passive cutaneous anaphylaxis, challenging with DNP$_{41}$-bovine serum albumin, and passive hemolysis, performed with tanned sheep erythrocytes coated with DNP$_{41}$-BSA]. . . .

Table III shows that 100 per cent of 40 strain 2 guinea pigs immunized consecutively with BPO$_{24}$-PLL$_{316}$ and with DNP$_{20}$-PLL$_{316}$ developed immune responses to these conjugates. In contrast, none of 11 strain 13 guinea pigs immunized with these conjugates showed evidence of an immune response to these conjugates. . . .

These data indicate that the genetic transmission of this trait (i.e., the ability to respond immunologically to hapten-PLL conjugates), is transmitted genetically as a unigenic autosomal Mendelian dominant trait. Consistent with this view is the finding that inbred guinea pigs strains 2 and 13 (which resulted from repeated full sibling breedings) were phenotypically (and probably also genotypically) homozygous with respect to this trait. Confirmation of this view would require study of the offspring of matings of homozygous and heterozygous responders with nonresponders. . . .

Individual antigenic specificity of isolated antibodies

1963 • Henry G. Kunkel, Mart Mannik, and Ralph C. Williams

Comment

Immunogenetic studies of immunoglobulins have faced colossal difficulties. All immunoglobulins contain constant regions and variable regions, which combine with the antigen. Within each individual, the unique sequences of amino acids in immunoglobulins potentially number in the hundreds of millions. The genetic origin of this astronomical assortment of DNA base sequences has puzzled immunologists since their acceptance of the clonal selection theory of antibody formation. That the genome directly codes for the horde of distinct immunoglobulins seemed a folly of inefficiency, and only some 300 to 400 genes for the variable regions are actually inherited. A generator of diversity, GOD(!), was therefore sought. After some 20 years, researchers discovered no single causative entity: Both genes and somatic chance events are responsible. Simplistically, genes from several loci are transcribed by RNA messengers, which are assembled for protein production by splicing, whose resulting chains are combined, all in a more or less random fashion. Foremost to clonal development is the unusually high rate of mutation among the genes of the variable regions. While a mutant of a similar gene might occur among 10^5 cells each generation, the H chain has a mutation rate of 2 to 4 percent.

Immunoglobulins are antigenically categorized as allotypes, isotypes, and idiotypes. Normal Mendelian inheritance and some constancy do occur among these characteristics. Allotypes refer to antibodies peculiar to different individuals. For instance, some 25 different allotypic IgG Gm groups on H chains and 3 Km (formerly Inv) groups on kappa chains are recognized. Isotypes, which concern the antibodies within a given individual having the same antigenic specificity, include the 5 classes of H chains, their subclasses (4 each of human and mouse IgG), the two types of L chains, and subtypes and subgroups. Idiotypes, however, are a far different matter. Idiotypes, which were discovered independently by Henry G. Kunkel (1916–1983) and Jacques Oudin, are the immunoglobulins within each allotype and isotype that vary in protein sequence and, more important, antigenic determinants.

Kunkel was a second-generation member of the Rockefeller Institute. In 1931 his father Louis O. Kunkel was invited to establish the Department of Plant Pathology at the Princeton facility at the Institute. When it came time to choose a college, the son conveniently selected Princeton University, where he completed his A.B. in 1938. Henry Kunkel, being more interested in the diseases of humans than those of plants, next went to the Johns Hopkins University School of Medicine. He became Assistant Research Physician at the Rockefeller Hospital in 1945, helping the investigation of infectious hepatitis. Two years later, on the death of Charles L. Hoagland, Kunkel was promoted to Associate and took charge of the liver research laboratory. In 1949 the Rockefeller Institute added him to its list of Associate Members. In 1953 he became a full Member, Professor of Immunology of the newly evolved Rockefeller University, and Senior Physician in the associated Hospital.

Kunkel was one of the masters of clinical immunology. He was known for his use of clinical material in basic research of immunological problems, and, in return, the development of immunological techniques for diagnosing disease. His year in Uppsala with Arne Tiselius (1950) was the turning point of his career. He discovered a flair for tools and technology. Paper electrophoresis was a wonder for him, but later dissatisfied with the poor yield of eluate, he developed the improved substrate of starch gel. Previously, he utilized antibodies to measure proteins. His next encounter with immunology was to suggest that myeloma proteins were an immunological model. Kunkel ascertained that these substances were immunoglobulins, if not functional antibodies. The molecules opened the door to the clonal selection theory, and were most valuable in comparative immunogenetics. He also established the pathology of immune complexes, discovering in 1957 autoimmune rheumatoid arthritic factors and in 1966 the complex of DNA and its antibody in cases of systemic lupus erythematosus.

He may not have been strictly an immunogeneticist, but Kunkel and his associates made some significant contributions to the field, including the following milestone on the discovery of antibody idiotypes, the linkage of complement C2 genes to the human major histocompatibility complex, and the existence of idiotypes on T cell leukemias. Kunkel was also a distinguished teacher, and this collection of milestones features his students Gerald M. Edelman, Thomas B. Tomasi, Jr., Eng M. Tan, Mart Mannik, and Ralph C. Williams.

Kunkel's team discovered in 1955 that myeloma proteins differed antigenically, and developed the conception of markers of individual antigenic specificity. In their milestone of 1963, they found that human antibodies against three different antigens were themselves antigenically unique in rabbits. Furthermore, the rabbit anti-antibodies were active only against the antibodies of the particular person. They would not couple with antibodies against the same immunogen isolated from different people. Thus, idiotypes were found to be clone-specific, and the findings with myelomas could now be expanded to all immunoglobulins.

Meanwhile, Jacques Oudin performed similar experiments in rabbits, which had the technical advantage of allotypy. He coined the term idiotypy to designate the marker for a given antibody, and organized the hierarchy of antibody antigens. In 1969 Oudin found that IgG and IgM molecules from a single rabbit that combine with the same antigen shared idiotypes. Eventually researchers discovered that, with the occasional exception of other but adjacent variable regions, the antigen-combining site is the source of idiotypy. Although they may be of similar configuration, the antigen-combining sites of antibodies from different individuals are antigenically unique. Cross-reactivity with anti-idiotype antisera, however, does occur, and inheritance of such a public idiotype reflects the common gene pool of a closely related population. Idiotypes, which are auto-immunogenic, are the basis of Jerne's network theory of immune regulation (see Part 5, Jerne, 1974).

For further information:

Bearn, A. G. (editor). 1985. Henry G. Kunkel 1916–1983. An appreciation of the man and his scientific contributions and a bibliography of his research papers. *Journal of Experimental Medicine* 161:869–896.

Greene, M. I. and A. Nisonoff (editors). 1984. *The Biology of Idiotypes.* Plenum Press, New York. 507 p.

Kindt, T. J. and J. D. Capra. 1984. *The Antibody Enigma.* Plenum Press, New York. 270 p.

Leder, P. 1982. The genetics of antibody diversity. *Scientific American* 246(5):102–115.

The Paper*

Numerous studies in the past have failed to show that isolated antibodies possess individual specificity

---

*Kunkel, H. G., M. Mannik, and R. C. Williams. 1963. Individual antigenic specificity of isolated antibodies. *Science* 140:1218–1219. [Copyright 1963 by the AAAS.]

as antigens. . . . However, observations from a number of laboratories have indicated that myeloma proteins and macroglobulins, with many of the characteristics of individual antibodies, do show antigenic specificity. Recently, this work has been extended to include "monoclonal" γ-globulins appearing in smaller amounts in certain presumed normal individuals, and to certain antibodies. In view of these findings a reinvestigation of the antigenicity of isolated antibodies was undertaken, particularly since new evidence for a close similarity between myeloma proteins and isolated antibodies has arisen from a variety of studies including starch-gel electrophoresis after reduction in the presence of urea and localization of genetic characters.

Anti-A antibodies were isolated from the serum of seven individuals who developed high titers after immunization with hog gastric A substance. Complement and natural anti-γ-globulin factors were removed by heating at 56°C for 30 minutes and absorption with aggregated γ-globulin. Specific precipitates formed at equivalence, with highly purified A substance, were washed and eluted with acetate buffer pH 3.8. After removal of residue precipitate, the supernatant was dialyzed rapidly against phosphate buffer, pH 7.5. These eluates were employed as antigens and were injected into rabbits primarily by the intraperitoneal route with complete Freund's adjuvants. Dextran and levan antibodies were prepared in a similar fashion from specific precipitates formed with the respective antigens. Subject Ka had produced antibodies to A substance, dextran and levan following immunization. . . .

Two of the seven anti-A antibodies produced individual, specific antibodies after injection into rabbits. The results with the antibodies from serum Th are representative. Three of six rabbits injected with Th antibody formed antibodies which still reacted strongly with the antigen after absorption with normal serum or normal γ-globulin. . . . Antiserum against Th antibody, after absorption with normal serum, failed to react with Fr II γ-globulin, normal and high γ-globulin sera, or with any of seven other isolated anti-A antibodies. Many additional γ-globulins and other isolated antibodies were tested [by Ouchterlony gel diffusion] but only the Th antibody showed the specific reaction with the three different antisera to Th antibody.

These antisera to Th antibody also showed the antibody in whole Th serum. . . . [A]n immunoelectrophoresis experiment [demonstrated] the sharp antibody line with both the absorbed and unabsorbed antiserum. The unabsorbed antiserum showed a strong reaction with 7S γ-globulin of the serum. . . . Clear identification of the sharp line as the anti-A antibody was obtained in two ways. First, ab-

sorption of Th serum with A substance completely removed the line. Second, immunoelectrophoresis experiments of Th serum with the antiserum in one trough and A substance in the other showed that the line with the rabbit antiserum corresponded exactly in position with the line obtained with A substance. Detailed studies of the antigenic character of isolated Th antibody demonstrated that it had the antigenic characteristics of ordinary 7S γ-globulin. Of particular significance was the finding that all the specificity could be precipitated by ordinary antisera to 7S γ-globulin and antisera to the F portion of 7S γ-globulin.

Antisera to five other isolated anti-A antibodies were also studied in detail. Only one of these showed similar individual specificity. This absorbed antiserum to Ka anti-A failed to react with Th anti-A or any other anti-A studied and reacted only with Ka antibody. Two antisera against other anti-A antibodies failed to show specificity despite the formation of extremely high titers of γ-globulin antibodies.

Two antisera to levan antibodies of Ka serum also showed strong individual specificity. These antisera, after absorption with normal serum, reacted only with the levan antibodies from this serum and not with the other antibodies or γ-globulins described above. Only one anti-levan antibody was available for study. As in the case of Th anti-A this antibody

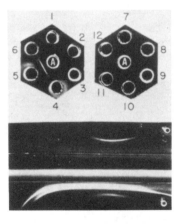

Figure 1 (Top) Agar plate analysis showing the specific reaction of isolated Th anti-A antibody with antiserum to Th antibody (central wells A). Outer wells: 1, normal serum; 2, Fr II; 3, 4, high γ-globulin sera; 5, isolated Th anti-A antibody; 6–12, other isolated anti-A antibodies. (Bottom) Immunoelectrophoresis pattern of serum Th developed against antiserum to Th antibody. With the antiserum absorbed with normal serum, a single sharp line is visible, representing Th anti-A antibody. With the unabsorbed antiserum the long γ-globulin line is seen with the unique short band below it.

could be detected in whole serum immunoelectrophoresis. Individual specific antibodies were also obtained with one of two anti-dextran antibodies, as well as with one cold agglutinin and two anti-γ-globulins. The latter were 19S proteins. Four other anti-γ-globulin factors failed to show individual specificity. Three antinuclear antibodies failed to show specificity.

Starch-gel electrophoresis of a number of the antibodies described above, after reduction with mercaptoethanol in the presence of urea, indicated a possible association between the specific antigenicity and sharp banding of the L chains. Anti-A Th and anti-levan Ka showed particularly sharp lines.

The present studies demonstrate that, contrary to accepted opinion, individual antibodies will elicit secondary antibodies in the rabbit which are specific for the antibody. This was shown with four antibodies of the 7S class, including anti-A, anti-dextran, and anti-levan antibodies; and with three proteins of the 19S class. There is some possible question about the antibody nature of the latter three despite their specific reactivity, because in contrast to the first group of antibodies they were not produced by intentional immunization. It is of interest that two of the antibodies showing antigenic specificity came from the same serum.

Thus far, the specificity obtained was found directed only against the individual antibody used for immunization. No cross-specificity between a large group of anti-A antibodies from different individuals was obtained. However, it must be stressed that further work is necessary to settle this point, particularly since many of the anti-A antibodies studied appeared to be extremely heterogeneous. . . . The accumulated evidence suggests that all antibodies might well serve as specific antigens, provided that those directed against individual antigenic sites are selected out.

The localization of the individual antigenic specificity of the γ-gloculin molecule is currently under study. The S fragment, obtained from papain- as well as pepsin-splitting of Th anti-A, contained all the specificity. This fragment is known to contain combining sites. It seems probable that previous data on the antigenic specificities of various myeloma proteins, Waldenstrom's macroglobulins, cold agglutinins, and certain other "monoclonal" γ-globulins are directly applicable to the antibody problem. These antigenic differences are marked and readily demonstrable. Their exact relationship to the antibody sites and to the L chains remains to be determined.

Part 8
Technology

Science is spectrum analysis. Art is photosynthesis. —Karl Kraus

Faith is a fine invention
For Gentlemen who see;
But microscopes are prudent
In an emergency. —Emily Dickinson

Our ride down the waterways of immunology has not been without the guidance of rudder, oar, and sail. Technology, no one will deny, has been an extremely significant influence in increasing our understanding of the functional behavior of immune systems. It opened the molecular world for inspection, and was instrumental in conceptualizing the mechanistic, reductive approach to phenomena. The limitations of technology also ultimately demonstrated the importance yet inadequacy of that philosophical approach.

Science begins with observation, curiosity, and hypothesis. The great body of descriptive works on botany and zoology has been sufficient for naturalists to generate some fundamental biological laws. Even their modern tools are mere extensions of the eye, such as the microscope, the camera, and the photon-amplifying nightscope, or of the simple caliper, as the image-analyzing computer. Beginning in the nineteenth century, however, science has meant attaining knowledge chiefly through manipulation and quantification and the ability to predict particular reactions. Nature is no longer watched; now it is tested under artificial circumstance: "What would happen if . . . ?" Variation, integral among both stars and life forms, and the recognition of population-related phenomena necessitated statistics and other quantitative analyses. The epitome of contemporary science has been chromatography, which permits separation, isolation, identification, and quantification of elements of the whole. This allowed us to create the interlocking but distinct subatomic, atomic, micro, macro, and cosmic realms. Western science thus is advancing from simply recognizing patterns to comprehending the web of changing arrangements. I emphasized Western, since Eastern science was founded on this philosophic conception, while Europeans built their scientific edifice on Cartesian principles. The difference, which is a matter of emphasis, took on dogmatic characteristics. Today a balance of both approaches is necessary.

This next series of milestones features many of the significant methods that propelled immunology forward. Again, it is not instruments, but methods. Immunologists have taken full advantage of the numerous devices created by chemists and physicists, modifying their function through the selective power of antibody-antigen reactions themselves. The earliest techniques were demonstrations of phenomena, which allowed the identification first of infectious agents and then of any antigenic substance. Herbert E. Durham and Max von Gruber described the generally specific agglutination of microorganisms by antisera in a test tube and on a microscope slide. The same technique was immediately used to diagnose typhoid fever. Within a year, Rudolf Kraus discovered flocculation and precipitation of cell-free soluble proteins, and although this was not a choice technique in the clinical laboratory, it provided the first glimpse into novel ways of differentiation and purification of the myriad of unknown, unseen chemical factors. Precipitation techniques also led to the concept of antibody valency. Jules Bordet and Octave Gengou mastered the puzzle of complement, demonstrating that it is not antigen-specific. They found, through the inhibition of hemolysis of antibody-sensitized erythrocytes, that complement can complex with antibodies and microorganisms that are resistant to tell-tale bacteriolysis. Competitive complement-fixation, which proved to be a highly sensitive technique for detecting antibodies as well as antigens, was adapted by August von Wassermann, Albert Neisser, and Carl Bruck to detect syphilis.

Quantitation of antibodies at first was based on convenient arbitrary standards and relative titers similar to those introduced by Paul Ehrlich in his studies on diphtheria antitoxins. The breakthrough came in 1929 when Michael Heidelberger and Forrest E. Kendall, using a pure carbohydrate antigen, could at last measure antibodies directly by determining the protein content of the precipitated complex. It was a boost to the young science of immunochemistry, allowing closer scrutiny of its dynamics.

An extraordinarily powerful tool to locate and identify fixed antigens in complex mixtures, such as in slide preparations of tissues, is fluorescein-tagged antibodies. Albert H. Coons, Hugh J. Creech, and R. Norman Jones developed that technique in 1941. Today every research and clinical laboratory makes use of such antibodies labeled by a variety of strategies, typically through tagged anti-IgG antibodies to a target-specific immunoglobulin.

Not every antigen readily triggers an immune response. This may be due to the similarity of the antigen to host configurations, and its low solubility, rapid elimination, or inadequate contact with immune cells. Certain materials, called adjuvants, can enhance the immune response by overcoming these and other obstacles. The most famous adjuvant is Freund's adjuvant. Many key experiments in the history of immunology depended on its use. Therefore, the paper of Jules Freund and his assistant Katherine McDermott is included.

If one tool must be singled out as central to immunogenetics, it would be the development of inbred, well-characterized strains of laboratory animals that differ in single characteristics, although perhaps it is a little crass to regard animals as tools. George D. Snell did most to develop this method, and for his contribution in furthering the study of histocompatibility genes he was awarded a share in the Nobel Prize.

Precipitation returns in the next two papers. Amazingly simple and inexpensive in design, precipitation techniques have become routine and commonplace. They offer both identification and quantitation. Örjan Ouchterlony, whose report is featured, and Stephen D. Elek discovered that antigen and antibody diffusing toward each other in agar gel can form a line of precipitate. Diffusion rates differ with each antigen, depending mainly on shape and size. The number and pattern of merging and crossing lines compared with controls indicated the purity of a preparation and the identification of an unknown sample. Other variations using standards can measure the concentration of the reagent. Pierre Grabar and Curtis A. Williams, Jr. with J. Courcon combined gel diffusion with the electrophoretic method of Arne Tiselius to invent immunoelectrophoresis, which adds electrical charge to the physical characteristics of diffusion. Sensitivity in detecting different antigens in a solution was thereby increased. Later, two-dimensional electrophoresis, borrowing from paper chromatography, produced an outstanding and graphically beautiful pattern of separated antigens.

Rosalyn S. Yalow and Solomon A. Berson are other Nobel winners in immunotechnology. They developed the first radioimmunoassay (RIA), which brought quantitative analysis its most sensitive but most complex and expensive technique. RIA allowed the measurement of trace levels of substances, which in physiology can nonetheless be crucial. Fortunately, newer techniques are replacing hazardous radioisotopes without sacrificing sensitivity.

In the examination of antibody formation, an in vitro means was needed to locate and quantify the antibody producing cells. Niels K. Jerne and Albert A. Nordin found it. Bordet's hemolysin was the indicator; agar was the medium. Like the viruses that cause plaques (lytic zones) in tissue cultures or in bacterial lawns on agar, single cells synthesizing antibody to erythrocytes can, in the presence of complement, cause the formation of clear plaques in the surrounding blood. Cellular immunology now had a useful model for study.

Immunogenetics and immunochemistry came together with the report by Tai Te Wu and Elvin A. Kabat. By utilizing natural monoclonal immunoglobulins from myelomas, they were able to determine and compare the sequence of amino acids. Their work and that of others using this approach precisely located the variable region of the antigen receptor and the constant domains specific to each class and type of chain, helped explain how immunoglobulins were assembled, determined why and where antibodies were autoimmunogenic, and allowed the creation of a detailed three-dimensional model of IgG. In short, this paper merged immunology and molecular biology.

The last report, which led to the Nobel Prize for George Köhler and Cesar Milstein, has given biotechnologists the ability to custom make monoclonal antibody. Such pure immunoglobulins, if of optimal avidity and specificity, may be the realization of Paul Ehrlich's Magic Bullets. They are the ultimate molecular probes, which already have reduced false positive results in diagnostic assays. Artificial monoclonal antibodies arise from a fusion of myeloma and plasma cells, replicating and forming a cell line called a hybridoma. The ability to culture and harvest kilogram amounts of pure, single idiotypic immunoglobulin has changed applied immunology and created a new industry of immunological engineers. The ramifications of biological engineering on ethics, human biology, evolution, and even metaphysics are just beginning to be recognized.

Presently, immunology and all other biomedical sciences are intently focused on molecular biology and the tools manufactured by genetic engineering. We live in the age of ultra-specialists, and the schism between them and the generalist has broadened. Some academic departments of medical microbiology and immunology have become de facto divisions of molecular biology, and the chemist and biological engineer are replacing the traditional biologist. However, the broad fields of psychobiology, in our case psychoneuroimmunology, are on the rise as a frontier science. Perhaps a more balanced scientific appreciation of molecule, cell, organism, and community; structure and process; and form and feeling will become the new mode. We await the novel techniques of the coming era of scientific fusions.

For further information:

Ackroyd, J. F. (editor). 1964. *Immunological Methods. A symposium organized by the Council for International Organizations of Medical Sciences established under the joint auspices of UNESCO & WHO.* Blackwell Scientific Publications, Oxford. 628 p.

Hudson, L. and F. C. Hay. 1980. *Practical Immunology.* Second edition. Blackwell Scientific Publications, Oxford. 359 p.

Mishell, B. B. and S. M. Shiigi (editors). 1980. *Selected Methods in Cellular Immunology.* W. H. Freeman and Company, San Francisco. 486 p.

Weir, D. M. 1978. *Handbook of Experimental Immunology.* Third edition. Three volumes. Blackwell Scientific Publications, Oxford.

On a special action of the serum of highly immunized animals

1896 • Herbert E. Durham

Comment

The first fruit of technical immunology was ripe in 1896. Independently, Sir Almroth E. Wright in England, Richard Pfeiffer and Wilhelm Kolle in Germany, Fernand Widal in France, and Max von Gruber in Austria gazed at the test tube or microscope slide holding a mixture of active bacteria and antiserum, observed the clumping of cells as noted by Albert Charrin and his assistant Roger in 1889, and realized that the reaction could be used diagnostically. Key to such an important decision was that the serum agglutinins seemed to be specific for the inducing agent and that the reaction was readily visible and unambiguous. The usefulness of this agglutination reaction often depends on the motility of the microorganism, specifically the presence of flagella. These protein structures are strongly antigenic. They also are highly susceptible to antibody cross-linking and immobilizing entanglement.

However, the author of the following milestone, the first analytical publication on specific agglutination, is none of the above famous pioneer immunologists; he is Herbert E. Durham (1866–1945). This report is actually a summation of his presentations before the London medical establishment. Durham was a student of Gruber (1853–1927), who shortly afterwards published his own full account of the agglutination phenomenon. Durham trained in zoology and bacteriology at King's College of Cambridge University and Guy's Hospital in London, where not so incidentally his father was senior surgeon. Having earned the degree of Sc.D. and begun working toward his Bachelor of Medicine, he received a studentship in pathology to study with Gruber in the Institute of Hygiene of the University of Vienna. One

morning in November 1894, Durham and Gruber were readying the culture of cholera vibrio and antiserum provided by Pfeiffer for studying his bacteriolytic phenomenon. Before injecting the mixture in guinea pigs, Gruber inspected the preparation under the microscope and was surprised to observe agglutination. Several days later, Durham set a test tube of the mixture aside for a short while and returned to find that the bacteria had formed a granular sediment. The micro and macro agglutination tests were born.

Gruber himself was an assistant to another Max, Max von Pettenkofer, before becoming a professor of physiology at his alma mater, the University of Vienna, in 1882. Between 1884 and 1887 he was professor at the University of Graz. He returned to the University of Vienna four years afterward to become the director of the Hygiene Institute, which was poorly equipped and housed in an old, run-down rifle factory. In 1902 he succeeded Pettenkofer as head of the eminent Institute of Hygiene at the University of Munich. Durham, whose name is linked by microbiologists to a small test tube that is inserted upside-down in a culture tube to demonstrate microbial gas production, later studied tsetse fly diseases in East Africa as part of a Royal Society expedition, yellow fever in Brazil under the aegis of the Liverpool School of Tropical Medicine, and beriberi in Malaya for the London School of Tropical Medicine. A significant loss of vision eventually forced him to leave research. In his later years he took up horticulture.

Gruber and Durham jointly published further results within months of the original announcement, and at the 13th Congress for Internal Medicine in Wiesbaden, Gruber passed example preparations and Durham's photographs among the audience of physicians. Gruber told the assembly that the serum of their patients could indicate a previous infection with cholera or typhoid. The original focus of Durham and Gruber was the development of the test as a simple means of identifying a bacterium, although they clearly recognized its potential for diagnosis. Widal was first to apply the test clinically by determining typhoid fever in a patient. He reacted a sample of the patient's serum with a laboratory culture of motile *Salmonella typhosa.* The serum typhoid test quickly became identified with him, but in deference to priority, it later was known as the Gruber-Widal test. Gruber himself, with another English student, Albert S. F. Grunbaum (who changed his name to Leyton after the start of World War I), published a more thorough clinical experiment six months after Widal.

Durham made the important observation that agglutination specificity was not absolute. Similar species, particularly among the vibrio, cross-reacted. In addition, variation in agglutination occurred among the cultures of *Escherichia coli* that were tested. This pointed to the limitation and risks of diagnostic tests: false positives and false negatives in qualitative analyses; questions of specificity, precision, and sensitivity in quantitative assays. In the instance of typhoid, some patients do not develop anti-flagella antibodies, and tests with cell wall antigens needed to be introduced as well. Also timing is important, since antibodies may not yet have formed when blood is collected. Other governing factors are antibody concentration, which, if too high, will hinder cross-linking, and repulsive electrostatics, which with neutral and weak ionic solutions may prevent cells from closing sufficiently for IgG, but not IgM, to span. Fortunately, the first typhoid agglutination tests were generally excellent, and they helped establish the clinical serology laboratory.

For further information:

Cabot, R. C. 1899. *The Serum Diagnosis of Disease.* William Wood and Company, New York. 154 p.

Foster, W. D. 1970. *A History of Medical Bacteriology and Immunology.* William Heinemann Medical Books, London. 232 p.

Schubert, J. H., P. R. Edwards, and C. H. Ramsey. 1959. Detection of typhoid carriers by agglutination tests. *Journal of Bacteriology* 77:648–654.

Zinsser, H. 1914. *Infection and Resistance. An exposition of the biological phenomena underlying the occurrence of infection and the recovery of the animal body from infectious disease.* Macmillan Company, New York. pp. 218–247.

The Paper*

1. A remarkable series of effects are produced on an emulsion of actively motile microbes by the addition of minute quantities of potent kinds of serum.

2. These effects have been observed with the cholera vibrio, a variety of other vibrios, the typhoid bacillus, the *Bacillus coli communis,* and the *Bacillus pyocyaneus.*

3. It is highly improbable that the phenomena are limited to the groups and species here named. . . .

4. The most prominent of the effects thus produced consists of an immediate aggregation of the bacteria into "clumps"; this is combined with loss of motility. Marked inhibition of growth also occurs.

5. The formation of clumps can be detected readily by the naked eye. Eventually they gravitate to the bottom of the tube containing them.

6. A "complete action" is obtained when all the clumps settle down, leaving a perfectly clear fluid. The time required for settling varies

---

*Durham, H. E. 1896. On a special action of serum of highly immunized animals, and its use for diagnostic and other purposes. *Proceedings of the Royal Society, London* 59:224–226. [With permission of the Society.] The full account appeared under the same title in the *Journal of Pathology and Bacteriology* 4:13–44 (1897).

somewhat with different organisms, as also according to the amount and potency of the serum used.

7. The least quantity of serum which will give a "complete reaction" in about one hour forms a convenient standard. A highly potent serum will react thus in 1 per cent solution, which is a convenient unit.

8. The more intense the action of the serum the more rapid and the more complete are the changes which ensue.

9. By means of the intensity of action in varying dilutions, two or more samples of serum, or of freshly drawn blood, may be gauged according to their potency.

10. Normal serum, and the serum obtained by immunizations with totally unrelated groups of organisms, do not interact upon the unrelated microbes, so far as present observation shows.

11. The action of cholera serum upon more or less closely related vibrios may be "complete" or nil. A series of gradations in intensity of reaction has been observed with cholera serum and vibrios of other species, and vice versa.

12. The action of such serum cannot therefore be regarded as "specific"; it is better named special or specialized.

13. The limit of the absolute value of such serum tests for the diagnosis of cholera vibrios has yet to be determined.

14. All the typhoid bacilli from nineteen different sources hitherto observed react with ty-

phoid serum; none of them react with the *B. coli* serum.

15. Of the *B. coli* varieties hitherto proved, some do not react with one sample of *B. coli* serum.

16. The agreement in action of the typhoid bacilli points to the use of the method for diagnostic purposes. Given a young culture and typhoid serum, diagnosis can be made in a few minutes.

17. As shown by serum experiment, the variation within the *B. coli* group is greater than that of *B. typhi* races.

18. By the method described, more delicate changes can be observed than with such methods as plate cultivations, and the fallacies thereof are avoided.

19. A vibrio and a vibrio serum which will give a "complete reaction" in vitro will also give a positive result in "Pfeiffer's reaction" (e.g., *V. iwanoffi* and *B. berolinensis* with cholera serum).

20. It is not worthwhile performing Pfeiffer's test unless a "complete reaction" has been obtained in vitro.

21. In the method described, the whole series of changes, if any, are before the eye the whole time. In Pfeiffer's method the changes can only be seen by removing samples from their hiding place in the guinea pig's peritoneal cavity. The extent of possible fallacy from using the peritoneal fluid of a living animal is not yet defined. . . .

On specific reactions in germfree filtrates of cholera, typhoid, and plague broth cultures produced with homologous serum

1897 • Rudolf Kraus

Comment

The discovery and application of specific agglutinins was immediately followed by the observation that unseen, dissolved antigenic particles can flocculate or precipitate with antisera. As we know now, the mechanism of both phenomena is essentially the same, and only the size and shape of the antigen differs. Ah, the simplicity and confidence of hindsight! However, in the 1890s the nature of antibodies was completely unknown, and the possibility of its bi- and multivalence for cross-linking would not even be proposed until 1934. Thus, antitoxins were considered to be different substances than agglutinins, and agglutinins were thought to be distinct from precipitins. Indeed, early immunologists thought that agglutinins were agents that changed the physical properties of cellular surfaces to allow mutual attraction and cohesion.

The first to examine precipitation was Rudolf Kraus (1868–1932), who was part of the serological school at the University of Vienna. The school had no single home, but was spread among the various loosely interacting theoretical research institutes in the School of Medicine. Its students and faculty included, besides Kraus and Max von Gruber, Clemens von Pirquet, Bela Schick, Karl Landsteiner, and Adriano Sturli. Kraus earned his M.D. at the University of Prague in 1893, and came to Vienna as an assistant in pathology and bacteriology at the Institute for Serum Therapy, which was then engaged in the production of diphtheria antitoxins. In 1903 he served as a resident in experimental pathology, and in 1910 he joined the medical faculty as an associate professor. Kraus crossed the Atlantic in 1913 to Buenos Aires, where he became Director of the Bacteriological Institute. Later he headed the Institute of Serology at Buatantan, São Paolo. Kraus enjoyed his work in Brazil, but accepted the appointment in 1923 of Director of his original laboratory, the Institute of Serum Therapy in Vienna. It was a short stay, since in 1928 he returned to South America, this time to Chile as head of a research institute in Santiago and in 1930 as Director-General of the National Health Service. Kraus was a careful, logical investigator and honored teacher and administrator. Respected also for his expertise in immunological technique, he served as editor and contributor of the first major handbooks and manuals of the science.

Kraus made his discovery of precipitation in 1897, using antiserum and a culture filtrate of cholera vibrio, which still contained flagella, membrane debris, and myriad globular proteins. In one of his experiments, he deliberately disrupted a bacterial preparation and extracted its antigens in broth, which was then filtered. Modern serological classifications of bacteria, notably streptococci, have utilized specific precipitins to cell wall antigens similarly extracted. Kraus ascertained the specificity of the phenomenon by mixing the filtrates in turn with normal sera and antisera to other bacteria made in a variety of animals. He then demonstrated the universality of the phenomenon by mixing filtrates of typhoid and plague bacteria with their respective antiserum. According to his report, a mixture of toxin and antitoxin did not form visible precipitates. This failure was a matter of technique rather than principle: the concentration of the antigen was probably too low. Excess antibody or antigen can hinder cross-linking, restrict the size of complexes, and maintain their solubility.

Precipitin methods are more difficult and less reliable than agglutination, and for many years they had comparatively little to offer for clinical diagnosis. One of the first innovations was the ring test developed in 1908 by W. Fornet, which called for layering the reagents in a narrow test tube. Through undisturbed diffusion after an extended period of time, a ring is formed at the interface. The significant advantages of precipitation in gels would not be known for several decades. Beginning in 1899, researchers observed precipitation with nonbacterial antigens as well. The trailblazers were Theodor Tchistovitch at the Pasteur Institute and later Jules Bordet, who found that rabbit antiserum to eel, horse, or chicken serum would yield precipitates. The first major investigative use of the precipitin reaction was a tedious phylogenic study of blood antigens by George H. F. Nuttall in 1904. Forensic applications were an immediate extension. Basic research centered on the characteristics of the precipitin-inducing and precipitating antigens, called at the time precipitinogens. Soon it was established that almost any soluble protein precipitated with antiserum under optimal conditions, which were met in part by preparing a series of serum dilutions. Mechanistic interpretations, however, were confused, since the chemistry, structure, and function of both antibody and antigen were unknown. Only the theoretical models of Paul Ehrlich provided a feeling for specificity and kinetic interaction. Precipitation methods, nevertheless, offered unique biological techniques to identify and, more important, specifically separate biochemicals in solution.

For further information:

Campbell, D. H., J. S. Garvey, N. E. Cremer, and D. H. Sussdorf. 1964. *Methods in Immunology. A Laboratory Text for Instruction and Research*. W. A. Benjamin, New York. 263 p.

Citron, J. 1914. *Immunity. Methods of Diagnosis and Therapy and Their Practical Application* (A. L. Garbat, translator). Second edition. P. Blakiston's Son and Company, Philadelphia. pp. 120–130.

Lesky, E. 1973. Viennese serological research about the year 1900. Its contribution to the development of clinical medicine. *Bulletin of the New York Academy of Medicine*. 49:100–111.

Lesky, E. 1977. Wassermann and the Vienna School of Serology. *International Journal of Dermatology* 16:526–530.

The Paper*

Issaeff and Ivanoff, Gruber and Durham, and Pfeiffer demonstrated agglutination, which has far-reaching significance in medical bacteriology. The principal value of this new method lies in its accuracy, which is not found in any chemical reaction. This method also proves the specificity of pathogenic microorganisms. It is the origin of a new classification scheme in bacteriology, and is the foundation of serum-diagnosis.

Subsequent work on agglutination was occupied with its practical use. Since the discovery of the reaction, there has not been any further information about the nature of agglutination.

In the beginning, Gruber had the idea that the bacterial wall, under the influence of specific serum, expands and becomes sticky. The surfaces then become glued together. Gruber believes that the expansion is a measure used by the microorganism against the attack of bactericidal serum. . . .

Bordet interprets agglutination as a process that can be explained by molecular attraction. . . .

Widal ascertained that the reaction is possible with killed bacteria as well. . . .

Widal's findings and E. Buchner's discovery of fermentation by zymase are the origin of the following experiments. On considering the previous facts, the thought arose that even solutions of dissolved bacterial substances can cause with antiserum as specific a reaction as the cultures themselves can provide.

The examinations were first carried out with cholera vibrio. . . . Broth cultures of different ages were filtered through bacterial filters. The clear filtrates then were checked for sterility either by reinoculation or by letting the filtrate sit at 37°C. After they were ascertained to be sterile, various amounts of also sterile goat antiserum were added and then incubated at 37°C.

Within 24 hr the following was observed: The filtrate that contained the specific serum became turbid with little flakes, which settled to the bottom. The liquid was totally clear above the sediment.

The turbidity of the liquid can appear light or heavy. The sediment can be plentiful or meager. What this variable reaction depends on could not be determined. Sometimes there was no reaction at all, even with large amounts of filtrate and added serum. The sediment itself appears grayish-white with a brown sheen. Shaking makes it fluffy and clouds the broth before it quickly settles again. . . .

To determine the specificity of the sediment, control experiments with heterologous serum were undertaken with the same filtrates in which sediment developed upon addition of specific serum. To the cholera filtrate were added various amounts of typhoid and coli [*Escherichia coli*] goat antiserum; normal horse serum; diphtheria, cholera, and streptococcal horse antiserum; and normal human serum. There was no sedimentation in these mixtures, except for the one with cholera antiserum. Even after 24 hr at 37°C, the different controls remained totally clear. . . . This reaction is as specific as agglutination with living or killed cultures.

For the present time I cannot decide whether the substances in the filtrates that were selected out by

*Kraus, R. 1897. Ueber specifische Reactionen in keimfreien Filtraten aus Cholera, Typhus und Pestbouillonculturen, erzeugt durch homologes Serum. *Wiener Klinische Wochenschrift* 10:736–738. [With permission by Springer-Verlag, Wien.]

specific antiserum were decomposition products of the bacteria. I only assume this. With the following experiment I believe that I can give a direct proof for my assumption.

Cholera vibrio, obtained partly from agar cultures and partly through filtration of broth cultures, were mixed with glass powder and subjected to a pressure of 300 atmospheres. The pressed mass was diluted with alkaline broth and filtered through bacterial filters. The filtrate then was checked for sterility, and afterward treated with cholera antiserum, as were the filtrates of cholera broth cultures. Within 24 hr at 37°C, turbidity and sedimentation could be observed.

The same result was reached through a modification of the experiment. Cholera cultures (2 days old) were scraped from agar plates, left at 37°C until dried, and then suspended in weak alkaline broth. The solution then was filtered through bacterial filters, and cholera antiserum was added. The result was the same as the one with the filtrates of cholera broth cultures and of the pressed culture masses. . . .

The same specific reactions . . . could also be observed with typhoid antiserum on germfree filtrates of typhoid broth cultures and with plague antiserum on germfree filtrates of plague broth cultures. The turbidity and sedimentation were similar to the ones described with cholera filtrates. The reaction sometimes appeared strongly, sometimes weakly, and sometimes not at all. . . .

Another point is that larger amounts of serum are necessary for the production of turbidity and sedi-

ments than for agglutination with cultures. I could not establish a quantitative proportion. The amount of the decomposition products of bacterial cells in the filtrates is most surely very dissimilar, dependent perhaps on the virulence of the culture and the age and alkalinity of the broth. This dependence possibly could be a reason for the variation in degree of sedimentation or the lack of a reaction. . . .

The following experiment ascertained whether filtrates of toxin-producing bacteria with the addition of specific antitoxic serum are capable of forming sediments. Various amounts of antitoxic horse serum were added to germfree filtrates of diphtheria broth cultures. After incubation for 24 hr at 37°C, the filtrates with specific serum were still totally clear. Even the control tests with the addition of cholera, typhoid, coli, and antistreptococcal serum did not cause any reaction.

These experiments offer the following conclusions:

1. Specific sediments can form in germfree filtrates of cholera, typhoid, and plague broth cultures with the addition of specific antiserum.

2. The substances in the filtrates that are separated with homologous serum are components of the bacterial cells.

3. There is no reaction when homologous antitoxins are added to germfree toxins (diphtheria toxin).

On the existence of sensitizing substances in the majority of antimicrobial sera

1901 • Jules Bordet and Octave Gengou

Comment

Sometimes a particular, popular application of a scientific method and its prominent proponent overshadow in fame the principle and the developer of the original test. Such a situation occurred with the serological test for syphilis. The disease is no longer the scourge and social horror it once was, thanks to education, public

health control measures, laboratory tests such as this, and, of course, penicillin. Nevertheless, this potentially lethal venereal disease still persists in the population. The first syphilis test was the Wassermann complement-fixation test, named after August von Wassermann, who developed it with his colleagues Albert Neisser and Carl Bruck. The Wassermann test became a generic name for this particular type of serum assay, even though improvements were made over the ensuing years by Hideyo Noguchi, John A. Kolmer, Reuben L. Kahn, and many others. The Wassermann test firmly established the usefulness of complement-fixation assays; however, this syphilis test was built upon the work of Jules Bordet and his brother-in-law Octave Gengou (1875–1957), who discovered the principle and method. It is their fundamental paper that follows.

In 1900 Bordet, who, as we have seen, determined the virtual mechanistic identity of hemolysis and bacteriolysis (Part 6/Bordet, 1898), desired to firmly establish that the complement involved in both reactions was nonspecific and, in fact, was one in the same. To some degree the experiment he performed was designed to answer a point raised by Paul Ehrlich, who believed that normal serum contained multiple specific complements. Bordet provided the first example of complement-fixation, whereby a limited amount of the agent in normal serum is first interacted with assumed antibody-sensitized antigen followed by the addition of sensitized erythrocytes. The blood cells serve as a clearly visible marker of activity. Hence, prior withdrawal of available complement (fixation) will leave the cells intact; excess or unaffected complement for lack of antigen-bound antibodies will trigger hemoglobin-releasing hemolysis. Bordet also reversed the sequence, using disrupted cholera vibrio as the marker of free complement.

Bordet knew that only a few microorganisms are susceptible to the lytic action of antibody and complement, but he offered the bold hypothesis that the complement fixes to other antibody-coated cells as well. His intent was to try to use the complement-fixation method to detect antibodies to infectious agents in the serum of convalescent patients and in laboratory animals. Bordet gave this project to Gengou. Since typhoid fever was then a major infectious disease, Gengou chose to test such patients first. Complement fixation was also

found with sera from animals immunized to the plague and anthrax bacilli and to *Proteus* species. Although Bordet and Gengou recognized that the concentration of each of the components in the test influenced the result, they at first did not consider the development of a quantitative assay. The principle behind the method was more important at the time. The following year Gengou discovered that antibodies, coupled to the soluble antigens of foreign serum, casein, and egg albumin, also fixed complement, but he regarded precipitins and sensitizing antibody to be different substances.

In 1903 Bordet observed the spirochete of syphilis in chancre tissue, but because their presence in preparations were variable, he could not rule out the possibility that they were part of the normal flora. The credit for discovering the syphilis spirochete thus went to Fritz Schaudinn and Erich Hoffmann, whose preliminary report appeared in April 1905. Shortly afterwards, Bordet tried his complement-fixation test as a possible aid in diagnosing syphilis. Unfortunately, the expected negative control was faulty. Although it consisted of healthy skin, the control, nevertheless, fixed complement and hence prevented hemolysis. The results indicated nonspecificity. He did not know that anti-syphilis antibodies cross-react with certain tissue lipids; normal human sera would not have sensitized the normal tissue of the control nor would it have reacted with syphilitic tissue. Wassermann's team by some quirk did not experience the problem of nonspecificity, and in May 1906 their findings were published. Since the spirochete can not be cultured on laboratory media, they used an aqueous extract of the liver from a syphilitic fetus. Wassermann, however, was not the first to apply the complement-fixation test successfully to human syphilis, as his original work was with a monkey model. The distinction of carrying out the first human test belongs to László Detre, alias Ladislas Deutsch, at the Jenner-Pasteur Institute in Budapest, whose account was issued two weeks after Wassermann's. Detre had previously studied with Elie Metchnikoff at the Pasteur Institute and had coined the terms antigen and immunogen. On the next page of the journal, following Detre's paper, Rudolf Kraus challenged the conclusions of Wassermann with his own findings of both false positive serum and false positive tissue. Others were similarly thwarted by the notorious cross-reactivities associated with syphilis. Then in 1907 Karl Landsteiner, Rudolf Muller, and Otto Potzl observed that an alcohol extract of normal guinea pig heart gave results equivalent to those of syphilitic tissue. The problem of cross-reactivity, with grave social consequences, engendered thousands of research papers over the next four decades.

Today syphilis is no longer diagnosed by laborious, expensive, and complicated complement-fixation methods. Qualitative screening of serum is now by simple flocculation of a standard cardiolipin-lecithin-cholesterol antigen or more specifically by fluorescein-labeled antibodies to human immunoglobulins that have been absorbed with indigenous saprophytic human spirochetes. The antigen is a killed preparation of an avirulent strain of *Treponema pallidum*.

For further information:

Balows, A. and W. J. Hausler, Jr. (editors). 1981. *Diagnostic Procedures for Bacterial, Mycotic and Parasitic Infections.* 6th Edition. American Public Health Association, Washington, DC. pp. 631–673.

Fleck, L. 1979 (1935). *Genesis and Development of a Scientific Fact* (T. J. Trenn and R. K. Merton, editors; F. Bradley and T. J. Trenn, translators). University of Chicago Press, Chicago. 203 p.

Kahn, R. L. 1942. *Serology in Syphilis Control. Principles of Sensitivity and Specificity.* Williams & Wilkins Company, Baltimore. pp. 38–52.

Silverstein, A. M. 1986. The Donath-Landsteiner autoantibody: the incommensurable languages of early immunologic dispute. *Cellular Immunology* 97:173–188.

Zinnser, H. 1914. *Infection and Resistance. An exposition of the biological phenomena underlying the occurrence of infection and the recovery of the animal body from infectious disease.* Macmillan, New York. pp. 168–217.

The Paper*

The serum of a number of animals contains alexine, a poorly defined material of unknown chemical constitution, the presence of which provides serum with the general property of exerting a destructive influence on various cells and certain microbes. Alexine loses its activity when serum is heated to 55°. This material is found in similar amounts in the serum of normal and vaccinated animals; artificial immunization apparently does not modify its quantity nor its character.

When an animal is vaccinated against the cholera vibrio, the body produces a particular substance, the preventive or sensitizing material, which can be detected in serum and which resists heating to fairly high temperatures. It itself is not in any way lethal for the vibrio. However, it considerably supports in a specific manner the destructive force that alexine exerts on this microbe. . . . In short, if the bacteriolytic or cytolytic serum possesses a destructive, however intense, power, it is because it contains, besides common alexine, a specific antibody, the sensitizer.

In the preceding lines, we have mentioned only cholera serum among the sera of animals vaccinated against microbes. In fact, it would have been risky to affirm the general presence of specific sensitizing material in antimicrobial sera. Indeed, until now, the existence of these substances has been demonstrated with complete certainty only in the sera of animals vaccinated against cholera vibrio or other similar vibrios.

This is easily recognized if one reflects on the method that at the time was able to demonstrate the sensitizing substance. . . .

Thus, this method requires, before declaring the existence of a sensitizer, that the given microbe on contact with active serum be susceptible of forming a lesion easily verifiable by the microscope; bacteriolysis must be observed. Likewise, for hemolytic serum the criterion is hemolysis.

However, all microbes do not satisfy this requirement. Most are not destroyed nor even visibly altered on contact with even highly immunized animal

---

*Bordet, J. and O. Gengou. 1901. Sur l'existence de substances sensibilisatrices dans la plupart des sérum antimicrobiens. *Annales de l'Institute Pasteur* 15:289–302. [With permission.]

sera. In such cases, the method that we have described is found faulty and ought to be replaced with another.

It is therefore a different procedure that we will offer in this work for demonstrating the presence of sensitizers in sera of animals vaccinated against microbes, such as the plague bacillus, the first anthrax vaccine, the typhoid bacillus, the bacillus of swine plague, and *Proteus vulgaris.*

First, we should recall an experiment related a year ago. . . .

These experiments have established . . . two distinct concepts: (1) Corpuscles or microbes acquire under the influence of sensitization the ability to avidly absorb alexine and remove it from the surrounding liquid; (2) In a given serum, the same alexine can initiate either hemolysis or bacteriolysis. . . .

To demonstrate the existence of a sensitizer in an antimicrobial serum, we can utilize the property of this substance of causing the microbe that it affects to absorb alexine.

As an experiment founded on this principle is almost always the same for any of various antimicrobial sera studied, we will describe in detail an example, antiplague serum. . . .

This [immune horse] serum and normal horse serum are heated to 56° for a half-hour to inactivate alexine. A 24-hour agar culture of the plague bacillus is suspended in a sufficient quantity of physiological saline to obtain a very turbid emulsion, rich in microbes. Also available is normal serum, free of corpuscles by centrifugation, that was obtained from a guinea pig bled the day before. This is the alexic serum. The six following mixtures are prepared in test tubes:

(a) 0.2 cc of alexic serum; o.4 cc of the emulsion of plague bacilli; 1.2 cc of antiplague serum previously heated at 56°C.

(b) As above, but with normal horse serum (previously heated at 56°) instead of horse antiplague serum.

(c) Same as "a", but without the emulsion of plague bacilli.

(d) Same as "b", but without the emulsion of plague bacilli.

These first four mixtures all contain the same amount of normal guinea pig alexine.

(e) 0.4 cc of bacterial emulsion; 1.2 cc of antiplague serum.

(f) 0.4 cc of bacterial emulsion; 1.2 cc of normal horse serum.

These two latter tubes are respectively like "a" and "b" except that they do not contain alexine.

The mixtures are held for about five hours at room temperature (15–20°). Then at the same time 0.2 cc of the following mixture is added to the various tubes: 2 cc of serum (previously heated for 1/2 hour at 55°) from a guinea pig previously immunized by three or four injections of 4–5 cc defibrinated rabbit blood; 20 drops of defibrinated rabbit blood. In other words, each tube receives two drops of very highly sensitized blood.

These are the results of the experiment:

Hemolysis appears very quickly with nearly the same speed in tubes "b", "c", and "d". In about 5–10 minutes these mixtures no longer contain intact corpuscles. In tube "a", which contains alexic serum, bacteria, and antiplague serum, hemolysis is not produced. . . . They also remain intact in tubes "e" and "f", which do not contain alexine. We see then that (1) the plague bacillus mixed in normal horse serum does not absorb alexine (or absorbs it only insignificantly); (2) this bacillus in the presence of antiplague horse serum fixes alexine with much avidity and removes it from the surrounding liquid; and (3) antiplague serum without the addition of bacteria leaves alexine perfectly free.

Consequently, we must conclude that the serum of a horse vaccinated against the plague bacillus contains a sensitizer that confers to this microbe the ability of fixing alexine. This sensitizer acts hence as the corresponding substances found in cholera and hemolytic sera.

It may be added that if a small quantity of bacteria is introduced into a mixture of alexine and antiplague serum, the microbes do not undergo after a period of 3 hours at 37° any perceptible morphologic alteration. Consequently, in this instance the presence of a sensitizer could be ascertained only through the fixation of alexine.

If the experiment described above is repeated with the same quantity of alexine (0.2 cc) but with much smaller amounts of the bacterial emulsion and antiplague serum, the fixation of alexine does not occur completely. The sensitized corpuscles that are then introduced undergo hemolysis, but after a more or less considerable delay. . . .

A quantitative study of the precipitin reaction

1929 • Michael Heidelberger and Forrest E. Kendall

Comment

Michael Heidelberger was becoming increasingly frustrated. Just before transferring from the Rockefeller Institute to Columbia University, he read and pondered Svante Arrhenius's *Immunochemistry* and Jules Bordet's *Treatise on Immunology in Infectious Diseases*. His previous work on pneumococcal antigens, so comparatively direct and fundamental in chemical approach, contrasted with the arbitrary and indefinite conditions these researchers were forced to impose upon the chemical nature of antibodies. The various agglutinins, precipitins, and other antibodies were measured by functional titers, whose endpoint in the series of dilutions was entirely subjective. Two researchers may agree one day that the reaction at a given dilution of serum is positive, but when the test is repeated, one may declare it negative and the other may read it plus-or-minus. Furthermore, what really is the difference between $+++$ and $++$? Even with the use of a standard preparation, itself relative and capricious, these unreliable assays were providing more confusion than answers. Titers of antisera to different antigens could not be fairly compared, because, as we know now, of the differences in avidity, specificity, and valence of the antibodies and in the number and distribution of epitopes of the antigen. A nagging possibility remained that antibodies were not even proteins, but substances of some other nature that simply adhered to serum proteins. How could the chemist Heidelberger, trained to treat invariable substances in exact terms of weight and mass, continue to deal with such a sorry state? The answer, of course, is that he could not. He knew that if progress was to be made on determining the true nature of antibodies, then the barrier of inexactitude had to be broken. Antibodies must be purified and weighed. At least they must be given a consistent value.

Heidelberger did not have much difficulty finding a way: He had already demonstrated that nitrogen-free pneumococcal polysaccharide combines with nitrogen-abundant specific antibody protein. By assaying the total nitrogen in a partly purified suspension of antibody before and after the addition of hapten, he was able to calculate the amount of specific antibody in the resulting precipitate. It was at last an unambiguous quantitative figure. With this method, the kinetics of antigen-antibody combination could be examined, quantitative precipitin curves plotted, and equations formulated. With such a quantitative tool, Heidelberger observed that the proportion of antibody and antigen varied with their respective concentration, but he did not at this time venture a guess about variable antibody valence or other mechanism. He was later able to identify agglutinins, precipitins, and protective antibodies as identical entities and, by showing that complement had weight, establish that it was not a change of property, but a unique chemical.

This striking milestone, which partly formed the foundation of John Marrack's lattice theory, was planted with the assistance of Forrest E. Kendall (1898–1975). Kendall had come to Heidelberger's laboratory at Columbia after having served two years as an instructor at Lafayette College in Pennsylvania. He had previously attended the University of Illinois, where he received his B.A. in 1921 and the Ph.D. in organic chemistry in 1926. The team of Heidelberger and Kendall produced a distinguished series of researches over a ten-year period. In 1938 Kendall was accepted into the faculty of Columbia University, advancing to Professor in 1955. Remarkably, his laboratory skills were handicapped by the loss of a hand, the result of a childhood accident with a threshing machine on his family's farm.

Heidelberger and Kendall had established the principle of quantitative immunochemistry, but their method was limited to peptide-free carbohydrates as antigens. To widen its usefulness to the vast majority of antigens, they set out to modify a protein antigen by giving it a distinguishing brand. Since ^{15}N had not yet been discovered and radioisotope technology was still in its formative stages, the team turned to dyes. Microbiologists and histologists had long differentiated bacteria and cells by their staining reaction; clinical chemists had made use of color changes in reagents to provide a diagnosis; now it was the immunochemists' turn. Heidelberger and Kendall sandwiched 2-naphthol-3,6-disulphonic acid between tetrazotized benzidine and egg albumin. They next designed the purification treatment to render the reddish protein nearly incapable of coupling to anti-albumin antibodies while remaining antigenic. Depending on the proportion of antibody to antigen, resulting complexes varied in hue from pink to red. Heidelberger and Kendall had to visually compare the color of the alkali-dissolved precipitate with standards, since photoelectric colorimeters had yet to be invented. The amount of nitrogen in the matched standards was then subtracted from total nitrogen to give the amount of antibody nitrogen and thereby weight of protein.

Today affinity chromatography and spectrophotometry have eased the purification and quantification of total and specific immunoglobulins to the advance of basic research and technology, but the weight or molecular mass of these biological chemicals do not fully quantify them. Two separate but parallel preparations containing equal concentrations of antibodies to a given antigen may differ in their capacity to bind the antigen. Monoclonal antibodies from different hybridomas are especially unique. Specificity and avidity, keenly important in biological assays, must be considered as well.

For further information:

Heidelberger, M. 1956. *Lectures in Immunochemistry.* Academic Press, New York. pp. 32–51.

Heidelberger, M. 1979. A "pure" organic chemist's downward path: Chapter 2—the years at P. and S. *Annual Review of Biochemistry* 48:1–21.

Kabat, E. A. and M. M. Mayer. 1948. *Experimental Immunochemistry.* Charles C Thomas, Springfield, IL. 567 p.

The Paper*

Of all the reactions of immunity the precipitin test is perhaps the most dramatic and striking. While other immune reactions are more delicate, the precipitin test is among the most specific and least subject to errors and technical difficulties. Attempts at its quantitative interpretation and explanation have been hampered either by the difficulty of finding suitable analytical methods or by the failure to separate the reacting substances from closely related, non-specific materials with which they are normally associated.

With the aid of recent work it has been found possible to avoid these difficulties to some extent. The isolation of bacterial polysaccharides which precipitate antisera specifically and possess the properties of haptens has not only afforded one of the components of a precipitin reaction in a state of comparative purity, but has greatly simplified the analytical problem. Since many of these polysaccharides contain no nitrogen, and antibodies presumably are nitrogenous, the latter may be determined in the presence of any amount of the specific carbohydrate. Moreover, Felton's method for the separation of pneumococcus antibodies from horse serum not only permits the isolation of a high proportion of the precipitin, freed from at least 90 per

---

*Heidelberger, M. and F. E. Kendall. 1929. A quantitative study of the precipitin reaction between Type III pneumococcus polysaccharide and purified homologous antibody. *Journal of Experimental Medicine* 50:809–823. [By copyright permission of the Rockefeller University Press.]

cent of the serum proteins and much of the serum lipoid, but is also applicable on a sufficiently large scale to furnish the amounts of antibody solution needed to make quantitative work possible. It is realized that antibody solutions of this type do not contain pure antibodies—indeed, only 40 to 50 per cent of the nitrogen is specifically precipitable—but since so small a proportion of the original serum protein remains with the antibody, a far-reaching purification actually has been effected. It should thus be possible . . . to obtain data of a preliminary character which should point toward the mechanisms of the reaction. The present paper is concerned with such data obtained in a quantitative study of the precipitin reaction between the soluble specific substance of Type III pneumococcus and Type III pneumococcus antibody solution. . . .

[T]he agglutination titer and the maximum amount of protein precipitable by the Type III polysaccharide (total N-N in supernatant $\times$ 6.25) are approximately proportional. The latter may therefore be taken as a more definite, though not necessarily more accurate, measure of the actual antibody content of the solutions. . . .

Analytical Procedure: . . . .5-cc portions of the "aged" antibody solution were pipetted into 15-cc Pyrex centrifuge tubes. Solutions of SSS III of the required concentrations were added and the volume was made up to 10 cc with 0.9 per cent salt solution. A blank containing 5 cc of antibody and 5 cc of saline was set up at the same time. The contents of the tubes were thoroughly mixed as quickly as possible. The mixtures were then incubated for 2 hours at 37°C, and allowed to stand over night in the ice-box. The precipitate was centrifuged off in the cold, and duplicate 2 cc samples of the supernatant were analyzed for nitrogen, using the Pregl micro-Kjeldahl method with N/70 acid and alkali. The amount of nitrogen in the precipitate was calculated as the difference between the nitrogen in the blank and nitrogen in the supernatant, and was multiplied by 6.25 to give the protein precipitated. The supernatant was tested for both SSS III and antibody by adding 0.5 cc 1:20,000 SSS III and 0.5 cc antibody solution to separate 0.5-cc samples of the supernatant. . . .

The ratios . . . are quite uniform over the fairly wide range of protein concentration from 7.1 to 16.5 mg per cc of antibody solution. . . . [A]t lower concentrations of protein (and antibody) a given weight of SSS III precipitates somewhat less protein. . . .

Combination of high protein/SSS III ratio precipitate with additional SSS III: 5 cc of antibody [solution], 1 cc of 1:20,000 SSS III, and 4 cc of 0.9 per cent saline were mixed and allowed to react as in the preceding experiments (Tube A). On the next day the mixture was centrifuged in the cold, yielding 0.2 cc of precipitate. Since this contained only about 6 mg of protein, its bulk was composed mainly of entrained supernatant. The supernatant liquid was carefully drained off and 0.2 cc added to another 15-cc centrifuge tube (check tube). To each of the tubes 1 cc of the 1:20,000 SS III solution was added, the volumes were adjusted to 10 cc with saline, and the mixtures were shaken mechanically at room temperature for 2 hours and allowed to stand overnight in the ice-box (Tubes A' and B'). In order to determine whether any effect observed might be due to adsorption rather than to chemical combination, the precipitate from a quantitatively similar Type I pneumococcus antibody-specific substance experiment was treated in the same way with 1 cc of the Type III SSS solution (Tube C'). The tubes were centrifuged in the cold and 5 cc from each were mixed with 5 cc of fresh antibody solution (Tubes A", B", and C"). Only a slight turbidity developed in the tube containing the supernatant which had been in contact with the high-ratio Type III specific precipitate, indicating that much of the second portion of SSS III added had combined with the precipitate to yield an insoluble product of lower ratio of protein to carbohydrate. Tubes B" and C" yielded immediate precipitates. After 2 hours at 37° and letting stand overnight in the ice-box, the tubes were centrifuged in the cold and nitrogen was determined in the supernatants on 2-cc aliquots.

It is thus seen that only in the Type III tube did combination occur, and that a high-ratio Type III specific precipitate actually does combine with more SSS III under the conditions of the precipitin test. . . .

Now it has been shown amply that the reactions of proteins may be explained according to the laws of classical chemistry and it also has been shown that the soluble specific substance of Type III pneumococcus is a salt of a highly ionized poly-aldobionic acid. It therefore would appear reasonable to test the experimental data by the law of mass action and thus to determine whether or not the precipitation of the hapten by its homologous antibody shows analogies to the behavior of simpler ionic reactions.

It is evident . . . that with constant amounts of antibody and increasing amounts of Type III soluble specific substance the ratio of the two components in the specific precipitate changes from approximately 120:1 at the smallest amount of precipitate which can be determined quantitatively with a fair degree of accuracy, to about 60:1 at the point of equilibrium, that is, at the point at which both antibody and SSS are demonstrable in the supernatant. It therefore would appear that a small amount of Type III polysaccharide in the presence of much antibody yields a precipitate of the composition 120:1 (in mg). This is capable of reacting further with increasing amounts of hapten up to the point at which both components are in equilibrium in solution when the composition of the precipitate is approximately 60:1. In other words, depending on the relative amounts of the reactants, the specific precipitate is a mixture of varying proportions of two compounds, or a whole series of compounds containing hapten and antibody in varying proportions whose limits may be expressed as:

$$A + S \rightleftharpoons AS \quad (120{:}1) \quad\quad (1)$$

$$AS + S \rightleftharpoons AS_2 \quad (60{:}1) \quad\quad (2)$$

in which S and A are equivalent amounts of Type III specific substance and antibody, respectively, entering into reaction to form the compound of ratio 120:1. . . .

At the point of equilibrium represented by Equation 2 both A and S are present in solution and either may be precipitated by addition of the other. Can this phenomenon, hitherto considered so baffling on account of the known insolubility of the specific precipitate, be quantitatively accounted for according to the law of mass action?

From Equations 1 and 2 may be derived the expression

$$\frac{[A]\ [S]^2}{[AS_2]} = K \quad\quad (3)$$

But AS_2 is a sparingly soluble substance and is present in excess at equilibrium, being mainly in the form of a precipitate, hence $[AS_2]$ = a constant and the equation may be written $[A]\ [S]^2 = K'$ (4). . . .

Now although the molecular concentrations of A and S are unknown, other units may be used provided they are comparable and may ultimately be expressed in terms of molecular concentration. If 1 mg of antibody protein be called 1 unit of antibody, then the smallest amount of hapten that will combine with it, namely 1/120 mg, may be called 1 unit of specific substance. . . . [O]n the average, about 1.5 mg of A per 10 cc are present in solution at equilibrium, or 0.15 unit per cc. Then the amount of S will be $0.15 \times 2 = 0.3$ units. Substituting in (4), $[0.15] \times [0.3]^2 = K'$ and $K' = 0.0135$ (5).

With this value of K' it should be possible to predict the smallest amount of Type III polysaccharide detectable with an antibody solution or serum of known antibody content. . . . It must be remembered, however, that with these proportions of A and S, the composition of the precipitate would be AS, not AS_2. Its solubility should, however, be of the same order of magnitude. . . .

The law of mass action thus supplies an adequate explanation of how appreciable, if small, quantities of Type III soluble specific substance and antibody can exist in solution in the presence of each other, although the solubility of either, especially of the hapten, is greatly diminished when an excess of the other is present. . . .

[M]aximum precipitation of antibody soon occurs as the concentration of specific substance increases beyond the equilibrium point, after which no further change takes place until at least ten times as much hapten is added as is required to cause complete precipitation. The inhibition zone phenomenon then comes into evidence, but at least a 100-fold excess of hapten over the amount required to reach the equilibrium point is necessary to prevent precipitation completely. . . .

This solution effect is as specific as the precipitating action of the specific substance. . . . Moreover, the solution, or inhibition zone, effect is reversible, in that AS_2 separates again when the concentration of soluble specific substance in the solution is reduced by dilution with saline. Therefore it should again be feasible to test the application of the law of mass action to the experimental data obtained in the inhibition zone.

If the precipitate at equilibrium again be considered as AS_2 and no assumption be made as to the composition of the soluble product or products formed, the reaction may be expressed as

$$AS_2 + nS \rightleftharpoons AS_p \quad (6) \quad\quad \text{Then}$$

$$([AS_2]\ [S]^n)\ /\ [AS_p] = K \quad (7)$$

Since $[AS_2]$ represents the concentration of the difficultly soluble AS_2 in solution, this would be constant at equilibrium provided precipitate were present. Hence, under these conditions

$$[S]^n\ /\ [AS_p] = K' \quad (8)$$

The amount of AS_p present can be calculated (as nitrogen $\times$ 6.25) by deducting the protein precipitated in the inhibition zone from the maximum precipitable, while free S may, for purposes of calculating n, be taken as the total S present, since the amount in combination is never more than 6 per cent of the total. . . .

It is therefore suggested that the inhibition zone effect is a chemical equilibrium which may be expressed by simplifying Equation (6) to

$$AS_2 + S \rightleftharpoons AS_3 \quad (9)$$

The equilibrium point evidently lies far to the left, since large amounts of S are necessary to cause the formation of appreciable amounts of the compound AS_3.

It therefore appears that the three phases of the precipitin reaction ... can be quantitatively expressed by the three equilibria:

$$A + S \rightleftharpoons \underline{AS} \quad (1)$$

$$\underline{AS} + S \rightleftharpoons \underline{AS_2} \quad (2)$$

$$\underline{AS_2} + S \rightleftharpoons AS_3 \quad (9)$$

in which the underlined products represent precipitates.

In (1) the reaction tends to proceed strongly to the right, as AS is very difficultly soluble. As the relative concentration of S increases, more and more AS_2 is formed at the expense of the AS, until a new equilibrium is reached. The product AS_2 has an appreciable solubility and dissociation tendency, hence at this point both antibody and specific substance may be detected in solution. Thus, when A is added, there will be a precipitate, since more AS will be formed; when a little S is added, reaction (2) will go further to completion and more AS_2 will be precipitated. When much S is added equilibrium (9) comes into play, and the precipitate redissolves. Moreover, in the three states of the reaction the proportions of S combined with A vary as 1:2:3. . . .

Immunological properties of an antibody containing a fluorescent group

1941 • Albert H. Coons, Hugh J. Creech, and R. Norman Jones

Comment

The scientist scans across the dark expanse, seeking the gloom-piercing photon signal. This tactic of high contrast is common to many sciences: An astronomer observes the night sky with a telescope for the light of a distant galaxy; a microbiologist uses the darkfield condensor of a microscope to detect among the tissue exudates the thin beam-reflecting spirochete of syphilis; and a physicist awaits the sign of a neutrino passing through a photomultiplier chamber in the depths of a mine. Albert H. Coons (1912–1978)—after being frustrated by the inadequacy of colored dyes, turning instead to fluorescent markers to tag his antibody probes—gazed into a specially designed fluorescent microscope, and also beheld a glowing splendor against a shadowy background. This event occurred in 1941. He had introduced the fluorescent antibody technique, soon giving biologists and clinicians a cytochemical and diagnostic tool that provides distinct, literally outstanding microscopic features and photographic images.

Coons came to the project with a solid medical education. After completing his undergraduate studies at Williams College in 1933, he entered Harvard University Medical School, where he was influenced by such distinguished researchers as Hans Zinsser and John Enders. The M.D., awarded in 1937, was followed by clinical training at Massachusetts General and Boston City Hospitals. Coons' career was centered at Harvard, one exception being the war years when he served in the South Pacific. On his return to Boston in 1946, he quickly rose from Instructor through the ranks to Professor in the Department of Bacteriology and Immunology. The origin of the following milestone took place in the summer of 1939. Coons was vacationing in Berlin, experiencing the eye of a hurricane moments before the Nazi outrage. A visit to the Pathological Institute at Charité Hospital returned his thoughts to medicine, and one afternoon shortly afterward he pondered a symptom of rheumatic fever, the

Aschoff nodule, and its possible association with streptococcal antigens. Perhaps, he thought, if he could locate the antigens in the tissue, then he could provide key evidence to the immunological origin of the disease.

On his return to Harvard, Coons tried to label antibodies by diazotization. As Michael Heidelberger, John Marrack, and others had discovered previously, pigmented antibodies do remain active, able to agglutinate and indirectly color bacteria. Unfortunately, the technique is only useful when antibody is highly concentrated; color is extremely weak when preparations are viewed by microscopy. To pursue the study, Coons switched from the clinic to the research bench, securing a National Research Council fellowship and space in Enders' laboratory at Harvard. He scuttled the dyes and turned to fluorescent microscopy, then a highly novel technique in which even the required microscope assembly had to be improvised.

Coons had the assistance of two chemists, who were already conjugating isocyanates to proteins. Hugh J. Creech (1910–   ) took his initial training at the University of Western Ontario, receiving the B.A. in 1933 and the Master's two years later. He completed his Ph.D. in biochemistry in 1938 at the University of Toronto: his postdoctoral position at Harvard was as Assistant Chemist. Through the war he was a professor at the University of Maryland, but in 1945 he became Immunochemist at Lankenau Hospital and Research Institute in Philadelphia. In 1947 he joined the Institute of Cancer Research, also in Philadelphia, rising to chairman of the Division of Chemotherapy in 1957. Coons' second associate was R. Norman Jones (1913–   ). Born in England, he received all his college degrees at the University of Manchester, with the Ph.D. in chemistry being awarded in 1936. At Harvard, Jones was a tutor in biochemistry. In 1942 he went to Queen's University in Canada first as a Lecturer and then as Assistant Professor. Between 1946 and 1977 he was a member of the National Research Council, advancing to Principal Researcher. Since then he has been a private consultant.

Coons and his colleagues first used anthracene, which fluoresced blue. Realizing that certain tissues had a similar natural fluorescent spectrum, they next conjugated fluorescein, whose emission spectrum is perceived as green. Once the war ended and economies stabilized, further improvements in the technique occurred rapidly. Methods of purification and conjugation increased product potency; frozen microtomy better preserved target antigens; labeled antibodies were cross-absorbed to tissues to reduce nonspecificity; control criteria were developed; and the fluorescent microscope itself evolved with special filtering and optic systems. New antibody labels also appeared, notably the red-fluorescing substances rhodamine and phycoerythrin.

Coons' procedure was direct, conjugating the tracer with the antibody to the target antigen. Although the procedure was fast and simple, it was soon found to be both expensive and often impractical, since a considerable amount of precious purified specific antibodies is lost in conjugation, and because labeling would be required for every antigen studied. The remedy, the indirect technique, was published in 1954. By this method, the fluorochrome is conjugated to anti-immunoglobulin antibodies. For example, rabbit anti-staphylococcus antibodies are reacted with the bacterium on a slide preparation. Next, labeled goat anti-rabbit IgG is added. The labeled antibodies, called second antibodies, are thus suited for any rabbit IgG, whatever the primary target. Concomitantly, sensitivity is increased by signal amplification, since more than one second antibody can attach to each anti-target immunoglobulin. In addition to locating and identifying antigens, fluorescent antibodies have also been applied to quantitative immunoassays and to automatic differential cell sorters. Coons' milestone indeed shines.

For further information:

Coons, A. H. 1961. The beginnings of immunofluorescence. *Journal of Immunology* 87:499–503.

Goldman, M. 1968. *Fluorescent Antibody Methods.* Academic Press, New York. 303 p.

Spink, W. W. 1962. The young investigator and his fluorescent antibody. *Journal of the American Medical Association* 181:889–891.

Sternberger, L. A. 1974. *Immunocytochemistry.* Prentice-Hall, Englewood Cliffs, NJ. 246 p.

The Paper*

Previous investigations involving chemical derivatives of antibodies usually have been planned either to establish the protein nature of the antibody molecule, or to elucidate the influence of specific polar groups on the mechanism of the antigen-antibody reaction. Reiner, however, prepared serologically active atoxyl-azo conjugates of antipneumococcus I and II antibodies, and suggested that they might be useful in quantitative studies of antigen-antibody reactions. Marrack allowed anti-typhoid and anti-cholera sera to react with diazotized benzidine-azo-R-salt, and demonstrated that homologous organisms were specifically colored pink by the chemically modified antibodies.

The objective of the present investigation is the development of a method by which antigenic substances could be revealed in mammalian tissues.

One of us (A.H.C.) has repeated Marrack's experiment with antipneumococcus II and III rabbit sera, and has found that suspensions of these organisms were agglutinated and colored by the specific azo-serum. The color obtained, however, was insufficiently intense to render the method suitable for the purpose in mind.

Conjugates prepared by the interaction of isocyanates of polynuclear aromatic hydrocarbons with several proteins have been shown to be highly fluorescent. Since such fluorescent labels might be easier to distinguish than colored groups, a β-anthryl-carbamido derivate of antipneumococcus III rabbit serum was prepared. Conjugation was obtained in an aqueous-dioxane medium by the interaction of β-anthryl isocyanate with the serum. Experimental conditions were chosen such that a minimum alteration of the protein molecule would occur. The an-

thracene content of the conjugate, determined by ultraviolet spectrophotometry, was two groups per molecule of protein (taking 160,000 as the molecular weight of the protein). This conjugate gives an optically clear solution in physiological saline in a concentration corresponding to 1/10th that of the original serum. It has a faint blue fluorescence in daylight, and an intense blue fluorescence in ultraviolet light, even in very dilute solution. Specifically precipitated by pneumococcus III carbohydrate, it agglutinates Type III organisms in the same titer as the original serum (1/800), fixes complement, and passively sensitizes the guinea pig to anaphylactic shock. Parallel opsonocytophagic tests with anthracene derivative and the original serum showed equal quantitative sensitization of the organisms. These tests, however, do not prove that the antibody molecules themselves are conjugated with the isocyanate, although the quantitative determinations suggest this.

Accordingly the conjugate (diluted 1:50 in terms of the original serum) was mixed in equal proportions with a similar dilution of unaltered Type II antipneumococcus rabbit serum of approximately equal agglutinating titer. Type II pneumococci were added to one aliquot of this mixture, and Type III pneumococci to a second. Agglutination occurred in both tubes. When these two suspensions were illuminated with ultraviolet light in the fluorescence microscope, the clumps of Type III organisms exhibited a bright blue fluorescence. No fluorescence was seen in the Type II clumps. After centrifugation the organisms were washed with 0.9% saline and recentrifuged. Again the Type III organisms showed a bright blue fluorescence macroscopically, where the Type II organisms did not. Moreover, when Types II and III organisms were dried on different parts of the same slide, exposed to the conjugate for 30 minutes, washed in saline and distilled water, and mounted in glycerol, individual Type III organisms could be seen with the fluorescence microscope, whereas the Type II organisms were invisible, although their presence was readily demonstrated at the same focus with visible light. Nonspecific adsorption and mechanical occlusion of fluorescent molecules during agglutination would thus seem to be eliminated. Although the isocyanate undoubtedly reacts with other protein molecules in the antibody solution, it seems clear that the antibody molecules also have undergone conjugation without demonstrable impairment of specific function.

Mammalian connective tissue normally exhibits a blue fluorescence which is enhanced by formalin fixation. This particular antibody conjugate, therefore, is inadequate for the demonstration of antigen in tissues, although it might well have other uses. . . .

---

*Coons, A. H., Creech, H. J., and R. N. Jones. 1941. Immunological properties of an antibody containing a fluorescent group. *Proceedings of the Society of Experimental Biology and Medicine* 47:200–202. [With permission of the Society.]

Sensitization to horse serum by means of adjuvants

1942 • Jules Freund and Katherine McDermott

Comment

In Bernard Shaw's satire *The Doctor's Dilemma*, Ridgeon, the character modeled on Sir Almroth Wright, defines opsonin as "what you butter the disease germs with," yet oddly, butter itself was actually once used to enhance the immunological response to bacteria. In 1897 Lydia Rabinowitsch, Robert Koch's only female student, mixed *Mycobacterium butyri* and other bacteria with dairy fat to produce a cellular response similar to that observed with *Mycobacterium tuberculosis*. Soon two adjacent parallel lines of research arose, begging to merge. First, since the appearance of Rabinowitsch's report, a small group of investigators, exploring the concept of lipoid adjuvants, had improved the method, including the substitution of butter by refined paraffin and mineral oils. Meanwhile, many others were observing the significant influence that tubercle bacilli, living or dead, have on increasing the immune response to a variety of subsequently introduced antigens. Then in 1940 Karl Landsteiner and Merrill Chase successfully combined the investigations by sensitizing guinea pigs to picryl chloride after injecting them first with a suspension of killed tubercle bacilli in paraffin oil. Materials of this sort, which are not antigenic in themselves, but enhance the antigenic response, came to be called adjuvants. Although adjuvants had been used earlier, today they are integrally associated with Jules Freund (1890–1960). Why?

Freund, who attained his M.D. in 1913 at the University of Budapest and then entered the Austrian Army for his internship, a year later found himself in the midst of World War I. With peace restored, he became Assistant Professor of Preventive Medicine at the University, but deteriorating economic and political conditions led him to emigrate to the United States in 1923. His first position in his new country was as Bacteriologist at the Von Ruck Research Laboratory in Philadelphia, which he held until 1926. He next was Associate Bacteriologist at the Henry Phipps Institute in Philadelphia. Freund returned to university life by joining the medical faculty of Cornell University in 1932 as Assistant Professor of Pathology. The additional duty as Assistant Director of the New York Department of Health began in 1938. He left these positions after World War II, remaining a lecturer until 1956 and switching to Chief of the Division of Applied Immunology at the Public Health and Research Institute of New York City. From 1956 until his death, he served as Chief of the Laboratory of Immunology at the National Institute of Allergy and Infectious Diseases.

In the early 1940s, Freund began a systematic study of immunological adjuvants, materials often able to boost antibody production 10- to 20-fold for up to two to three years. His interest in adjuvants was a result of his earlier experiments on tuberculin sensitivity. In 1935 as part of a research team at Cornell, he verified a French report that a mixture of paraffin and killed tubercle bacilli can induce delayed sensitivity in guinea pigs. The use of the same animals a year afterwards for another study led to his chance discovery that the previous immunization had enhanced antibody formation to the new bacterium as well. In the following milestone, which firmly linked his name to oil adjuvants, Freund made a key addition in composition and a change in procedure that allowed adjuvants to be used for any antigen. Oil and tubercle bacilli are compatible in mixture because the cell wall of this bacterium contains waxes and waxy glycopeptides. Lipophobic protein antigens injected with oils show no immune enhancement. Therefore, Freund emulsified water in oil with the assistance of a water-miscible lanolinlike material (itself later found to be an adjuvant) to incorporate both the tubercle bacilli and the target antigen in a single aggregate preparation. This original Freund's complete adjuvant was crude but generally effective, and it clearly established the principle. The materials were impure, causing irritation, and the droplets were far too large to maintain the emulsion. Later a mannide monoleate detergent was added to the adjuvant for improved oil dispersion and the formation of a fine milky emulsion.

Oils are not the only materials that can be used in an adjuvant. The wide variety of helper substances include aluminum salts, silica, and kaolin; vitamin A; tapioca; bacterial endotoxins; the glycolipids and peptoglycolipids of *Corynebacterium acnes,* the common skin bacterium, and its cousin *Mycobacterium* and *Brucella* species; and synthesized ribonucleotides, such as polyinosinic-polycytidylic acid (poly I:C). Freund's adjuvants do their deeds by slowly releasing the antigen like a continuous booster shot, yielding greater levels of increasingly more specific and avid antibodies. Adjuvants also protect labile antigens from rapid destruction or elimination. They nonspecifically attract inflammatory cells, including macrophages and lymphocytes, forming, especially with tubercle bacilli, a granuloma. Alternatively, the droplets are dispersed to regional lymph nodes. Other adjuvant mechanisms may directly affect lymphocytes, probably by inducing cellular replication, by breaking tolerance through the selective increase of helper over suppressor cells, and by simply improving opportunities for T and B cells to contact antigen-presenting macrophages.

Freund gave immunology an uncomplicated general tool for inducing antibody formation and cellular immune responses to weakly antigenic substances and for producing models of autoimmune disorders. Artificial adjuvants have also offered some insight into the natural augmentation of immune responses to certain microbial infections. Since their development, adjuvants have been used countless times by thousands of researchers, and will probably remain—by whatever modification or type—a fundamental immunological technique.

For further information:

Adam, A. 1985. *Modern Concepts in Immunology. Volume 1. Synthetic Adjuvants.* John Wiley & Sons, New York. 239 p.

Freund, J. 1956. The mode of action of immunologic adjuvants. *Advances in Tuberculosis Research* 7:130–148.

Jollès, P. and A. Paraf. 1973. *Chemical and Biological Basis of Adjuvants.* Springer-Verlag, Berlin. 153 p.

White, R. G. 1976. The adjuvant effect of microbial products on the immune response. *Annual Review of Microbiology* 30:579–600.

The Paper*

Lewis and Loomis discovered that tuberculous guinea pigs produce more antibodies when injected with various antigens not related to tubercule bacilli than nontuberculous guinea pigs. Dienes and Schoenheit made the interesting observation that when egg white or horse serum is injected into tuberculous foci, sensitization to these antigens is different from that usually seen in guinea pigs free of tuberculosis. Some aspects of the difference are: In tuberculous guinea pigs the cutaneous reactions to animal proteins appear and disappear slower; in tuberculous guinea pigs the reactions are often necrotic but in the nontuberculous pigs very rarely if ever. . . . Dienes reported that he was able to reproduce his experiment when killed tubercle bacilli were substituted for living ones. Three different methods of sensitization were partly or wholly successful. The first technic

---

*Freund, J. and K. McDermott. 1942. Sensitization to horse serum by means of adjuvants. *Proceedings of the Society for Experimental Biology and Medicine* 49:548–553. [With permission of the Society.]

requires repeated injections of killed tubercle bacilli into a lymph node and after a lapse of a few weeks the repeated injections of a mixture of killed tubercle bacilli and egg white into the site of previous injections. The second method consists of two intraabdominal injections. Twenty mg of killed tubercle bacilli are injected into the peritoneal cavity and 10 days later 20 mg of tubercle bacilli mixed with egg white. Some of the guinea pigs so treated die after the second injection from shock. The third method, which uses the testicles for the site of injections, does not yield consistent results.

In view of the advantages of employing killed tubercle bacilli instead of living ones we attempted to sensitize guinea pigs with killed tubercle bacilli and egg white. We made a single injection of killed tubercle bacilli into the subcutaneous tissue of the groin and 2 days later we injected egg white into the same site. The sensitization to egg white was not of the tuberculin type.

Since the addition of paraffin oil to killed tubercle bacilli enhances both the lesion and sensitization to tuberculin produced by killed tubercle bacilli, we injected egg white into lesions produced by killed tubercle bacilli suspended in paraffin oil. Sensitization to egg white was not different from that observed in control guinea pigs. Landsteiner and Chase, however, found that "sensitization to a simple chemical, picryl chloride, can be satisfactorily attained by means of intraperitoneal injections of the compound when killed tubercle bacilli suspended in paraffin oil were used as an adjuvant." These authors later, using the same adjuvant, produced sensitization of the contact-type to conjugates made with homologous erythrocyte stromata. In the experiments just mentioned Landsteiner and Chase injected into the peritoneal cavity killed tubercle bacilli suspended in oil once or twice and soon afterwards the sensitizing substance.

It occurred to us that the difficulty of influencing sensitization to proteins (like egg white) by means of killed tubercle bacilli suspended in paraffin oil might be overcome by combining the antigen in the aqueous phase with a lanolin-like substance and in turn suspending the combination in paraffin oil containing tubercle bacilli. . . .

Aquaphor and heavy paraffin oil were sterilized in the autoclave. Tubercle bacilli of human type, a strain designated Jamaica No. 22, were grown on glycerol broth and heated in the Arnold sterilizer at 100°C for half an hour. They were dried in vacuo over phosphorus pentoxide, weighed and suspended in paraffin oil.

Horse serum was chosen for these experiments and was combined with the adjuvants in the following way. Ten ml of horse serum were added in small amounts to 10 ml of Aquaphore in a mortar and the two blended thoroughly. Twenty ml paraffin oil containing 40 mg killed tubercle bacilli were mixed in the mortar with the combination of horse serum and Aquaphore. The whole was shaken in a test tube and 0.5 ml injected into guinea pigs. One dose contained 0.125 ml horse serum, 0.125 ml Aquaphore, 0.5 mg killed tubercle bacilli and 0.25 mg paraffin oil. The guinea pigs weighed from 690 to 920 g. Five animals were injected intramuscularly into the back of the neck about 1 cm laterally from the midline and 5 intramuscularly into the thigh. They were tested by intracutaneous injection of various concentrations of horse serum 7, 13, and 19 days later and again 6 and 12 months after injection. Another 10 guinea pigs were injected with 0.125 ml of horse serum diluted with saline solution into the back of the neck. They were tested with horse serum in exactly the same way as the animals sensitized with horse serum and the adjuvant 1, 2, 3 weeks and one year after sensitization. The cutaneous reactions were observed 3 to 4 hours after the injection and then every day until they disappeared. The experiment was repeated; 6 guinea pigs were injected with horse serum and the adjuvants into the neck and 6 with horse serum alone.

The adjuvants modified sensitization in several respects. (1) The rate of appearance of the reactions to undiluted horse serum was similar in all groups of pigs, i.e., conspicuous swelling was present in 3 hours; but in the first experiment with the higher dilutions of horse serum there was a difference in the rate of appearance of reactions. In the group with tubercle bacilli the swelling was noticeable only one day after the injection except in the test one year after the sensitization, whereas it was seen in the control group within 3 hours. With the former animals all the reactions reach their maximum in 48 hours, in the latter group in 24. However, in the second experiment all the reactions appeared within 3 hours in both groups of animals. (2) The disappearance of the reactions was strikingly different in the two groups. In the group with tubercle bacilli the reactions persisted for 72 hours or longer and in the control group disappeared within 48 hours. (3) There was a sharp difference as to the presence or absence of necrosis. Necrosis occurred frequently at the site of injection of undiluted and occasionally diluted (1:10) horse serum in the group with the adjuvants but never in the group injected with horse serum alone. (4) Reactions to higher dilutions of horse serum occurred more frequently in the group sensitized with the aid of adjuvants. In this group 6 to 10 pigs reacted to a 1:100 dilution of horse serum whereas in the control group only 2 of 10 (in the test one week after sensitization). . . .

TABLE III.
Precipitin-titers 28 Days After the Injection of

Guinea pig	Horse serum and adjuvants				Horse serum alone			
	1:10	1:100	1:1000	1:5000	1:10	1:100	1:1000	1:5000
1	+++	+	Trace	Faint trace	Trace	+	0	0
2	+++	++	+	0	+	Trace	0	0
3	+++	++	Trace	0	+	Trace	0	0
4	+++	++	+	0	+	Trace	0	0
5	+++	++	+	0	Trace	Trace	0	0
6	—	—	—	—	0	0	0	0

+++ Precipitate on the bottom of the tube.
— Not done.
0 Negative.

Table III Precipitin titers 28 days after the injection of horse serum and adjuvants and horse serum alone.

In the second experiment 28 days after the initial injection precipitin-titrations were made using 1 ml horse-serum dilutions and 0.1 ml guinea pig serum. The results are shown in Table III.

The repeated intracutaneous test-injections probably contributed to the sensitization and precipitin-formation.

The mechanism of the effect of the adjuvants used is a complex one. Killed tubercle bacilli probably play the same role as living ones, though their role has not been elucidated; paraffin oil enhances the cellular reaction caused by tubercle bacilli and protects the bacteria from destruction and sustains sensitization and antibody-formation. Aquaphore may have two effects. It may retard the possible separation of the horse serum, thus delaying destruction and elimination. . . .

Methods for the study of histocompatibility genes

1948 • George D. Snell

Comment

What could be more basic to bacteriology than the microscope? A test tube is the fundamental instrument of the chemist; the mathematician is incomplete without a chalkboard. When the great knot of DNA was not yet unravelled, how then could a geneticist explore immunity or an immunologist study the inheritance of specificity? The answer is cross-breeding of inbred animals with defined characteristics. Often crossings of dissimilar strains yield complicated, abstruse data. Numerous matings and backcrosses are required before gene linkages are recognized and satisfactory chromosome maps can be constructed. However difficult it may be to examine even relatively simple genetic expressions like hair color, the multiple gene activity of such broad phenomena as graft rejection normally defies individual analysis. Experimental circumstances, however, would be much improved, to say the least, if animal strains were isogenic except for one particular narrow and easily observable genetic expression. George D. Snell (1903–) accomplished the deed, and helped determine the major histocompatibility complex, the keystone of immunity (see Part 7/Gorer, 1937).

Snell began his studies at Dartmouth College, receiving his B.S. in 1926. His graduate training in genetics was at Harvard University. In 1930 with his newly earned Sc.D., he became a zoology instructor at Brown University, but took a postdoctoral position as a National Research Council fellow at the University of Texas the following year. Snell studied with Herman Muller, who would receive the Nobel Prize of 1946 for his work with X-ray induced mutations of fruit flies. Snell next joined the faculty of Washington University as an assistant professor. In 1935 he left academic life to concentrate on experimental science, becoming a Research Associate at the Roscoe B. Jackson Memorial Laboratory at the rustic island community of Bar Harbor, Maine, where he has remained. The Laboratory was founded in 1929 by Clarence C. Little as a center for the study of mammalian genetics. In 1957 Snell rose to Senior Staff Scientist and has served in emeritus standing since 1969. In 1980 he shared the Nobel Prize with two other immunogeneticists, Baruj Benacerraf and Jean Dausset.

Snell focused his studies at the Jackson Laboratory on the control of tumor transplantation, a subject that had influenced Little himself when he was a graduate student at Harvard. In 1944 Snell considered two strategies to examine individual genetic loci on chromosomes. The first was derived from the standard repertoire of genetic techniques: He could use visible markers of genes that are juxtaposed on the same chromosome with a single histocompatibility gene. The second was novel with the promise of uncertainty, complexity, and difficulty: This technique involved the transfer to another inbred strain of a chromosome segment containing a single histocompatibility gene. The progeny of such an effective series of cross-matings would thus be its own unique strain and possible future parent of a subline.

Snell decided to first try the method using marker genes, since it seemed faster and easier. He selected 18 markers grouped into six mouse colonies. For instance, one histocompatibility gene is associated with a fused tail. When Peter Gorer visited the laboratory in 1946, they compared notes and performed confirmatory experiments establishing that Gorer's histocompatibility-related blood antigen II segregated with Snell's fused tail gene. They had been studying the same locus. The two investigators decided on a common nomenclature, and thus the mouse H-2 histocompatibility system was born. Later studies by Snell and others determined that H-2 contained at least two loci, K and D, with numerous alleles, since chromosomal crossovers occur at this region. Over 90 recombinants have thus far been recognized. The H-2 complex today consists of three class I loci (K, D, and L), five class II loci, and one class II locus, which codes for complement component C4.

Snell next commenced the production of congenic strains, which are inbred animal lines that are genetically alike except for single characteristics. The breeding of such congenic mice required 14 to 15 generations, and in 1947 as he was making significant gains in developing the colonies, the Laboratory suffered a disastrous fire. Although the flames forced him to start over, they did not take away his new knowledge or will. The following milestone describes the methods for producing these unique animal populations. Fifty-four congenic lines were established by 1953, and their number has increased substantially over the ensuing years. The importance of these living laboratory assets is indicated by the shipping of over 100,000 congenic mice to researchers each year. Classical immunogenetics as pioneered by George Snell and others has now been augmented by molecular biology, which is translating the chromosomal foci associated with particular recombinant frequencies of phenotypic expression into the nucleic acid sequences of genes. The advent of modern biochemical techniques in genetics is analogous to the great increase of resolution and magnifying power provided by electron microscopy over that of the finest light microscope.

For further information:

Klein, J. 1975. *Biology of the Mouse Histocompatibility-2 Complex. Principles of immunogenetics applied to a single system.* Springer-Verlag, New York. 620 p.

Snell, G. D. 1981. Studies in histocompatibility. *Science* 213:172–178.

Snell, G. D., J. Dausset, and S. Nathenson. 1976. *Histocompatibility.* Academic Press, New York. 401 p.

The Paper*

Genes of the type postulated in the genetic theory of tumor transplantation will be here referred to as histocompatibility genes. The prefix "histo" is used because the same genes which determine susceptibility or resistance to tumor transplants probably also determine susceptibility or resistance to tissue transplants in general. These genes will be symbolized, as a group, by the letter H and h; where specific genes are indicated, by H or h followed by a number (H-1, H-2, etc.).

The available data do not permit an accurate estimate of the total number of loci in all stocks of mice concerned in causing compatibility or incompatibility of transplants, but they do permit an approximate estimate. . . . The results are tested against two hypotheses: (1) that histocompatibility genes are either completely dominant or completely recessive, (2) that, like the blood type genes A^m and A^n, the heterozygote shows the characteristics of both pure types. . . .

Taking the data as a whole, it appears that there are at least five and more probably six or seven dominant H alleles present in the dba stock of which the A stock carries the recessives or h alleles, and conversely certainly not less than three and probably four or more H alleles in the A stock where the dba stock carries the h alleles. Hence at least eight and more probably 10 or 11 loci are indicated. . . .

While most experiments in the genetics of tumor transplantation have utilized the A × dba cross, there is sufficient other evidence to indicate that the results obtained with this cross are not exceptional. . . .

The above calculations have been based on the assumption that genes for resistance are completely recessive. This is the assumption that has usually been made, but as pointed out to the writer by Dr. Gorer

it is not necessarily correct; in fact by analogy with the human blood-group genes a completely recessive condition should be the exception rather than the rule. . . .

Several other factors must be taken into consideration in attempting to estimate the total number of histocompatibility loci causing susceptibility or resistance to transplanted tumors in inbred strains of mice. If there are some 7 histocompatibility loci for which the A and dba stocks carry different alleles, these are most probably also loci for which they carry the sample allele. Specifically, if we assume, for simplicity, that for each histocompatibility locus half of all inbred stocks carry the H allele and half the h allele, then for any pair of stocks picked at random, both will be HH one-quarter the time, both hh one-quarter of the time, and one HH and other hh one-half the time. In other words, any given cross will segregate on the average for only one-half of all histocompatibility loci. Hence if we take 7 as the number of loci differentiating the A and dba stocks, the estimate for the total number of histocompatibility loci becomes 14.

The assumption that half of all inbred stocks carry the H allele and half the h allele for each locus is an over-simplification. Actually in some cases the distribution would certainly be quite uneven, one allele being rare. . . .

Working in the opposite direction is the probable existence of multiple alleles at some of the loci. Such alleles would increase the chance of segregation for any given locus in any given cross and hence increase the proportion of all loci revealed by the cross. While the widespread occurrence of multiple alleles is an accepted genetic fact, there is a complete lack of evidence as to what multiple alleles may exist in the case of histocompatibility genes. . . .

Tending again to increase the estimate of gene number is the probable existence of linked histocompatibility loci. Since there are twenty pairs of chromosomes in the mouse, our estimate of 14 loci would indicate that some linkage must almost certainly occur. Two closely linked genes would of course tend to appear as one.

Another possible factor is the existence of tissue-specific antigens which would be revealed only by transplantation of tumors arising in the specific tissues concerned. . . . If different tissues possess different gene-determined antigens, studies with different types of tumors should reveal different histocompatibility loci. While this factor may well necessitate an important upward revision of our estimate of 14 histocompatibility loci, the probable extent of this revision is very uncertain.

Also bearing on the problem of histocompatibility gene number are . . . cases in which immunity has

---

*Snell, G. D. 1948. Methods for the study of histocompatibility genes. *Journal of Genetics* 49:87–108.

been induced to a given tumor in animals of the strain in which the tumor arose. . . .

There would appear to be three possible explanations for this immunity to transplants within an inbred strain:

(1) Inbred strains are continuously undergoing minor genetic changes as a result of mutation. . . .

If this be the correct explanation, it follows that there are h genes whose effect is so weak that they can be detected only when special experimental methods are used. Homozygous hh mice in the case of such genes will grow H tumors in 100% of all cases unless, through the use of small initial doses or the special treatment of implants, the weak natural resistance is given an especially favorable opportunity to express itself. Such genes may be alleles of other "stronger" h genes, or may be located at separate loci. If such genes exist and are at least in part separately located, they call for an important upward revision of any estimate of histocompatibility gene number based on strictly genetic evidence.

(2) In certain specific cases, animals can form autoantibodies, i.e., antibodies against their own tissue. . . . If this be the explanation . . . it emphasizes the importance of tissue-specific antigens in such immunity. . . .

(3) A final possible explanation of immunity phenomena in intra-strain transplantation is that tumors contain antigen not present in the tissue from which they arise. . . .

To facilitate further genetic and physiological studies of histocompatibility genes, a method has been developed for the introduction into an established inbred strain (E), homozygous for the gene H, of its recessive allele h, so that a new stock is produced of the genotype hh but otherwise identical or isogenic with the original strain. This method is shown in Fig. 1. . . .

The method . . . consists essentially of the production of F_2 individuals from the cross E × any other strain, followed by the recrossing of the resistant (hh) F_2 individuals to the E strain to produce again F_1 and F_2 generations.

The continued repetition of this process results in the production of a strain increasingly like strain E in its genotype, but hh instead of HH. After ten generations, the chromatin of the isogenic resistant (IR) subline is 96.9% derived from strain E. Moreover, in the great majority of IR individuals all but one of the originally segregating h genes will have been eliminated. Specifically, if 2 histocompatibility genes, h and k, incompatible with the growth of a given tumor, originally segregated in the cross, then by the tenth generation the odds are 0.952 to 0.048, or approximately 20 to 1, that any given IR individual will carry only one of them. . . .

There are several other systems of mating by which isogenic resistant (IR) stocks can be produced. An alternative method is shown in Fig. 2. While this method is more rapid than the one just described in the sense that it requires fewer generations to accomplish the same result, it is also more laborious. . . .

A complicating factor in the above scheme is the possibility or probable existence of certain h factors which, when homozygous, are unfavorable to the development of certain tumors, yet fail to prevent their progressive growth in 100% of inoculated animals. . . .

Gorer has shown that the gene for his erythrocyte antigen II, of which the A strain carries the dominant allele, is necessary for the growth of an A strain sarcoma in crosses with the C57 black stock. This establishes the identity of a histocompatibility gene and a specific blood group gene. . . .

The following question thus arises. Given an established inbred stock, E, genetically H-1H-1, and a resistant isogenic subline, IR, genetically h-1h-1, how can we determine if a third inbred stock, Q, is H-1H-1 or h-1h-1? . . . If the F_1 from the cross IR × Q is resistant to an E strain tumor, the Q stock is h-1h-1 (or at least carries an allele different from H-1); if it is susceptible, the stock is H-1H-1. By using this test, any stock can be diagnosed for all genes that have been isolated in isogenic resistant sublines.

A special case arises when a recessive gene h-1, introduced into an established inbred stock A, is to be tested for identity or nonidentity with a gene h-? introduced into a second inbred stock. . . . The crosses and inoculations are: F_1(A × BIR) inoculated with B-strain tumor, F_1(AIR × B) inoculated with A-strain tumor, F_1(AIR × BIR) inoculated with both A- and B-strain tumors. . . .

[Examples are next given which illustrate how a systematic search for linkages between histocompatibility genes and known marker genes can be conducted through crosses of multiple recessive and multiple dominant stocks.]

While the identification of individual histocompatibility genes, made possible through the development of isogenic resistant stocks, should be of considerable interest in itself, the principal value of the stocks lies in their applicability to other purposes. There are two main fields of research to which they can be applied. The first is in connection with studies in tumor immunity.

When a tumor transplanted into a foreign strain grows and regresses, the host animal is thereby partially or completely immune to a second transplant of the same tumor. . . . In a number of instances a similar immunity has been produced by injection of nonliving tumor material. Considerable progress has

Gen.	Fraction E chromatin in IR mice	If 2 genes, fraction of IR individuals of types **HHkk** or **hhKK**	If 2 genes, fraction of odd generation matings of types **HHKk** × **HHKk** or **HhKK** × **HhKK**
0	0	0	
1			0
2	0·500	0·286	
3			0·428
4	0·750	0·627	
5			0·729
6	0·875	0·811	
7			0·875
8	0·937	0·905	
9			0·942
10	0·969	0·952	
11			0·974

Figure 1 Method of introducing a histocompatibility gene (h) into an established inbred strain (E), genetically HH, to produce a resistant strain (IR) homozygous hh but otherwise isogenic with strain E. Mice of lines IR and IS are inoculated from generation 2 on with a transplantable tumor of strain E origin. The survivors (line IR) are mated to strain E mice. Column 2 shows the fraction of strain E chromatin in successive generations of IR mice. The figures in this column apply strictly only to chromosomes not carrying genes for resistance to the particular tumor used, since the gene h will carry in with it a chromosome segment of undetermined length.

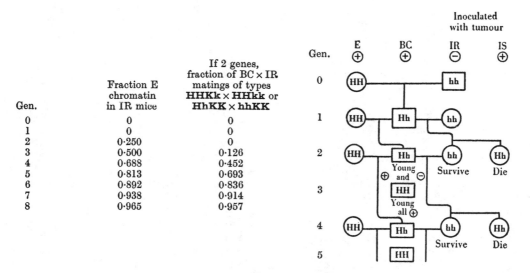

Gen.	Fraction E chromatin in IR mice	If 2 genes, fraction of BC × IR matings of types **HHKk** × **HHkk** or **HhKK** × **hhKK**
0	0	0
1	0	0
2	0·250	0
3	0·500	0·126
4	0·688	0·452
5	0·813	0·693
6	0·892	0·836
7	0·938	0·914
8	0·965	0·957

Figure 2 Alternative method of introducing a histocompatibility gene (h) into an established inbred strain (E), genetically HH, to produce a resistant strain (IR) homozygous hh but otherwise isogenic with strain E. Same procedure as Figure 1, except the survivors (line IR) are mated to their half-brothers (line BC) to produce the next generation of IR and IS mice. Some BC mice produce only susceptible (IS) young. These are discarded. Column 2 shows the fraction of strain E chromatin in successive generations of IR mice. The figures in this column apply strictly only to chromosomes not carrying genes for resistance to the particular tumor used, since the gene h will carry in with it a chromosome segment of undetermined length. This method requires fewer generations than that shown in Figure 1 for the production of an isogenic stock, but is more laborious.

been made in the isolation of the antigens responsible for this immunity. . . .

In view of the very clear genetic basis of tumor immunity, it can hardly be doubted that these antigens are a more or less direct product of histocompatibility genes. . . . Our knowledge of the relation of gene to end product is much too limited to permit any positive inference from gene number to antigen number. By analogy with the blood groups, however, it would seem that the number may be something of the same order as the number of genes. . . .

If the antigenic picture is as complex as this estimate would indicate, further progress in its analysis will surely be facilitated by, and perhaps almost require, the use of controlled genetic material. . . .

Through the use of the isogenic resistant (IR) stocks described in this paper the elimination of all but one antigen (on the probable assumption that one gene produced no more than one antigen) as a factor in any given study is accomplished once and for all by genetic methods.

When a tumor originating in an established inbred strain of mice (genetically HH) grows and regresses in a mouse of an isogenic resistant (IR) subline (genetically hh), the regression can with some assurance be attributed to the action of a single antigen produced by the gene H. It is, further, a reasonable working hypothesis that extracts or concentrates prepared from the tumor contain only one protein foreign to the IR sublines, although relative to distinct mouse strains some half-dozen of the proteins might be foreign. An acquired immunity to the tumor, or any serological reactions demonstrable because of this immunity, thus become specific tests for a single substance rather than for a group of substances. . . .

The second major use to be made of isogenic resistant (IR) sublines is in the study of somatic mutation. . . .

In vitro method for testing the toxin-producing capacity of diphtheria bacteria

1948 • Örjan Ouchterlony

Comment

The brain is a pattern analyzer. Everything we perceive is processed through "learning" into patterns, sets of archetypic characteristics, including dimensional and abstract shape, activity, and organization. A table does not become a table until some other entity is put on its top surface (dimensional arrangement plus function) and, equally important, until the elementary form is encountered again and recognized. We are thus conditioned or educated to find significance in forms. We learn to "connect the dots" or fill in spaces to produce recognizable, learned configurations or patterns, such as the constellations of the night sky. The first observer of a polymorphonuclear neutrophil seen through the microscope only noted an indistinct blob until its attributes were systemized through analysis and insight; later an instructed observer had little difficulty recognizing the blood cell when first encountered. Memory thus is a store of patterns, and identification requires pattern comparison and matching. Some people proclaim it a miracle when an image of Jesus appears, for instance, on a heat-discolored steel plate; what is miraculous is that such a pattern can be recognized at all.

As pattern analysis is the underlying essential mechanism of life, be it at the most primitive chemical level of cellular metabolism or in the transcendent domain of mind, it is also the fundamental basis of certain immunological techniques. Most precipitin techniques are acutely dependent on the patterns produced by the interacting reactants. The formation of precipitins at the interface of solutions of antibody and an unknown antigen layered in a narrow or capillary tube allows the identification of that antigen. This arrangement of immunological reagents in a tube, called the ring test, also can conversely reveal the existence of a particular antibody specificity in a serum. When researchers performed the reaction in solid agar medium, especially in a plate rather than a tube, they observed new patterns of lines. The recognition of the meaning of these patterns was a technical advance of the highest order. The single method of double diffusion of antigen and antibody has the power to not only identify an unknown complementary reagent, but also to indicate the approximate number of substances in a preparation, or the number of epitopes of an antigen, and their cross-reactivity to similar material.

The milestone that follows is not the first example of solid phase immunoprecipitation; it is, however, the first such report by the immunologist whose name has become synonymous with the test: Örjan Ouchterlony (1914–).

The early development of immunodiffusion tests does not follow a connected course. It is noted by several missed opportunities. Why immunologists did not quickly stumble on to such a simple technique remains a wonder. Burnt laurels of ignominious distinction for discovering the immunodiffusion test without recognizing its significance goes to the chemist H. Bechhold. In 1905 he incorporated rabbit anti-goat serum in 1 percent gelatin and poured the mixture into test tubes. The addition of goat serum on top of the cooled gel eventually yielded two bands of precipitate. Unfortunately he was concerned more with colloidal states of precipitates than with antigen-antibody specificity.

Two years later, the immochemists Svante Arrhenius and Thorvald Madsen, considering that variation in the rate of diffusion of mixed antigens through gels might offer a possible method for their separation, sectioned for analysis the gelatin mixtures in test tubes after incubating them for one to four weeks. They did not apply antiserum to the intact solid gel. In 1920 Maurice Nicolle and his colleagues at the Pasteur Institute at least logically reproduced the interfacial ring test using gelatin-incorporated diphtheria or tetanus toxins and overlays of various dilutions of antisera. They did not, however, take the next step.

G. F. Petrie in 1932 found a bacteriological twist to immunodiffusion. In a one-step process of isolating and identifying microorganisms in broth, he plated a sample onto agar containing antiserum to a suspected bacterium. A halo of precipitate around the developing colony would indicate its identity. Petrie was able to antigenically type pneumococci and meningococci by this procedure, and also observed that the precipitin halos forming around closely adjacent colonies coalesced, establishing the characteristic pattern of antigenic identity.

R. Brown made the closest approach to distinguishing multiple antigen-antibody bands within the same vessel. Layering a mixture of pneumococcal soluble capsule substance and somatic C polysaccharide over gelatin with antipneumococcus antisera, she misinterpreted the double bands as an artifactual temperature-related phenomenon. Jacques Oudin is credited with the first understanding of the independent precipitin reactions and the effects of reagent concentration. His preliminary report appeared in 1946, and made use of existing test tube systems. The significant advance of double diffusion in plates belong to Stephen Elek and Ouchterlony, who independently analyzed the problem.

The serological methods of Ouchterlony were rooted in his bacteriological research. When he was running out of guinea pigs for the then standard animal toxicity test for diphtheria bacilli, he sought a suitable in-vitro substitute, discovering the gel precipitation technique. The featured report is a preliminary account, which was presented at a Scandinavian congress. The expanded manuscript which should have appeared first, was rejected in 1947 by the journal of choice, the editors deeming the work of little interest! It appeared in another journal two years later.

Ouchterlony has had a career affected by wars and epidemics. His medical studies, begun in 1932 at the Karolinska Institute in Stockholm with additional courses at Uppsala University, were interrupted by volunteer service as an army hygienist and bacteriologist in Finland between 1939 and 1942 during the Russo-Finnish war, after which he received his medical license. His M.D. came in 1949. Ouchterlony's first research position was at the State Bacteriology Laboratory in Stockholm, where earlier, between 1935 and 1938, he was an unpaid assistant, and where later, in 1949, he headed the diagnostic department. His international service began in 1945 as Red Cross epidemiologist assisting the evacuation of concentration camps in Germany. In 1947, again under the Red Cross, he traveled to Egypt to investigate the epidemic of cholera. Later, in 1959, he was the Infection Officer of the World Health Organization in Hyderabad, India, and spent short periods between 1968 and 1981 as a consultant to the SEATO Cholera Research Laboratory in Dacca, Bangladesh. Ouchterlony came to the Pasteur Institute in Paris in 1950 as a research fellow. Three years later he lectured at Harvard Medical School and Massachusetts General Hospital. He returned in 1955 to Sweden for a professorship in the Department of Medical Microbiology of Guteborg University, but in 1972 he was again in the United States, this time at the University of Montana as a Visiting Scientist. He is now Professor Emeritus at Goteborg University.

For further information:

Crowle, A. J. 1961. *Immunodiffusion.* Academic Press, New York. 333 p.

Ouchterlony, Ö. 1968. *Handbook of Immunodiffusion and Immunoelectrophoresis.* Ann Arbor Science Publishers, Ann Arbor. 215 p.

The Paper*

There exist at present several methods for testing the toxin-producing capacity of diphtheria bacteria, and some are very well known and minutely elaborated. Roux, Ehrlich, Romer, Ramon and Claus Jensen are all names connected with this field of investigation where the experiences also many a time have opened a way to investigations of other kinds of toxin-producing bacteria. Much theory and speculation concerning antigen-antibody reactions in general and toxin-antitoxin reactions in particular are also based on observations of diphtheria toxin-antitoxin. . . .

These tests have been made in Petri dishes with serum agar (1% agar, 50% serum). In test 1, two so-called penicillin cups were placed on the surface of the medium, about 3 cm from each other. Diphtheria toxin (27 FIU/ml) was poured into one of the cups and antitoxin (45 FIU/nl) into the other. The plate was then incubated at 37°C. After two days a thin streak could be observed between the cups and it grew sidewards little by little. Beside the primary distinct streak, a couple of adjacent streaks, somewhat less distinct, were also observed. Test 2 was arranged in the same way, but here the toxin was first heated (70°C, ½ hour). A distinct primary streak as in test 1 was, however, not to be seen in this test.

In test 3, diphtheria immune serum [10 FIU/ml of medium] was added to the serum agar in the plate. Three cups placed on the medium were filled with diphtheria toxin of the concentrations 25, 20 and 15 FIU/ml, after which the plate was incubated at 37°C. After 48 hours a halo formation, whose diameter was larger the lower the toxin strength in the cup had been, could be observed around each cup. On continued observation it could be seen that the diameter of the halo increased and that multiple halo phenomena appeared.

In test 4, a series of immune serum plates with falling quantity of antitoxin (10, 5, 2.5, 1.25 FIU/ml of medium) was made. On each plate was placed a cup containing toxin of strength 25 FIU/ml and the plates were incubated at 37°C. After one or two days there appeared around the cups a halo. The larger the diameter of the halo, the lower the content of immune serum of the plate. The first halo observed was formed in the plates with a high content of immune serum.

In test 5, a smearing of the strongly toxin-producing strain PW 8 was made on an immune serum

*Ouchterlony, Ö. 1948. In vitro method for testing the toxin-producing capacity of diphtheria bacteria. *Acta Pathologica et Microbiologica Scandinavica* 25:186–191. [With permission.]

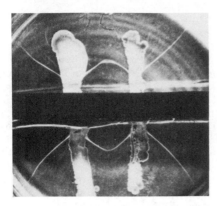

Figure 1   Serum agar plate with a trench containing immune serum agar as in model test 7. Two strokes of the strain PW 8 demonstrating interference phenomena.

plate (5 FIU/ml of medium), which was then incubated at 37°. After 24 hours there appeared around the growing strain a halo, which increased in strength during the following days.

In test 6, some diphtheria strains, which had shown themselves toxic or atoxic in guinea pig tests, were smeared on a plate as in test 5. After some days there could be seen halo formations around the smearings of the toxic strains, but not around the smearings of the atoxic strains.

In test 7 finally, a transversal trench was cut out of a serum agar plate and immune serum agar was poured into this trench. Across the plate, at right angles to the trench, the strain PW 8 and some diphtheria strains, toxic and nontoxic to guinea pigs, were smeared. The plate was then incubated at 37°. Between 24 and 96 hours afterwards there could be observed moustach-like streaks, going out from the

bacterial growth, in the angle between the trench and the growth. The first strain to produce this streak was PW 8. The primary distinct streaks originating from this strain and the toxic strains gradually turned off to the corresponding streak of the adjacent strain and finally joined it. Weaker streaks, appearing somewhat later, were observed, above all from the atoxic strains. These streaks did not interfere with the primary, more distinct streaks but crossed them, apparently without being affected. . . .

If an antigen and the corresponding precipitating or flocculating antibody diffuse towards each other in an indifferent gel of suitable consistency, e.g. gelatin or agar, there will appear, under certain circumstances, a streak- or band-like precipitation in the gel between the two diffusing components. The reaction is probably of the same nature as that between an antigen and antibody. The position of the band of precipitin in relation to the two diffusion centers depends inter alia upon the initial concentration and diffusion velocity of the two reacting substances. A similar reaction is obtained if antigens are allowed to diffuse in gels with a suitable constant content of antibodies or vice versa. In these cases the reaction appears at varying distances from the diffusion center, depending partly on the concentration conditions, the diffusion velocity and the time elapsed before the reaction becomes visible.

If different antigens and antibodies have been mixed, multiple reactions appear and the different systems react independently to one another. In these cases it is possible through a special procedure to obtain interference and crossing phenomena, which may be of help in the qualitative analyses (test 7). The diffusion method can also be arranged so as to allow quantitative estimations within certain limits (tests 3 and 4). . . .

Immunoelectrophoretic method for the analysis of mixtures of antigenic substances

1955 • Pierre Grabar, Curtis A. Williams, Jr., and J. Courcon

Comment

Arne Tiselius proved the advantage of electrophoresis, introducing a powerful tool of chromatography. The variation in electric charge of

particular proteins in a mixture allows their separation along a plane; their presence is detected typically by staining. The identity of any of the spots, however, is not usually self-evident (radioactive and fluorescent labels are example exceptions), requiring known standards to be run alongside for site comparison. Resolution is also a problem. On the other hand, Örjan Ouchterlony's immunodiffusion technique allows immediate identification, although it is even poorer in resolution than electrophoresis. M. Dave Poulik published in 1952 the first report that attempted to merge the two methods. He electrophoresed diphtheria toxoid on a paper strip, covered it with agar, and placed over the gel another filter paper strip that was saturated with antiserum. This crude approach was no match to the simple and wholly visible agar slab method of Pierre Grabar (1898–   ) and Curtis A. Williams, Jr. (1927–   ). Beginning in 1952, with the assistance of J. Courcon, they independently developed—and coined— the technique of immunoelectrophoresis, incorporating the benefits of both techniques. Closely situated proteins that would otherwise appear as a confluent smudge by electrophoresis or as a thick confluent band with polyspecific antisera now could be discerned as discrete arcs of precipitate. The method is so clear and straightforward that their first experiment, completed one week after considering the concept, left no doubt.

Later variants of this technique permit improved quantitative analysis. One such method is rocket electrophoresis, so called from the stretched, pointed appearance of precipitate. The radius of the halo precipitate developed in single radial immunodiffusion of antigen in antibody-incorporated gel is proportional to the concentration of the antigen. With the addition of electrophoresis, the halo becomes a rocket, whose height correlates with antigen concentration. Another technique combines standard immunoelectrophoresis with the rocket technique. It is termed crossed immunoelectrophoresis, since it involves two-dimensional electrophoresis. The principle of double electrophoresis was originally described in 1959 by B. Blanc in Grabar's laboratory with the practical effect of shifting apart nearly overlapping arcs. The result of cross immunoelectrophoresis, however, is far more spectacular. With the second electrophoresis, the separated antigens migrate into an adjacent and fused gel layer containing antibody. Thus, the single assay but multistage technique, which creates a beautiful array of overlapping fans of precipitate, enhances antigen separation and both identifies and measures them.

Such technical tinkering often originates with someone with extensive training in the physical sciences. Grabar is no exception. His first home was Kiev in Czarist Russia, but he began his college education in the Faculty of Sciences at the University of Strasbourg and later the University of Paris. He completed his Sc.D. at Lille with a specialty in chemical engineering. In 1926 Grabar was a lecturer in the faculty of medicine at Strasbourg, but in 1938 he came to the Pasteur Institute. He rose from laboratory chief to department head in 1945. In 1969 he assumed emeritus status. Grabar's concurrent position between 1961 and 1968 was Director of the Cancer Research Institute at the National Center for Scientific Research in France. In 1983 he was elected honorary fellow of the Royal Society of Medicine in London, and he is also an officer of the Légion d'honneur.

His American associate Williams earned his Bachelor's degree in 1950 at the Pennsylvania State University and his Ph.D. in zoology four years afterward from Rutgers University. He worked with Grabar between 1952 and 1954 as a Waksman and United States Public Health Service fellow. The next year took him to the Carlsberg Laboratory in Copenhagen. Later in 1955 he joined the Rockefeller Institute first as a research associate in microbiology and, after a three-year interruption at the National Institute of Allergy and Infectious Disease, a professor of biochemical genetics. Williams next went to the State University of New York at Purchase in 1969 to serve as Professor of Biology and the Dean of Natural Sciences. Since 1980 he has been the chairman of the Department of Biology there.

While its development was not based on a new technical principle, immunoelectrophoresis was a novel combination of two unrelated useful assays. Because of its ability to separate and distinguish amounts of protein as low as a few micrograms, and especially after Jean Jacque Scheidegger at the University Polyclinic in Geneva miniaturized the test in 1955 to gel slabs on microscope slides, it rapidly became a routine research procedure. Immunoelectrophoresis has entered the clinic as well, particularly in the analysis of individual classes and light chains of immunoglobulins. The immunology laboratory, which was once characterized by its arrays of serological test tubes, was now beginning to be filled with gadgets adapted from the physics department. The process has not abated; indeed, it has accelerated.

For further information:

Clausen, J. 1970. Immunochemical techniques for the identification and estimation of macromolecules. In: *Laboratory Techniques in Biochemistry and Molecular Biology. Vol. 1* (T. S. and E. Work, editors). North-Holland Publishing Company, Amsterdam. pp. 404–572.

Grabar, P. 1964. Immunoelectrophoretic analysis. In: *Immunological Methods* (J. F. Ackroyd, editor). Blackwell Scientific Publications, Oxford. pp. 79–91.

Johnstone, A. and R. Thorpe. 1982. *Immunochemistry in Practice*. Blackwell Scientific Publications, Oxford. 298 p.

Williams, C. A., Jr. 1960. Immunoelectrophoresis. *Scientific American* 203(3):130–140.

The Paper*

In a preliminary note we have described the principle of a method that permits in the same small

---

*Grabar, P., C. A. Williams, Jr., and J. Courcon. 1955. Méthode immunoélectrophorétique d'analyse de melanges de substances antigéniques. *Biochemica et Biophysica Acta* 17:67–74. [With permission of Elsevier Science Publishers.]

sample both electrophoretic separation and immunochemical reactions. After the publication of this note, numerous experiments using this method had led us to introduce a few improvements, and had allowed us to ascertain their utilization in the study of natural mixtures of proteins and eventually polysaccharides. . . .

For demonstrating differences in two proteins, even if very slight, immunochemical reactions are of particular interest, because their sensitivity and specificity are very much greater than those of most chemical reactions or physical measurements. This is because immunochemical methods have been for a long while used for the identification of proteins, but this is especially thanks to the quantitative studies on the antigen-antibody reactions by the Heidelberger school, which have entered current use. In the past few years, techniques based on specific precipitation in gel medium have been described. These techniques allow the enumeration and in certain conditions direct comparison of different constituents in a mixture. However, when attempting to define a constituent detected by an immunochemical method, difficulties have been encountered, unless samples are of pure substances. Thus, when fractions of serum proteins, obtained by salting out or by precipitation in alcohol, are compared by the method of Ouchterlony, one could identify certain precipitin lines thanks to such pure samples, whereas others could not be characterized. . . .

In order to overcome this disadvantage, we have sought to focus on a method that allows the definition of constituents in a mixture by their speed of electrophoretic migration and their manifestation by specific precipitation with appropriate immune sera. This method consists of electrophoresing a mixture of agar gel and then allowing the antiserum to diffuse perpendicularly to the axis of the electrophoretic migration. Each constituent, giving a fine precipitin band with its corresponding antibody, can be characterized by its position on the axis of migration, whereas the number of precipitin lines reveal the minimal number of components in the initial mixture.

Four stages can be distinguished: preparation of agar plates in which the product to be analyzed is introduced; electrophoresis in the agar; specific precipitation; and recording of results. . . .

The strict specificity of immunochemical reactions, and particularly those where the antigen is a protein, provides that in a mixture of antigens each constituent reacts independently with its corresponding antibody. However, one should also consider the eventuality of crossed reactions. Under the effect of an electric field different constituents of the initial mixture move within the gel, and at the

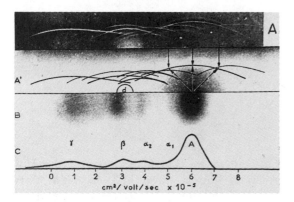

Figure 3 Comparison of various methods of electrophoresis. A, photograph of the results of analytical immunoelectrophoresis with normal human serum; A', diagram explaining the formation of specific precipitin lines; B, electrophoresis on paper; C, electrophoresis in liquid medium of the same human serum in the same buffer.

end of electrophoresis they are found at different locations according to their mobilities. The space that they occupy in the gel should have a volume nearly superior to that of the initial hole in which the product to be analyzed was deposited, because during the time of electrophoresis they also had the possibility to freely diffuse. They then continue to diffuse in the gel in all directions. Antibodies, on their side, diffuse perpendicularly to the axis of electrophoretic migration. Specific precipitation occurring where the antigens and antibodies are found in appropriate proportion, it is evident that the precipitins form regular ellipsoidal arcs. Conversely, if this precipitate does not form a regular arc, one can conclude that the substance in question does not have a uniform dispersion of electrophoretic mobilities.

The number of independent precipitin bands discloses the minimal number of different antigens present in the mixture, if the antiserum utilized contains antibody against all these antigens, whereas the position of these bands permit the characterization

of these antigens by their relative electrophoretic mobilities. . . .

Actually, the method is not quantitative, but by conducting tests with different quantities of a mixture, we were able to set limits on dilutions by which certain precipitin lines disappear. For some purified serum proteins and with horse antisera we have found a limit of sensitivity on the order of 3 to 10 μg.

The principal problem of the method, as with all immunological methods, is the difficulty of preparing identical antisera. . . .

Another disadvantage of the method is electroosmosis. In practice, we have observed electro-osmotic displacement of immobilized constituents almost as significant as the electrophoretic transport of serum albumin. . . .

Despite these few difficulties, we believe that the method presents some advantages in comparison with classical electrophoresis as well as immunological reactions in agar medium.

Indeed, thanks to specific immunological reactions, one can distinguish constituents in a mixture even if their mobilities are identical or very nearly so, which would not be possible with common electrophoretic methods, particularly when the constituents occur in small concentrations. Furthermore, thanks to the dispersion of components in a mixture by the electrophoretic field, the precipitin bands are separated and thus there is very little chance for the superposition of two bands, as could occur when one employs precipitation techniques in agar medium. From these facts, it is easier to distinguish between an eventual splitting of a precipitin band and the presence of two distinct bands: In the first instance, division starts at the central part of the precipitin arc, that is to say, the site where the eventual excess of antigen can interpose most rapidly. In contrast, when there are two independent precipitates, their maxima generally will not have the identical position because of differences in the electrophoretic migrations. Even if the latter are identical, the precipitin bands will be parallel but independent, if the diffusion constants of the studied substances or the relations between the respective quantities of antibodies and antigens are different. . . .

Immunoassay of endogenous plasma insulin in man

1960 • Rosalyn S. Yalow and Solomon A. Berson

Comment

Radioactivity, a word full of cultural consequence and emotion, is apt to send a shiver of dread or awe down the back. Optimistic fantasy creator Walt Disney likened radioisotopes to a genie in a bottle, a provider of profound benefit as well as the more familiar terror of death and destruction that keeps the world population in hostage. Even the biologist or physician who altruistically has harnessed these isotopes as analytical, diagnostic, and therapeutic tools recognizes the inherent biological hazards, the colossal expense of supplies and equipment, and the need for extraordinary precautions, training, and safety monitoring, all controlled by volumes of bureaucratic regulations. The use of radioisotopes in the laboratory hence must be clearly advantageous to warrant the great bother, and today new hazard free and far more simple immunological techniques, particularly the enzyme-linked immunosorbent assay (ELISA) first developed by Eva Engvall and Peter Perlmann in 1971, is rapidly replacing most radioisotope-based biological assays. However, in 1960 medical science thirsted for an exquisitely sensitive quantitative method to detect and measure minute levels of metabolites and drugs. Rosalyn S. Yalow (1921–) and Solomon A. Berson (1918–1972) quenched that craving with their development of the radioimmunoassay. Their report is the next featured milestone.

Yalow, who has been since 1972 a Senior Medical Investigator with the Veterans Administration Hospital in the Bronx, New York, is not a physician, nor is she even a biologist by formal education. She came to immunology as a physicist. After receiving her A.B. in physics and chemistry from Hunter College in 1941, she went to the Urbana campus of the University of Illinois, where in 1943 she attained the Ph.D. in physics. Yalow remained in the Department as an Instructor, but returned to Hunter College in 1946 as a Lecturer and Acting Assistant Professor. Her consulting relationship with the mentioned VA hospital between 1947 and 1950 led to the position of Physicist and Assistant Chief of the Radioisotope Unit. In 1970 the titles of both person and laboratory changed: she became Chief of the Nuclear Medical Service, with additional posts in related reference and research laboratories. Her hats also included that of Research Professor at the Department of Medicine of the Mt. Sinai School of Medicine between 1968 and 1974, Distinguished Professor-at-Large since 1979 at the Albert Einstein College of Medicine, and Chief of the Department of Clinical Sciences at Montefiore Hospital in the Bronx since 1980. In 1977, Yalow shared the Nobel Prize in medicine, which focused on hormones.

Berson would probably have been included in that honor were he still alive. He was the medical anchor of the research team. With his undergraduate program at the City College of New York completed in 1930, he entered New York University for his Master's, awarded in 1939. While serving two years as an assistant in anatomy in the College of Dentistry, Berson decided to enter medical school. The war increased the need for physicians. While engaged in medical studies, he helped support himself by becoming a lecturer at Hunter College. With his medical degree in 1945, and having completed his internship, he took his residency in internal medicine at the Bronx VA Hospital between 1948 and 1950. He next received an appointment as Internist in Yalow's Radioisotope Unit. Thus, collaboration began, and he rose to Assistant Director of the unit in 1952 and two years afterward Chief of the Service. In 1968, while maintaining his connection with the VA as Senior Medical Investigator, he became Professor of Medicine and later Chairman of the Department at the Mt. Sinai School of Medicine.

The subject of their difficult report is not related to immunology, except, of course, for its technological principle. They desired to measure insulin in a patient's plasma using the tactic of competitive inhibition or displacement, so that an increase of insulin would be indicated by a decrease in the amount of radioactive iodine-labeled animal insulin complexed to cross-reacting animal antibodies. The sensitivity of radioimmunoassay, a result largely of photomultiplying scintillation detectors but also dependent on antigen, covers the range of nano- to picograms, and thanks to antibodies, prior extraction or purification of test material is often not required. These advantages contributed greatly to the advance of all the medical and biological sciences; radioimmunoassay became indispensable to the modern laboratory. However, the technique had significant practical problems in its acceptance, such as the production of suitable isotopes at optimal level, the necessity to develop sophisticated electronic counters, and the ability to obtain exceedingly pure proteins and suitable antisera. Other considerations, which remain a thorn in clinical settings, are that an analysis often takes days, the shelf-life of reagents is short because of normal radioactive decay, and waste disposal, the bane of the nuclear industry, is a nuisance.

Technology is ephemeral, and it seems that, like automobiles and military aircraft, by the time a particular test leaves research and development for mass production, it becomes obsolete. Few tests and instruments are so fundamentally practical and, more significantly, popular to endure the span of decades even in modified form. Radioimmunoassay has ably served thirty years, but it will likely become an anachronism soon. Nevertheless, it established the power of the antibody as a molecular probe of the highest specificity, suitable as a general scientific tool. The replacement of radiotracers will still be an immunologically based assay.

For further information:

Abraham, G. E. (editor). 1977. *Handbook of Radioimmunoassay*. Marcel Dekker, New York. 822 p.

Odell, W. D. and P. Franchimont (editors). 1983. *Principles of Competitive Protein-Binding Assays*. 2nd edition. John Wiley & Sons, New York. 311 p.

Wang, C. H. and D. L. Willis. 1965. *Radiotracer Methodology in Biological Science*. Prentice-Hall, Englewood Cliffs, NJ. 382 p.

The Paper*

For years investigators have sought an assay for insulin which would combine virtually absolute specificity with a high degree of sensitivity, sufficiently exquisite for measurement of the minute insulin concentrations usually present in the circulation. Methods in use recently depend on the ability of insulin to exert an effect on the metabolism of glucose in vivo or in excised muscle or adipose tissue.... [T]hese procedures ... are of doubtful specificity for the measurement of insulin per se.

Recently it has been shown that insulins from various species (pork, beef, horse and sheep) show quantitative differences in reaction and cross-reaction with antisera obtained from human subjects treated with commercial insulin preparations (beef, pork insulin mixtures).... In preliminary communications we have reported that the competitive inhibition by human insulin of binding of crystalline beef insulin-I[131] to guinea pig anti-beef insulin antibodies is sufficiently marked to permit measurement of plasma insulin in man, and to be capable of detecting as little as a fraction of a microunit of

*Yalow, R. S. and S. A. Berson. 1960. Immunoassay of endogenous plasma insulin in man. *Journal of Clinical Investigation* 39:1157–1175. [By copyright permission of the American Society for Clinical Investigation.]

human insulin. Preliminary data on insulin concentrations in man before and after glucose loading have been reported. The present communication describes in detail the methods employed in the immunoassay of endogenous insulin in the plasma of man, and reports plasma insulin concentrations during glucose tolerance tests in nondiabetic and in early diabetic subjects and plasma insulin concentrations in subjects with functioning islet cell tumors or leucine-sensitive hypoglycemia. . . .

The antiserum employed in the present study was obtained from a guinea pig immunized with protamine zinc beef insulin without adjuvant and was selected for its relatively high antibody concentration and other suitable characteristics. . . .

Because of the desirability of keeping the concentration of added insulin-I^{131} as low as possible and yet assuring an adequate counting rate, it is necessary to prepare the insulin-I^{131} with a high specific activity. The lots of insulin-I^{131} employed in this study had specific activity of 75 to 300 mc per mg at the time of use. The preparation of such highly labeled preparations entails difficulties not encountered when the specific activity is very much lower. The Newerly modification of the Pressman-Eisen method was used for labeling with several further modifications designed to increase specific activity and to minimize damage to the insulin from irradiation and other causes. . . .

Considerable sacrifices in total yield are made to expedite the procuring of a highly labeled preparation which usually contains no more than 4 to 6 per cent damaged components. . . .

The basis of the technique resides in the ability of human insulin to react strongly with the insulin-binding antibodies present in guinea pig anti-beef insulin serum, and by so doing, to inhibit competitively the binding of crystalline beef insulin-I^{131} to antibody. The assay of human insulin in unknown solutions is accomplished by comparison with known concentrations of human insulin. The use of I^{131}-labeled animal insulin as a tracer is necessitated by the lack of a crystalline preparation of human insulin.

The determination of antibody-bound insulin-I^{131} and free insulin-I^{131} by paper chromato-electrophoresis has been described previously. Briefly, the separation of antibody-bound insulin from unbound insulin in plasma results from the adsorption of all free insulin (when present in amounts less than 1 to 5 μg) to the paper at the site of application ("origin"), while the antibody-bound insulin migrates toward the anode with the inter-β-γ-globulins. Thus, in the presence of insulin-I^{131} there appear two separate peaks of radioactivity: measurement of the areas beneath the two peaks (by planimetry) yields the

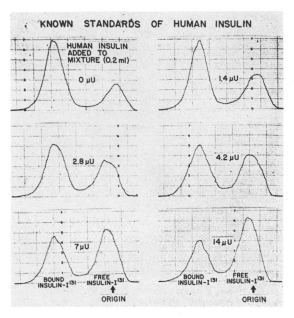

Figure 2A Radiochromato-electrophoretograms of antiserum/insulin mixtures. Mixtures contained the same concentrations of guinea pig antibeef insulin serum and beef insulin-I^{131} but varying concentrations of human insulin as indicated.

relative proportion of bound insulin-I^{131} (migrating with serum globulins) and free insulin-I^{131} (remaining at origin). The ratio of bound insulin-I^{131} to free insulin-I^{131} (B/F) is a function of the concentration of insulin-binding antibodies, of both insulin concentrations, and of the characteristic kinetic and thermodynamic constants for the reactions between the insulins and the particular antiserum. Selection of an antiserum for purposes of this assay is determined primarily by the desirability of obtaining a relatively marked decrease in B/F ratio with small increments in the concentration of human insulin. Although the antibody concentration is of only secondary importance, it should be high enough to permit at least 1:100 dilution of the antiserum (preferably 1:1000 dilution or greater). On the basis of preliminary tests the antiserum is diluted appropriately to yield an initial B/F ratio between 2 and 4 for tracer beef insulin-I^{131} alone, in the absence of added human insulin. Provided that the amount of the beef insulin-I^{131} used is truly a tracer quantity, the initial B/F ratio is inversely proportional to the dilution factor. In the presence of human insulin, the B/F ratio decreases progressively with increase in insulin concentration: with sensitive antisera the B/F ratio is reduced by about 50 per cent in the presence of 15 μU per ml human insulin.

Two preparations of human insulin were employed as standards. The first is reported to have a potency of 1.8 U per mg crude preparation; the second was assayed at 6.8 U per mg in 1956. . . .

The demonstration that unlabeled insulin could displace insulin-I[131] from complexes with insulin-binding antibody and that the fraction of insulin-I[131] bound to antibody decreases progressively with increase in insulin concentration laid the foundation for the immunoassay of insulin employing isotopically labeled insulin. In initial reports describing results with the present method for immunoassay of beef insulin it was emphasized that species differences in the reaction of insulin with insulin antisera exist and that human anti-beef, pork insulin serum is useful for microassay of animal insulins. However, the human antisera react too weakly with human insulin to serve as a basis for assay of the latter hormone in plasma. Fortunately, however, the serum of guinea pigs immunized with beef insulin was reported to react sufficiently strongly with human insulin for purposes of assay. . . .

To our knowledge there have been only two other immunologic methods employed for the assay of insulin. Arquilla and Stavitsky developed an assay for insulin based on the inhibition of hemolysis of insulin-sensitized red blood cells; however, the lower limit of detectability by this technique was approximately 0.1 μg (2.8 mU) making it unsuitable for determination of plasma insulin. Loveless has used certain normal human subjects, in whom the skin can be locally sensitized to insulin (by the intracutaneous injection of human anti-insulin serum) to assay insulin by the whealing response obtained. Aside from the inconvenience associated with this method, the lower limit of detectability was 200 μU beef insulin per ml and human plasma insulin was not detectable, a result attributed in part to the lesser reactivity of human insulin. . . .

Plaque formation in agar by single antibody-producing cells

1963 • Niels K. Jerne and Albert A. Nordin

Comment

An experiment is said to be elegant if it establishes a key fact or principle with an approach that is lucid, direct, often narrow or specific, but especially clever. Thus, it is the method itself, rather than the actual data, that merits such rare praise. Typically, the method is an amalgam of established procedures from diverse sources. The following milestone, which describes the detection of individual antibody-secreting cells, is an example. The technique is simple in design yet powerful in its application. Superficially, results bear resemblance to the already familiar phenomenon of viral plaques, the circular, clarified zones of infected and destroyed cells on tissue cultures or bacterial lawns. The method thereby has the benefit of rapid identification and quantification. The plaque-forming agent, however, is not infectious; indeed, it is the opposite, the defending lymphocyte.

The authors of this inspired technique are Niels K. Jerne and Albert A. Nordin (1934–   ). Theoreticians, who step away from the laboratory bench to gain a wider perspective, can sometimes see connections and correlations from different researches. Some remain at this vantage point. Jerne, however, being more than an armchair theoretician and a conceptual tinkerer (see Part 5/Burnet, 1959, and Jerne, 1974), saw technologically useful models and jumped back into the laboratory to meld them into a new method that could be applied to testing a novel postulate.

The basis of the system is the hemolysis of erythrocytes, usually coated with the test epitope or antigen, incorporated in agar with lymphocytes from immunized animals. The formation of 10^3 to 10^6 molecules of corresponding antibody in the area surrounding a single B cell is indicated by the subsequent application of complement. Jules Bordet and Elie Metchnikoff would have loved it! The method requires no modern equipment, no special apparatus at all.

Jerne's associate Albert Nordin went to the University of Pittsburgh for his undergraduate training. After the award of the B.S. in 1956, he remained at the campus, receiving his Ph.D. in microbiology in 1962. Graduate student became faculty member, as he rose from Instructor to Assistant Professor between 1963 and 1966. Nordin then transferred to the University of Notre Dame. He left the faculty in 1972 to become Research Chemist at the National Institute of Aging, National Institutes of Health, where he continues his investigations. His work in developing the plaque technique occurred when he was a junior faculty member in the Department of Microbiology in Pittsburgh; the new chairman of the Department was Niels Jerne. Jerne's directorship of the Basel Institute of Immunology in 1969 supported Nordin's appointment as Visiting Scientist at the Swiss Institute of Experimental Cancer Research in 1969 and Visiting Professor at the Basel Istitute in 1975, 1980, and 1981.

The hemolytic plaque technique came at the beginning of the immunological renaissance, and was instrumental in ascertaining the validity of Sir Macfarlane Burnet's clonal selection theory, to which Jerne himself had significantly contributed. The technique figured prominently in the Cold Spring Harbor Symposium on antibodies in 1967. The technique also assisted in the study of stimulation and suppression of antibody-mediated responses, including their components, processes, and kinetics, even to locate the original splenic site of the immune clones. The isolation of a given actively antibody-secreting cell was a brilliant in-vitro method to further the awakening and growth of cellular immunology.

Many variations and improvement of Jerne's plaque technique have since appeared. For instance, microscope slides rather than Petri dishes are sometimes more practical when reagents need to be conserved and large numbers of assays are required. Agarose has been used instead of regular agar because it does not inhibit complement; alternatively, DEAE dextran may be added to agar to block the anticomplementary activity. Since the original method chiefly detects the more hemolytic-efficient IgM, indirect amplifying procedures utilizing xenogenic anti-IgG antibody help to locate lymphocytes that secrete the weakly or non-complement-fixing classes and subclasses of immunoglobulin. To detect the many clones of lymphocytes that are secreting antibody to different antigens, erythrocytes have been coated with protein A from *Staphylococcus aureus,* which binds to the nonspecific Fc portion of IgG. Anti-IgG followed by complement then initiate hemolysis. Another alteration is to substitute erythrocytes with certain target tissue cells for examining antibody responses to H-2, Thy-1, tumor-associated antigens, and other cell surface markers. The mark of a successful technique is its ability to be adapted for sundry studies using a variety of tactics. Jerne and Nordin's borrowing of microbiological technical strategy has thus proved itself to be a triumphant insight of immunological methodology.

For further information:

Jerne, N. K., C. Henry, A. A. Nordin, H. Fuji, A. M. C. Koros, and I. Lefkovits. 1974. Plaque forming cells: Methodology and theory. *Transplantation Reviews* 18:130–191.

Mishell, B. B. and S. M. Shiigi. 1980. *Selected Methods in Cellular Immunology.* W. H. Freeman and Company, San Francisco. pp. 69–123.

Sell, S., A. B. Park, and A. A. Nordin. 1970. Immunoglobulin classes of antibody-forming cells in mice. I. Localized hemolysis-in-agar plaque-forming cells belonging to five immunoglobulin classes. *Journal of Immunology* 104:483–494.

The Paper*

We have developed a simple technique for scoring individual antibody-forming cells among a mixed cell population. The following experimental example describes the procedure.

From a rabbit that had received three injections, each of 5 times 10^9 sheep red cell stromata, in the footpads during the preceding three weeks, a popliteal lymph node was removed and its contents of

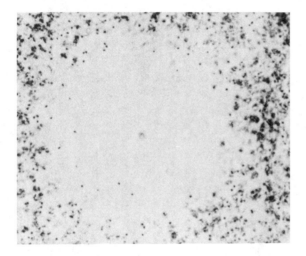

Figure 1 Rabbit lymph node cell producing a plaque.

*Jerne, N. K. and A. A. Nordin. 1963. Plaque formation in agar by single antibody-producing cells. *Science* 140:405. [Copyright 1963 by the AAAS.]

cells teased out into tissue culture medium containing no serum. Microscopic examination of the cell suspension obtained after washing by three centrifugations and resuspension in this medium in the cold showed the presence of nonaggregated lymphoid cells of various types. One million of these cells in 0.1 ml as well as 200 million sheep red cells in 0.1 ml were added to 2 ml of a 0.7-percent Difco-agar solution in the culture medium that was kept fluid at 45°C, and the mixture was poured onto a supporting 1.4-percent agar bottom layer in a petri dish so as to form a thin, semisolid top layer. After incubation at 37°C for 1 hour this layer was covered with 1.5 ml of complement (guinea pig serum 1:5). Further incubation for 15 minutes revealed about 100 clear plaques of about 0.25 mm diameter that stood out sharply against the uniformly red background.

Experiments of this type with rabbit lymph node cells as well as with mouse spleen cells have shown that the number of plaques obtained is proportional to the number of lymphoid cells plates. This suggests that each plaque is due to the activity of an individual cell. Microscopically, a plaque shows up as a circular hemolytic clearance in a field of closely scattered red cells, and in the center of most plaques a lymphoid cell is seen which presumably is the cell that released the sensitizing antibody. Larger plaque sizes are obtained by using a lower red cell concentration, though this diminishes the color contrast. Plaque formation did not occur in the presence of 0.01 molar potassium cyanide.

By using red cells coated with other antigenic determinants, the technique may be extended to other antigen-antibody systems, whereas multiple antibody production by individual cells could be studied by using mixed red cells. . . .

An analysis of the sequences of the variable regions of Bence Jones proteins and myeloma light chains

1970 • Tai Te Wu and Elvin A. Kabat

Comment

Technology, as the previous articles have demonstrated, includes more than specialized instruments and common laboratory apparatus.

A unique experimental procedure or method may be the blade that cuts a path through the jungle of entangled conceptions. Mathematical approaches, particularly statistical analysis, are also tools that, for instance, can disclose the highly significant influence of some previously overlooked or once thought minor variable, in addition to the customary evaluation of core experimental data. The determination of the entire sequence of amino acids on a protein is a profound technological achievement. The comparative examination of amino acid sequences of equivalent proteins from different species and occasionally individuals, or their blueprint codes on chromosomes, may offer insight into evolution and ontogenic development. While differences in but a single amino acid locus will in the strict sense alter the shape of the protein and thereby render it unique, the symbolic mathematical rather than the subtle spacial patterns are a far more practical means of analysis.

Antibodies are extraordinarily complex protein units, being composed of at least two pairs of chains, each variety directed by multiple genes (see Part 3/Edelman, 1961, and Part 7/Kunkel, 1963). Amino acid substitutions, additions, or deletions in areas comprising the antigen receptor are required to physically define variation in antibody specificity. In order to discover the root cause of unique antigen receptors and other antibody properties that are largely dependent on three-dimensional structure as well as physical chemistry, purified monoclonal antibody must be obtained for comparisons. In the days before hybridoma fusions, the only source of large amounts of singular immunoglobulin was the rare natural myeloma, particularly the light chain form, which is secreted in the urine as Bence-Jones protein. Thus, as collections, myeloma immunoglobulins, which were eventually established to be comprised of the normal lymphocyte proteins, became a critically important immunogenetic tool for the study of the archetypical antibody.

Among the leaders of this statistical form of structural analysis are Tai Te Wu (1935–   ) and Elvin A. Kabat. Wu is a scientist at home in physics, mathematics, and biochemistry. Born in Shanghai, he began his college education at the University of Hong Kong. After receiving a B.S. in 1956, he came to the University of Illinois, Urbana, completing a second B.S. in 1958. He obtained his Ph.D. in engineering in 1961 at Harvard University. He remained at Harvard, becoming a research associate in biological chemistry within the medical school. In 1967 he joined the faculty of the Cornell University Graduate School of Medical Sciences to teach biomathematics. Wu held a concurrent position with the Sloan-Kettering Institute. In 1970, now an Associate Professor, he switched to Northwestern University first as a professor in the departments of physics and engineering science and then since 1974 as Professor of Biochemistry, Molecular and Cellular Biology, with additional appointments in engineering science and applied mathematics. Wu's research continues on the three-dimensional structure of macromolecules and their evolutionary relationships. When the following milestone appeared, Kabat, whose career was outlined in an earlier section (Part 3/Tiselius, 1939), was at Columbia University also holding titles in a variety of departments: microbiology, neurology, and human genetics and development.

Wu and Kabat's paper, itself a key contribution to immunogenetics and immunochemistry, is featured as a representative of the numerous reports that examine the sequence of the amino acids in immunoglobulins. These investigations have correlated the fine structure of the antibody with its biological and physicochemical activities. Comparisons of the sequences of the over 400 amino acids of the heavy chain and some 200 amino acids of the light chain allowed the discovery that the positions in which amino acids vary among allotypes and idiotypes especially are congregated in particular sections. The largest clusters by far are at the nitrogen-terminal of both the heavy and light chains, indicating that these sites form the antigen receptor. Immunoglobulin classes and subclasses, seen to be a result of the variation of amino acids in otherwise constant regions, has provided rich information on the discrete sets of antibody genes. Analysis has also disclosed the hinge area of immunoglobulins, whose flexibility permits bridging of antigenic molecules or like epitopes of a single antigenic particle. Further studies have allowed the inspection of those domains associated with the J chain, with complement-binding, and with macrophage attachment. Finally, these studies have assisted the determination of the genetic-somatic origin of immunoglobulins and antibody specificity. Wu and Kabat's report is an often cited example. They proposed that the immunoglobulin light chains are assembled from two genes, then a radical idea. One of the set of genes for the variable region, initially extrachromosomal like bacterial plasmids, would then be randomly inserted into the chromosome during cellular differentiation or after antigen contact. While it did not prove to be correct in its later expanded details, the highly original hypothesis had much merit in its principles of multiple genes and combinations.

For further information:

Kindt, T. J. and J. D. Capra. 1984. *The Antibody Enigma.* Plenum Press, New York. 270 p.

Solomon, A. 1976. Bence-Jones proteins and light chains of immunoglobulins. *New England Journal of Medicine* 294:17–23; 91–98.

Low,T. L. K., Liu, Y-S. V., and F. W. Putnam. 1976. Structure, function, and evolutionary relationships of Fc domains of human immunoglobulins A, G, M, and E. *Science* 191:390–392.

Kabat, E. A., T. T. Wu, and H. Bilofsky. 1979. *Sequences of Immunoglobulin Chains. Tabulation and analysis of amino acid sequences of precursors, V-regions, C-regions, J-chain and β₂-microglobulins.* National Institutes of Health, Bethesda. 185 p.

The Paper*

The extraordinary versatility of the antibody-forming mechanism in producing an almost limitless number of specific receptor sites complementary for almost any molecular conformation of matter within a size range represented by a hexa- or hepta-saccharide as an upper and a mono- or disaccharide as a lower limit, is almost certainly related to the unique structural feature of immunoglobulins and differentiates them from all other known proteins. These antibody-combining sites are formed as a consequence of the interaction of two polypeptide chains, a light and a heavy chain. . . .

The large body of sequence data related to immunoglobulin structure comes from the analysis of urinary Bence Jones proteins and from the monoclonal immunoglobulins found in large amounts in the sera of patients with multiple myeloma and Waldenstrom macroglobulinemia. While a substantial body of evidence was available relating these proteins to immunoglobulins, the recent demonstration that many myeloma globulins have specific ligand-binding properties like those of many antibodies provides increasing confidence that myeloma globulins represent homogenous populations of antibody molecules. . . .

The unique finding that distinguishes the immunoglobulins from all other proteins is that the N-terminal half of the light chains and the N-terminal quarter of the heavy chains vary in sequence in samples obtained from individual monoclonal immunoglobulins and that indeed no two such variable regions of any chain and no two myeloma immunoglobulins or Bence Jones proteins have thus far been found to be identical in sequence. The constant region, however, is essentially no different from other proteins in that the variation in the amino acids found at any position is ascribably to species and class variation or to genetic variants such as Inv factors. By comparison of sequence data on the variable and constant regions of Bence Jones proteins with amino acid composition of purified human antibodies, it could be shown that most of the compositional variation could only originate in the variable region. . . .

The present communication is an extension of earlier efforts from this laboratory to locate more precisely those portions of the variable region which

---

*Wu, T. T. and E. A. Kabat. 1970. An analysis of the sequences of the variable regions of Bence Jones proteins and myeloma light chains and their implications for antibody complementarity. *Journal of Experimental Medicine* 132:211–250. [By copyright permission of The Rockefeller University Press.]

are directly responsible for antibody complementarity, that is which make direct contact with the antigenic determinants, and to explain the unique capacity of these proteins to have so many complementary regions.

As in the earlier studies, all human κ, human λ, and mouse κ Bence Jones protein and light chain sequences are aligned for maximum homology and all variable regions are considered as a unit and compared with the constant regions. The earlier studies had called attention to the following:

(a) The variable regions had few if any species-specific positions while the constant regions of the human and mouse proteins had 36 species-specific amino acid substitutions per 107 residues. . . .

(b) When the invariant residues of these two regions were compared, the latest tabulation showed the variable regions to have 10 invariant and almost invariant glycines and no invariant alanines, leucines, valines, histidines, lysines, or serines while the constant regions had 3 each of invariant alanine, leucine, or valine, and 2 invariant histidines, 23 invariant lysines, and 5 invariant serines. It was suggested that the invariant glycines were important in contributing to the flexibility needed by the variable region in accommodating the numerous substitutions at the variable positions. It was also suggested that the invariant glycines near the end of the variable region at positions 99 and 101, plus the almost invariant glycine at position 100, provided a pivot upon which the complementarity-determining regions might move to make better contact with the antigenic determinant just as the walls of the lysozyme site have been shown to adjust somewhat to accommodate its hexasaccharide substrate. The hydrophobic residues in the constant region were hypothesized to be involved in noncovalent bonding to the heavy chain.

(c) From an examination of sequences of the κI, κII, and κIII subgroups of the human Bence Jones proteins in which many of the proteins in a subgroup had an identical sequence for the first 20–24 residues, it was postulated that there are two kinds of residues in the variable regions, those making direct contact with the antigenic determinant and those which are involved only in three-dimensional folding. . . . It was hypothesized that these first two regions might represent the complementarity-determining regions and that complementarity might be acquired by the insertion of small linear sequences into the light and heavy chains by some episomal or other insertion mechanism. It is striking that the differences in chain length seen in the Bence Jones proteins are confined to those two regions of the chain. The remaining portions of each chain would be essentially under the control of structural genes.

The inserted sequences would be drawn from a large but finite set and either inserted under the influence of antigen, if antibody-forming cells are multipotent, or individual sequences might be distributed to immunoglobulin-forming cells during differentiation if the capacity of individual cells to synthesize antibody is restricted.

This working hypothesis offers several advantages:

(a) It is capable of providing the evolutionary stability and accounts for the universality of the antibody-forming mechanism throughout the vertebrates. . . .

(b) It offers a substantial simplification to the problem of producing a very large number of complementary sites. While it is known that in all proteins with specific receptors the site is formed by residues from widely separated portions of the chain, these sites are all formed by single chains. Thus, forming a three-dimensional site must involve residues from various regions. The antibody site being formed by a heavy and light chain need not necessarily be so restricted. . . .

Complete and partial sequence data have been published on 77 Bence Jones proteins and immunoglobulin light chains as well as on a number of heavy chains [of various human and mouse subgroups]. . . .

The accumulation of such large numbers of sequences makes it possible to use statistical criteria in defining the types of residues. . . . The definition of an invariant residue used in this paper is taken as a position at which 88–90% or more of the samples contain the same amino acid. . . .

The basic property that differentiates glycine from all other amino acids structurally is the absence of a side chain. As a result, glycine can have many sterically allowable configurations. This has been verified experimentally in the case of lysozyme and tosyl-α-chymotrypsin. . . . This unique property of glycine thus may permit relative motion of the chains attached to the two ends of the molecule. With immunoglobulins, flexibility of the protein backbone can be one of the major factors that permit substitution of the various amino acids at the variable positions; it also may allow movement of the site to make most favorable contact in combining with an antigenic determinant. Though a glycine residue confers maximum flexibility over all other amino acids, it might also arise from a random mutation in which the difference between glycine and other amino acids is not adverse for the overall structure. In addition, some glycines might be complementarity determining. . . .

For the variable region of the light chains of human and mouse immunoglobulins and of Bence Jones proteins, alignment of amino acid sequences serves to identify the glycines which may be conferring flexibility. . . . The frequencies, expressed as per cent, can roughly be divided into three categories:

A. 94–100%: Positions 16, 41 (or 39), 57, 64, 68, 99, and 101. Since glycine occurs at these positions in nearly all the proteins studied, it must have a fundamental structural significance and has been preserved in the evolution to man and mouse. . . .

B. 35–62%: Positions 25, 66, 77, and 100. A careful examination indicates that glycines at these positions are at least group specific. . . .

C. 4–24%: Positions 9, 13, 24, 26, 27f, 28, 29, 30, 50, 51, 55, 74, 81, 84, 92, 93, 95, and 107. These glycine residues are at variable positions. They therefore play a distinctly different role from those of the other two categories. They might either be related to antibody complementarity or, if not involved in the site itself, could have arisen from random mutation and be nevertheless compatible with three-dimensional folding.

Thus there are about 8 (human κ and mouse κ) to 10 (human λ) glycines in the variable region of the light chains of all proteins for which sequence data are available. . . .

A parameter, HO_{ave}, based on the free energies of transfer of amino acid side chains from an organic to an aqueous environment has been introduced by Tanford and applied by Bigelow to the study of various proteins. HO_{ave} is expressed in kilocalories per residue and varies from 3.00 for Trp to 0.45 for Thr and is very small, zero, or negative for Gly, Ser, His, Asp, Glu, Asn, and Gln; these have been taken as zero. . . .

Of the 35 invariant residues in the constant region, 11 have values of 0.00 or 0.45, 13 have values of 2.40 to 3.00, and 11 have values of 0.75 to 1.70. Thus the constant region has invariant residues which appear to be relatively uniformly distributed with respect to HO_{ave} while in the variable region they are generally either very high or zero.

The average hydrophobicity for invariant residues of the variable region is about 1.09 while that of invariant residues of the constant region is 1.39. . . .

In considering the nature of the variable region, it is of importance to ascertain whether the variability is uniformly distributed or is confined to small segments of the variable regions. Thus, a quantity is defined for each amino acid position in the sequence in which the denominator is the number of times the most common amino acid occurs divided by the total number of proteins examined. . . .

Plotting variability against position for the 107 residues of the variable region shows three main peaks in the regions of residues 28, 50, and 96, two of these 28 and 96, are the highly variable regions (7, 45, 47, 49) in which insertions occur, while position 50 has not been associated with an insertion. . . .

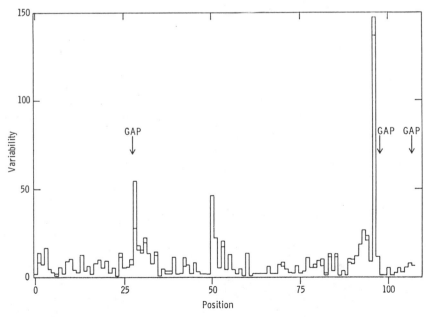

Figure 2 Variability at different amino acid positions for the variable region of the light chains. GAP indicates positions at which insertions have been found. Variability = Number of different amino acids at a given position ÷ Frequency of the most common amino acid at that position.

The overall sequence data were also examined to ascertain whether amino acid substitutions at each position were reflected in changes in hydrophobicity confined to certain stretches of the variable region. The findings . . . showed that the same three regions associated with high variability were those with the greatest variation in HO_{ave}. . . .

For the moment, if one accepts (a) the tendency of the positions of unaccountably high variability to be concentrated in the two short stretches of the chain at which insertions are found, (b) the finding that subgroup and group specificity occurs in the variable regions and indeed probably over substantial portions of it, one might formulate the following working hypothesis extending the earlier concept: The light chains of immunoglobulins except for the regions of unaccountable variability, 23, 34, and 89–97, are governed by a number of structural genes, each chain being the product of two linked genes, one for the variable and one for the constant region. These structural genes are free to mutate and are limited only by the requirement that their product be capable of assuming the proper three-dimensional structure to permit an antibody site to be formed. By hypothesis the complementarity-determining residues are considered to be the result of the insertion into the DNA of the two short linear sequences, 23, 34, and 89–97, which specifically determine what kind of antibody site will be formed. In the light chain the two insertions would be brought into close proximity by the disulfide bond I_{23}–II_{88}. . . .

The suggestions put forward are admittedly speculative as is the case at the moment with all other hypotheses. They do however present the problem of the antibody-combining site and of immunoglobulin structure in a different way, but in a way which is susceptible to verification or disproof by further data. Whether the model proposed ultimately stands or falls, the effort to assign each amino acid residue in the variable region a definite role by the statistical analysis employed should prove useful.

Continuous cultures of fused cells secreting antibody of predefined specificity

1975 • Georges Köhler and Cesar Milstein

Comment

The last milestone of this section is ahead high on the left bank. We land our raft, observing that the ever wider and faster river of immunology bends sharply to the right and disappears into a greenish mist. The unmistakable roar of a large cataract deafens our ears. In the far distance between two hills we can just discern an immense body of water. Not a clue can be found to judge whether it is a great flow as the Amazon, a basin with exit as Lake Albert on the Nile, the limitless ocean, or a mocking mirage. It may also be, as once pessimistically envisioned by Gunther Stent, a shallow, evaporating lake. Consulting our charts, we find that we are at the precipice of biological engineering.

One of the greatest advances in modern immunology was the discovery that human myeloma proteins were monoclonal immunoglobulins, often antibodies. Since they were of pathological origin, the specificity of these antibodies was singular but random. Normally, the introduction of an antigen in a human or animal elicits antibodies from multiple clones that collectively, as in serum, vary in specificity and avidity. Building on the clonal selection theory of Burnet, the authors of the featured milestone developed a technique so ingenious and so important that it has virtually revolutionized immunology. The paper describes a method for the artificial production of monoclonal antibodies to potentially any given antigen; it involves the fusion of a B-cell myeloma and a plasma cell from animals immunized to a target antigen. The prize committee of the Karolinska Institutet in Stockholm quickly recognized the significance and profound consequence of the method, and recommended that the Nobel Prize in Physiology or Medicine for 1984 be awarded to its developers Cesar Milstein (1927–   ) and Georges J. F. Köhler (1947–   ). Niels Jerne shared the honor for his theoretical contributions.

Milstein, who was born in Argentina, attended the National University of Buenos Aires between 1945 and 1952, attaining his diploma in chemical science. Continuing his studies, he earned a doctorate in chemistry in 1957, and joined the staff of the National Institute of Microbiology. On leave in 1958, Milstein traveled to Cambridge University as a British Council Fellow, and two years later received his Ph.D. from Fitzwilliam College. Over the next year, he served on the staff of the Department of Biochemistry at Cambridge. Milstein returned to Argentina to head the Division of Molecular Biology, but his stay was short. When political persecution of liberal intellectuals precipitated an attack against the Director of the Institute, Milstein resigned and returned to Cambridge, this time to the Medical Research Council Laboratory of Molecular Biology. His research brought him fellowship in the Royal Society in 1975. In 1981 he served as a Fellow of Darwin College, and in 1983 he became Head of the Division of Protein and Nucleic Acid Chemistry.

Köhler was born in Munich. His college education at the University of Freiburg led to the diploma in biology in 1971 and the Ph.D. in 1974. His doctoral research actually took place at the Institute for Immunology in Basel. When Milstein visited Basel in 1973 for a seminar, he invited Köhler to come to Cambridge in 1974 as a postdoctoral fellow with Milstein. In 1976 Köhler returned to Basel as a member of the Institute.

Köhler and Milstein's discovery was not a result of a specific campaign, nor was it an ac-

cident. In 1962 Michael Potter developed a method to produce mouse myelomas, and the art of their care and feeding soon followed. Milstein with Richard G. Cotton had already fused rat and mouse myelomas to determine whether the variable and constant regions of immunoglobulins are directed by different chromosomes. Their analysis of the subsequent secreted antibodies showed that both regions were always of one species, although hybrids of heavy and light chains were encountered. Köhler, whose dissertation demonstrated that some 1000 different mouse immunoglobulins can react with a single epitope, accepted a project with Milstein on mutations of antibody genes. When the research stalled, Milstein suggested that he try to discover which antigen couples to myeloma P3 immunoglobulins, but Köhler was reluctant, deciding to turn the question around, i.e., to find a way to produce myeloma antibodies of known specificity. The hybridoma idea came to him around Christmas 1974 while in bed in that familiar creativity-releasing state of consciousness between wakefulness and sleep. Milstein, learning about the notion the next morning, encouraged Köhler to experiment and offered suggestions. The first assay of activity was delayed until they felt that the hybrid cells were stable and synthesizing antibody. The experiment succeeded; however, after the initial studies both Milstein and Köhler, now back in Switzerland, had six months of experimental failures. Eventually a toxic batch of reagent was found to be the culprit. Milstein wrote the report, and at first received most of the honors and credit.

Monoclonal antibodies provide the ultimate specificity, although cross-reactivity to very closely related antigenic configurations does occur. If equally optimal in avidity and complement-binding ability, monoclonal antibodies become the Magic Bullet of Paul Ehrlich and the perfect diagnostic and research probe. The mass production of pure, singular immunoglobulin is an immunogeneticist's and an immunochemist's delight. However, monoclonal antibodies are sometimes too specific for assays. Unless the antigen is a polymer, lattices are unable to form and, therefore, antigen-monoclonal antibody complexes do not precipitate in gels. Also monoclonal antibodies labeled with enzymes or fluorescent dyes do not yield an adequate signal; labeled polyclonal anti-immunoglobulins are better suited for the task. In addition to the conjugation of toxins with monoclonal antibody to produce cancer therapeutic immunotoxins, recombinant DNA techniques have replaced the Fc portion of immunoglobulins with enzymes. Thus, the antigen receptors are the homing device of these peculiar medical torpedos; the tail is the cellular explosive. Recombinant procedures have further achieved what Milstein failed to do: the production of immunoglobulins with the variable region of one species (mouse) and the constant domains of another (in this case, human). As Milstein has observed, when genetic engineering is coupled with the eventual knowledge of the rules of protein folding and the effects of amino acid sequences, antigens will one day direct the formation of antibodies, as in the old instruction theory, through the manipulative intermediacy of humans. The industrial manufacture of antibodies may become a totally chemical process, the B cell no longer necessary.

Once more scanning our charts, we note that the cartographer has also drawn a sea serpent in the adjacent margin to warn that hazards lie ahead. The rainbow over the monster, however, tempers that fear with hope, since every technological revolution has two faces, which are manifested sooner or later. Tools are neither good nor bad; it is their application and product that take on moral overtones. The deliberate manipulation of the genome is of the highest ethical concern, for it could and will improve the public health and vastly enhance the efficiency of both industrial and agrarian economies, but it likewise has the potential to alter evolution and human biology as extensively and darkly as the aftermath of a global nuclear war. Genetic engineering, the most ominous of the new biotechnologies, is limited

only by imagination, and has so far been beneficial. Biological engineering will probably continue this happy course for many more years; however, it will surely affect society in negative ways as well, some as already predicted by pundits and others yet unforeseen. Humans, already lords of Earth, have, with the power of transformation, become biological alchemists and gods of life.

For further information:

Goding, J. W. 1986. *Monoclonal Antibodies: Principles and Practice. Production and application of monoclonal antibodies in cell biology, biochemistry and immunology.* Second edition. Academic Press, London. 302 p.

Hurrell, J. G. R. (editor). 1982. *Monoclonal Hybridoma Antibodies: Techniques and Applications.* CRC Press, Boca Raton, FL. 240 p.

Milstein, C. 1986. From antibody structure to immunological diversification of immune response. *Science* 231:1261–1268.

Wade, N. 1982. Hybridomas: The making of a revolution. *Science* 215:1073–1075.

The Paper*

The manufacture of predefined specific antibodies by means of permanent tissue culture cell lines is of great interest. There are at present a considerable number of permanent cultures of myeloma cells and screening procedures have been used to reveal antibody activity in some of them. This, however, is not a satisfactory source of monoclonal antibodies of predefined specificity. We describe here the derivation of a number of tissue culture cell lines which secrete anti-sheep red blood cell (SRBC) antibodies. The cell lines are made by fusion of a mouse myeloma and mouse spleen cells from an immunized donor. To understand the expression and interactions of the Ig chains from the parental lines, fusion experiments between two known mouse myeloma lines were carried out.

*Köhler, G. and C. Milstein. 1975. Continuous cultures of fused cells secreting antibody of predefined specificity. *Nature* 256:495–497. [By permission, copyright 1975 Macmillan Journals Limited.]

Each immunoglobulin chain results from the integrated expression of one of several V and C genes coding respectively for its variable and constant section. Each cell expresses only one of the two possible alleles. When two antibody-producing cells are fused, the products of both parental lines are expressed, and although the light and heavy chains of both parental lines are randomly joined, no evidence of scrambling of V and C sections is observed. These results, obtained in an heterologous system involving cells of rat and mouse origin, have now been confirmed by fusing two myeloma cells of the same mouse strain, and provide the background for the derivation and understanding of antibody-secreting hybrid lines in which one of the parental cells is an antibody-producing spleen cell.

Two myeloma cell lines of BALB/c origin were used. P1Bu1 is resistant to 5-bromo-2'-deoxyuridine, does not grow in selective medium (HAT), and secretes a myeloma protein Adj PC5, which is an IgG2A (κ). Synthesis is not balanced and free light chains are also secreted. The second cell line, P3-X63Ag8, prepared from P3 cells, is resistant to 20 μg/ml 8-azaguanine and does not grow in HAT medium. The protein secreted (MOPC 21) is an IgG1 (κ) which has been fully sequenced. Equal numbers of cells from each parental line were fused using inactivated Sendai virus and samples containing 2 $\times$ 10⁵ cells were grown in selective medium in separate dishes. Four out of ten dishes showed growth in selective medium and these were taken as independent hybrid lines, probably derived from single fusion events. The karyotype of the hybrid cells after 5 months in culture was just under the sum of the two parental lines. . . . The hybrid cells give a much more complex [isoelectric focusing, IEF] pattern than either parent or a mixture of the parental lines. The important feature of the new pattern is the presence of extra bands. These new bands, however, do not seem to be the result of differences in primary structure; this is indicated by the IEF pattern of the product after reduction to separate the heavy and light chains. The IEF pattern of chains of the hybrid clones is equivalent to the sum of the IEF pattern of chains of the parental clones with no evidence of extra products. We conclude that, as previously shown with interspecies hybrids, new Ig molecules are produced as a result of mixed association between heavy and light chains from the two parents. This process is intracellular, as a mixed cell population does not give rise to such hybrid molecules. The individual cells must therefore be able to express both isotypes. This result shows that in hybrid cells the expression of one isotype and idiotype does not exclude the expression of another: both heavy chain isotypes (γ1 and γ2a) and both V_H and V_L regions (idiotypes) are

expressed. There are no allotypic markers for the $C\kappa$ region to provide direct proof for the expression of both parental $C\kappa$ regions. But this is indicated by the phenotypic link between the V and C regions. . . .

We conclude that in syngeneic cell hybrids (as well as in interspecies cell hybrids) V-C integration is not the result of cytoplasmic events. Integration as a result of DNA translocation or rearrangement during transcription is also suggested by the presence of integrated mRNA molecules and by the existence of defective heavy chains in which a deletion of V and C sections seems to take place in already committed cells.

The cell line P3-X63Ag8 described above dies when exposed to HAT medium. Spleen cells from an immunized mouse also die in growth medium. When both cells are fused by Sendai virus and the resulting mixture is grown in HAT medium, surviving clones can be observed to grow and become established after a few weeks. We have used SRBC as immunogen, which enabled us, after culturing the fused lines, to determine the presence of specific antibody-producing cells by a plaque assay technique. The hybrid cells are cloned in soft agar and clones producing antibody were easily detected by an overlay of SRBC and complement. Individual clones were isolated and shown to retain their phenotype as almost all the clones of the derived purified lined are capable of lysing SRBC. The clones were visible to the naked eye. Both direct and indirect plaque assays have been used to detect specific clones and representative clones of both types have been characterized and studied.

The derived lines (Sp hybrids) are hybrid cell lines for the following reasons. They grow in selective medium. Their karyotype after 4 months in culture is a little smaller than the sum of the two parental lines but more than twice the chromosome number of normal BALB/c cells, indicating that the lines are not the result of fusion between spleen cells. In addition, the lines contain a metacentric chromosome also present in the parental P3-X67Ag8. Finally, the secreted immunoglobulins contain MOPC 21 protein in addition to new, unknown components. The latter presumably represent the chains derived from the specific anti-SRBC antibody. . . .

The hybrid Sp-1 gave direct plaques and this suggested that it produces an IgM antibody. This is confirmed in [an agarose well assay] which shows the inhibition of SRBC lysis by a specific anti-IgM antibody. IEF techniques usually do not reveal 19S IgM molecules. . . .

The above results show that cell fusion techniques are a powerful tool to produce specific antibody directed against a predetermined antigen. It further shows that it is possible to isolate hybrid lines producing different antibodies directed against the same antigen and carrying different effector functions (direct and indirect plaque).

The uncloned population of P3-spleen hybrid cells seems quite heterogeneous. Using suitable detection procedures it should be possible to isolate tissue culture cell lines making different classes of antibody. To facilitate our studies we have used a myeloma parental line which itself produced an Ig. Variants in which one of the parental chains is no longer expressed seem fairly common in the case of P1–P3 hybrids. Therefore selection of lines in which only the specific antibody chains are expressed seems reasonably simple. Alternatively, non-producing variants of myeloma lines could be used for fusion.

We used SRBC as antigen. Three different fusion experiments were successful in producing a large number of antibody-producing cells. Three weeks after the initial fusion, 33/1,086 clones (3%) were positive by the direct plaque assay. The cloning ef-

ficiency in the experiments was 50%. In another experiment, however, the proportion of positive clones was considerably lower (about 0.2%). In a third experiment the hybrid population was studied by limiting dilution analysis. From 157 independent hybrids, as many as 15 had anti-SRBC activity. The proportion of positive over negative clones is remarkably high. It is possible that spleen cells which have been triggered during immunization are particularly successful in giving rise to viable hybrids. It remains to be seen whether similar results can be obtained using other antigens.

The cells used in this study are all of BALB/c origin and the hybrid clones can be injected into BALB/c mice to produce solid tumors and serum having anti-SRBC activity. It is possible to hybridize antibody-producing cells from different origins. Such cells can be grown in vitro in massive cultures to provide specific antibody. Such cultures could be valuable for medical and industrial use.

Part 9
Systems

A system . . . is exactly the opposite of a machine, in which the structure of the product depends crucially on strictly predefined operations of the parts. In the system, the structure of the whole determines the operation of the parts; in the machine, the operation of the parts determines the outcome. —Paul Alfred Weiss

In their attempts at finding scientific substitutes for what they called disparagingly "metaphysics," the scientific philosophers very often fell into metaphysical difficulties of their own. For although they might with some justice reject the metaphysical speculations of philosophers, they were prone to forget that scientific enquiry itself proceeds on the basis of certain presuppositions. —Bertrand Russell

---

The final part of this book returns the scale of our immunological examination from the molecular and cellular levels to the entire organism. For most of this century, the thrust of science has been to dissect, disintegrate, and divide in the hope that the reduction to simpler forms will permit or facilitate the determination of the mechanisms by which the whole, be it organism or atom, behaves (functions) and gains its structure. The strategy has been extraordinarily successful, but it affords only partial understanding of the subject, and restricts the scope of approved methodology. An appreciation of systems—and the system of systems known as an organism—has lagged until recently. Indeed, some of the attributes of higher organisms, especially the psychological aspects, still remain out of the mainstream of science because of their apparent inconsistency or randomness and the lack of appropriate models and "objective" techniques and recording instruments. Science is both limited and defined by its tools.

While the interactions or the combinations of basic physical, chemical, and biological units can synergistically create systems or networks with properties greater than can be predicted from the sum of their parts, systems regulate and coordinate downward the activities of their components. These principles may be found across the hierarchies of order, such as (1) the upward formation of a protein from the sequential linkage of amino acids and the downward folding of the chain into the biochemically active configuration of an enzyme; and (2) the development of a society from a group of individuals, whose behavior is regulated by an evolved culture and system of laws.

The organism, whether a life form or a government, to some degree may also produce its systems. A vertebrate, for instance, will develop organs, tissues, and cellular and molecular agents from the single cell of fused gametes. Biologists have logically yet arbitrarily organized these body features into digestive, reproductive, nervous, endocrine, immune, and other systems based on apparent common function. Reproduction and digestion on first glance are clearly differentiated activities; however, drawing boundaries within the body is not as simple as it appears in elementary textbooks. The growing fetus in the womb is an obvious complication. Nevertheless, these and other body systems have traditionally been treated apart from each other, except for physical proximity. Evidence over the recent decades is at last changing the picture to a holistic, ontogenetically correct perspective: at least some of the systems communicate and interregulate. The association of the neurological and endocrine networks was soon recognized, followed by their conjunction with the immune system. Researchers now speak of particular axes of function across tissues, organs, and traditional systems, as a traveler plots a route across the network of highways.

In the scientific journals today one may easily find reports of macrophage-secreted mediators of lymphocytes, such as interleukin-1, also acting upon liver cells, neural cells, and pituitary cells. Macrophages and lymphocytes in turn have receptors for mediating neuropeptides. Endocrine gland-secreted adrenocorticotropic hormone (ACTH), thyroid-stimulating hormone (TSH), and endorphins modulate lymphocytes; lymphocytes, themselves, secrete ACTH, TSH, endorphins, and gonadotropins. The thymus, lymph nodes, and spleen are innervated, and neuropeptides can regulate mast cells. The idiotypic network of antibodies with its "internal images" of antigens may have enzyme- and hormone-like activity. Our knowledge of the connections continues to expand. Therefore, science has essentially fused the once differentiated and isolated neurological, endocrine, and immunological systems into the neuroendocrinoimmunological system, a mutual feed-back regulating organization. However, this scientific treatment, while providing key molecular and cellular insights for totally interconnected and coordinated organismal responses, remains on the safe, material side of the philosophical coin. The neurological branch of the new supersystem forces the question of mind, consciousness, awareness, and will, which most biologists are reluctant to discuss in scientific journals.

Such a consideration is a giant leap into the metaphysical abyss, according to some scientists, but into the brilliant sunrise of scientific-philosophical fusions for others. Discomfort in some researchers stems from current technology, which permits only correlative or representational physiological and physicochemical data; no device exists that can display a mental image or convey a particular feeling. Although the present volume of research articles suggest that the problem of mind and matter with respect to experimental immunology is new, the study began over 60 years ago. In 1926 Serge Metalnikov carried the teachings of Ivan Pavlov into immunology. The conditioned response, the placebo effect, and the detrimental influence of mental stress on immunological cells were opened for investigation, if only temporary, by Metalnikov's series of experiments. His first report on the immunological effect of stress is the following and final milestone. Now deemed a pioneer of a new discipline, psychoneuroimmunology, Metalnikov integrated immunology with the intangible—consciousness and mind.

However, the field began to fade in the 1940s with the advance of reductive molecular investigations of antibody formation. The traps of this scientific approach were not yet appreciated. For instance, several researchers, interpreting certain quantitative serological data, concluded that stress or corticosteroids have no influence on secondary antibody responses. Interest further abated when another scientist denervated lymph nodes without apparent effect on antibody formation, dismissing the neurological connection to the immune response.

The inquiry, however, was not completely ignored. In late 1950s, the increasing public interest in hypnosis spilled over into the laboratory of John Humphrey, a distinguished English immunologist at the National Institute of Medical Research. His research team discovered that a posthypnotic suggestion could inhibit both the clinical manifestations of immediate hypersensitivity and the positive tuberculin hypersensitivity reaction in volunteers. Their experimental design, involving the Mantoux tuberculin test, was drawn with great care, requiring thorough standardization of procedures and histological examination of biopsies of injected sites. The inhibited sites, while apparently normal by eye, demonstrated by microscopy the expected cellular infiltration; however, fluid exudate was absent. In the United States at the same time, Robert A. Good's research group was conducting similar studies, testing the ability of subjects under hypnosis to react to simple protein antigens in the Prausnitz-Küstner test. Volunteers were injected in both forearms with serum from a highly allergic donor. The next day, while the volunteers were under hypnosis, the suggestion was made that a given arm should not react to the challenge injection of antigen. The striking result was that the specified arm indeed displayed only a minimal response while the opposite arm was strongly reactive. Despite such remarkable findings, these and the few related reports scattered about the scientific literature had no significant effect on the course of immunological research.

The interdisciplinary science of psychoneuroimmunology has arisen seemingly overnight. One of the hallmarks of the Western cultural revolution (circa 1964–1975) was the profound interest in mind, including its identity and its hitherto unrecognized or poorly developed powers, especially from the perspective of Asian psychology. The holistic health and ecology movements can be attributed largely to this psychosociological foundation. Systems theory and the other related emerging paradigms of self-organization and nondualistic models of quantum reality also stem from this epoch. With the general sociological, psychological, and philosophical underpinnings in flux, moving away from compartmentalization and independence of phenomena, researchers have become open to interpret their data of cross-system mediators and receptors as more than just an interesting but insignificant coincidence. Today, the subject of the mind-immunity relationship is at the leading edge of science.

To explore immunology or even the atom without considering mind is to obtain an incomplete and distorted picture of existence. As time and space are inseparable, brain (matter) can not be parted from mind. Science, therefore, faces its greatest challenge in the comprehension of mind-matter and its probable interpenetration and interaction. As some biologists are now merging organ and tissue systems back into their original organismal unit, some theoretical physicists are speculating on dimensional units of time-space-mind. The final answers probably will (or should) not be attained, but the scope of immunology, indeed all science—for the various fields are not truly separate—is again harmonious with the deepest questions of philosophy.

For further information:

Ader, R. (editor), 1981. *Psychoneuroimmunology.* Academic Press, New York. 661 p.

Goetzl, E. J. (editor). 1985. Neuromodulation of immunity and hypersensitivity. *Journal of Immunology* 135:739S–863S.

Grossman, C. J. 1985. Interactions between the gonadal steroids and the immune system. *Science* 227:257–260.

Korneva, E. A., V. M. Klimenko, and E. K. Shkhinek. 1985. *Neurohumoral Maintenance of Immune Homeostatis* (S. A. and E. O'L. Corson, translators and editors). University of Chicago Press, Chicago. 253 p.

Locke, S., R. Ader, H. Besedovsky, N. Hall, G. Solomon, and T. Strom (editors). 1985. *Foundations of Psychoneuroimmunology.* Aldine Publishing Company, New York. 480 p.

The role of continued reflexes in immunity

1926 • Serge Metalnikov and V. Chorine

Comment

It did not go away. Ignoring it was convenient. Scientists could thereby remain secure in their tangible, orderly temple-fortress. When a colleague, however, dared to tie the loose end by a radically different model of nature, a shiver ran through the establishment, and the fine edge of reality blurred and disappeared into a metaphysical haze. Depending on its ramifications and foundation, a paradigm shift can be a long and traumatic process or a brief sigh of relief. The reaction of scientists to the unorthodox, however well-grounded, is no different or less variable than any human population facing revolutions and upheavals. The "it" of physics was the photoelectric effect and black-body radiation. The "it" of medicine and immunology remains the placebo effect and the related stress or conditioned reflexes. In both cases science is dragged screaming to the inevitable confrontation of the awesome philosophical question of mind-matter.

The scientific roots of psychoneuroimmunology are deep. The ancient linkage of mind and health acknowledged by physicians, shamans, and folk healers received its first modern scientific treatment by Ivan Pavlov in his discovery of the conditioned reflex. During the 1920s and 30s, fueled by the pioneers of psychoanalysis and psychotherapy, unsophisticated psychological and psychosomatic conceptions were in vogue, but steadily declined in societal awareness. Biologists, who were initially interested, also became disenchanted after inconsistencies and failures according to their new gods, quantification and reductionism. Furthermore, experimental science was continuing to pull away from its religious and formal speculative, philosophical origins; besides being difficult to quantify and control results, any biological study of the mind (in contrast to the brain) would be reversing the path to materialistic independence. An era of avoidance and hence ignorance had begun.

One of the main wellsprings of psychoneuroimmunology is the 1926 opus of Serge Metalnikov (1870–1946), who at the Pasteur Institute adapted Pavlov's procedures of stimulant conditioning to activate and enhance cellular and antibody immune responses to foreign substances, particularly otherwise lethal doses of cholera and anthrax bacteria. Metalnikov's extreme modesty and quiet charm contrasted with the heroics of his mentor Elie Metchnikoff, in whose laboratory at the Pasteur Institute in 1901–1902 he investigated phagocytosis and acquired immunity in invertebrates, mainly insects. Metalnikov had previously worked in Heidelberg with the protozoologist Otto Bütschli and visited the Naples Zoological Station. He returned to Russia for studies with Metchnikoff's friend and zoological colleague Alexander Kovalevsky. In 1907 Metalnikov became Professor of Zoology at the University of St. Petersburg and Director of the Lesgaft Institute. After the revolution, he left Russia and in 1919 he was welcomed back to the Pasteur Institute by Emile Roux. Among Metalnikov's varied fields of microbiological and immunological research were some worthy achievements: the cure of tuberculous guinea pigs by intestinal secretions of a moth caterpillar that

dissolved the bacterium's waxy coat; the use of microbial spores to kill insect pests; the first artificially produced antiserum to autogenous cells, i.e., sperm, which are normally found in an immunologically privileged site; work on the heredity of immunity in insects; the effects of radioactivity on multiplication and structure of microorganisms; and the previously mentioned psychological and neurological influences on immunity.

Metchnikoff himself in 1892 first realized the regulatory association of the nervous system with immune and inflammatory responses, even characteristically leaping to the bold premise that our conscious efforts in developing measures for host defense are an evolutionary extension of somatic nerve-immune cell interactions. Today the familiar influence of stress has been affirmed by depressed in-vitro responses of immune cells taken from such animal and human subjects. More remarkable is the observation of allergic states unique to each "person" in patients with multiple personality disorders, consistent with the alteration of hypersensitivity reactions in normal subjects by hypnotic suggestion described earlier. Psychoneuroimmunological responses resemble and may indeed be associated with memory characteristics, information transfer, and pattern recognition.

Many progressive immunologists feel that they are on firmer ground with the materialistic study of chemical mediators of the now merged neuroendocrine and immunological systems. Others are fascinated by the idea of a precursor gene responsible for the homologies of thymocyte and neural cell surface antigen Thy-1, of domains of antibodies, and of histocompatibility β_2-microglobulin, and the similarity of neural and immunological mediators, further exploring Metchnikoff's notion of the evolutionary union of self, self-awareness, and the immunological defense of self. Still other researchers travel the professionally hazardous high mountain road of consciousness studies and the deliberate mental control of emotions and physical responses to stress by such transforming powers as biofeedback, visualization, and meditation. Also the influence and origins of circadian rhythm are being examined. Therefore, we are witnessing the development of a more encompassing theoretical framework in biology as revolutionary as was general relativity and, later, quantum mechanics in physics. Physician-mystics throughout the world and adepts of Tao, Tantra, and Zen are not surprised.

For further information:

Herbert, N. 1985. *Quantum Reality. Beyond the New Physics.* Anchor Press/Doubleday, Garden City, NY. 268 p.

Laudenslager, M. L., S. M. Ryan, R. C. Drugan, R. L. Hyson, and S. F. Maier. 1983. Coping and immunosuppression: inescapable but not escapable shock suppresses lymphocyte proliferation. *Science* 221:568–570.

Metalnikov, S. 1934. *Role du Système Nerveux et des Facteurs Biologiques et Psychiques dan l'Immunité.* Masson et Cie., Paris. 166 p.

Riley, V. 1981. Psychoneuroendocrine influences on immunocompetence and neoplasia. *Science* 212:1100–1109.

Russell, M., K. A. Dark, R. W. Cummins, G. Ellman, E. Callaway, and H. V. S. Peeke. 1984. Learned histamine release. *Science* 225:733–734.

The Paper*

The importance of the study of conditioned reflexes has been brought to light thanks to the remarkable work of I. Pavlov and his students. . . .

We have attempted to apply Pavlov's method to the study of immunity.

In a series of works, we have demonstrated that the defensive reactions of various cells of the organism are the basis of immunity.

Defensive reactions can occur either external to the organism (in the mucosa of the nose, the eyes,

the throat, etc.) or internal (in the blood, the body cavities, and the organs). Not only do the free cells of the blood react, but also all the other cells: connective and reticulo-endotheial cells, vessels, hematopoietic glands, nerves, etc. The formation and secretion of different antibodies are also manifestations of these cellular defensive reactions.

Since all these reactions are involuntary, we can state that they are very complicated internal reflexes. These defensive reflexes can vary greatly under the influence of different stimuli, i.e., of various microbes, toxins and foreign bodies that are introduced into the organism.

Thus, we can always produce a typical reaction by injecting a suspension of a given microbe into the peritoneal cavity of a guinea pig. The duration and the strength of these reactions depend on the quantity and quality of the injected substances. We can repeat these injections several times, always obtaining the same typical reflex.

A question arises: Would it not be possible, by repeating these injections 10 to 20 times successively and by associating them to some external stimuli, to create a reflex similar to the conditioned reflexes of Pavlov? To solve this question, we undertook a series of experiments on 24 guinea pigs.

Each guinea pig received intraperitoneally a small daily dose of tapioca, or of *B. anthracis,* or of filtrates of staphylococci. This injection was always associated with an external stimulus: scratching the same area of the skin or bringing the skin in contact with a heated metal plate.

After 15 to 20 injections and external stimulations of this sort, we let the guinea pigs rest some 12 to 15 days, until the exudate of their peritoneal cavity returned to normal. On that day, we applied the external stimulus (scratching or heating) several times, but we did not inject anything into the peritoneal cavity. Next, we examined the peritoneal exudate several times during a 24- to 48-hour period.

It is appropriate to remember that in a normal, untreated animal the peritoneal exudate is transparent and contains only very few elements, particularly lymphocytes and monocytes.

Almost immediately following the injection of a foreign substance into the peritoneal cavity, leucocytes appear in great numbers and the amount increases hour by hour.

Polynuclear cells especially begin to appear in the first hours after the injection. Toward the end of the first or second day, the number of polynuclear cells diminishes rapidly. Afterwards, monocytes appear in large quantity, reaching their maximum toward the third or fourth day after the injection. Finally, lymphocytes arrive, which are the most numerous toward the fifth to seventh days.

---

*Metalnikov, S. and V. Chorine. 1926. Role des réflexes conditionnels dans l'immunité. *Annales de l'Institute Pasteur* 40:893–900. [With permission.]

For further clarification, the results of some experiments are given [See tables].

On examining the results of experiments II, III, and IV, we observed that guinea pigs 42, 98, and 16, which had not received anything intraperitoneally, but which have been externally stimulated, yielded the same leucocyte reaction in the peritoneal cavity.

This reaction is weaker and more transitory than in the animal that received the suspension in the peritoneal cavity, but it is highly convincing. While in the normal guinea pig the reaction of monocytes always appears later (two to four days) monocytes in the guinea pigs with conditioned reflexes often react sooner than polynuclear cells.

If the external conditioned stimuli are capable of initiating an internal defensive reaction, would it not be possible to utilize these stimuli as a means of defense against a lethal infection? To solve this question, we undertook a series of experiments:

Experiment V. Two guinea pigs, Nos. 95 and 96, had 12 times intraperitoneally received filtrates of staphylococci associated with an external stimulus (scratching of the skin); 6 hours after the last injection, the same spot of skin was scratched several times. The following day the two guinea pigs, as well as a control, received intraperitoneally lethal doses of the cholera vibrio. While the control died in six hours, the two guinea pigs with conditioned reflexes remained alive.

Experiment VI. Two guinea pigs, Nos. 20 and 75, had 24 times received intraperitoneally *B. anthracis* associated with an external stimulus (scratching). Fifteen days after the last injection, the same region of skin was scratched on guinea pig No. 20. The next day, guinea pigs No. 20 and 75, as well as a control, received a lethal dose of cholera. The control died after 7 to 8 hours. No. 75, which had not been stimulated, died after 6 hours. No. 20 died after 36 hours (the dose was too strong).

Experiment VII. Two guinea pigs, Nos. 21 and 16, had intraperitoneally received 18 injections of *B. anthracis* associated with an external stimulus. Seventeen days after the last injection, the two guinea pigs were scratched several times. The following day, guinea pigs Nos. 21 and 16, as well as a control, received a lethal dose of cholera. While the control died, guinea pigs Nos. 21 and 16 remained alive.

Experiment VIII. The two guinea pigs Nos. 21 and 16 are again tested (a month after the last injection of cholera). Only guinea pig No. 16 is exposed to conditioned stimuli; guinea pig No. 21 remains as is. The next day, guinea pigs Nos. 16 and 21, as well as two controls, receive intraperitoneally lethal doses of virulent streptococci. The two controls and guinea pig No. 21 die; guinea pig No. 16 remains living.

Of the 24 guinea pigs which had been subjected to these experiments, 10 died from causes unrelated to the experiments; of the 14 remaining, 10 yielded typical defensive reactions, the other 4 being insignificant.

All these experiments demonstrate that in guinea pigs with conditioned reflexes, the influence of a corresponding external stimulus can produce defensive reactions, which in certain instances may protect them against a lethal infection. . . .

All these experiments demonstrate that conditioned reflexes can play a very important role not only in immune reactions, but also in different diseases.

Everything that surrounds the patient can act as conditioning stimuli, initiating the same disease as the original cause. From this point of view, the sensations of pain and of discomfort can occur not only under the influence of a natural cause (virus, intoxicant, etc.), but also through the action of various stimuli that accidentally become associated during the disease. It is possible that in many chronic and nervous diseases (asthma, heart troubles, neuroses,

Experiment I   Cellular reactions in the peritoneal cavity of guinea pig No. 42 which received an emulsion of tapioca (2 cc).

| | Leucocyte formula | | | |
	Polynuclears	Monocytes	Lymphocytes	Quantity of cells
Before the injection	0	35	65	+
30 minutes after the injection	4	16	80	+ +
2 hours after the injection	26	14	60	+ +
5 hours after the injection	90	8	2	+ + +
24 hours after the injection	82	16	2	+ + + +
48 hours after the injection	47	35	8	+ + + +
3 days after the injection	29	50	21	+ + + +
5 days after the injection	12	37	51	+ + +

Experiment II   Guinea pig No. 42 received 21 injections of tapioca. Before each injection a warm metal plate was placed upon the skin; 30 days after the last injection the same area of the skin was heated several times.

	Leucocyte formula			Quantity of cells
	Polynuclears	Monocytes	Lymphocytes	
Before stimulation	0.6	29	69.6	+
2 hours after stimulation	9.3	78.2	12.5	+ +
5 hours after stimulation	62	32	6	+ + +
24 hours after stimulation	24.5	53	22	+ +

Experiment III   Guinea pig No. 16 received 18 injections of a suspension of *B. anthracis* associated with an external stimulus (heating). Fifteen days after the last injection, the same area of skin was heated several times.

	Leucocyte formula				Quantity of cells
	Polynuclears	Monocytes	Lymphocytes	Eosinophiles	
Before stimulation	0	35	54.5	10.5	6,300
3½ hours after stimulation	41.6	26.6	20.4	10.8	8,650
24 hours after stimulation	1.5	30.5	58	15.5	13,300
48 hours after stimulation	0.4	46.9	45.8	7.3	9,500
3 days after stimulation	0.5	50.9	38.8	9.5	11,920

etc.) attacks and episodes occur under the influence of conditioned stimuli that have nothing in common with the fundamental cause of the disease.

For this reason, such patients need not be treated with some remedy, but by the suppression of conditioned stimuli that developed during the illness. A simple change in living conditions (i.e., the suppression of some conditioned reflexes) is often sufficient to produce a beneficial effect on the patient. On the other hand, during convalescence and immunization, conditioned reflexes are also formed that are very useful, because they initiate defensive reactions. As we have seen in our experiments, these conditioned reflexes are often capable of protecting the organism against a lethal infection and produce a beneficial effect.

Epilogue

Any body of scientific knowledge may contain a significant component that is socially determined, and hence relative to the particular social group that has created this knowledge. —John Ziman

Science is not a logical process, it is rather a dialectic experience where we grapple with our innate inability to envisage Nature's true complexity. —Baruj Benacerraf

Reality, as the Latin word "res" indicates, is what "resists". What does it resist? Trials of strength. If, in a given situation, no dissenter is able to modify the shape of a new object, then that's it, it is reality, at least for as long as the trials of strength are not modified. —Bruno Latour

---

Zen koans:

1. A monk asked, "Since all things return to one, where does this one return to?"
   The master replied, "When I was in the city, I purchased a robe weighing seventy ounces."
2. A monk asked, "What is my true self?"
   "Have you finished your breakfast?" asked the Master.
   "Yes, I have finished it," replied the monk.
   "Then go and wash your dishes," said the Master.

Scientific enigmas:

1. Is a virus alive? (What is life?)
2. Is a photon a wave or a particle? (What is matter?)
3. How can stress cause disease? (What is mind?)
4. What is immunology? (What is self?)

This immunological journey has ended with the questioning Hydra having more heads than when we began, which is what science is about. Our insatiable appetite to know grows with each addition to the data bank, such that the present era has been called the Information Age. However, we have been swamped by the deluge, and desperately fight to locate and snatch from the

317

now rising ocean that particular datum that meets our requirement before it floats away to some nearly inaccessible archive. We have become so splintered in our knowledge that everyone by necessity has become an expert on something but a tyro on nearly everything else. This collection of historical milestones, as does any broad historical approach, can only touch on the principles, conceptions, turning points, and trends, and simply point to more explicit sources for the scholarly seeker. Nevertheless, what an overview loses in fine detail, it gains in high order.

I have attempted to draw the reader to the heights for a fresh sight of the field. Since exposition has its limits, I have frequently resorted to metaphor as a tactical and strategic device for rapid communication of common information and philosophical perspectives. Experimental interpretations are creating the new paradigm, and as this paradigm is becoming established, it is shaping experimental designs and analysis. Before our raft is secured to its moorings, the questions of self and the purpose of the immune response, which have weaved immunological history, should again be considered.

A thorough, comprehensive study and practice of any natural science requires examination of the subject at every intermeshing level—the environment, biosphere, community, organism, organelle, molecule, atom, quantum entity—including its association with the humanities, the social sciences, even the fine arts, but that encyclopedic pursuit is, of course, inexhaustible. However, as in the web of Indra's jeweled beads, each facet of existence is reflected by all others. For instance, human intellectual history was irrevocably transformed when lunar astronauts delivered photographs of our spaceship Earth. Some of these intrepid travelers experienced mystical insights as they silently floated in space gazing at their shrunken planetary abode. Likewise, when the specialist steps back for a universal view or the generalist dives into the particular, an intellectual sense of wholeness and interconnection can develop. What may also occur is a comprehension of operations and epistemology. I have asked questions in my commentaries that challenge certain models of immunology; I did not answer them, since any inference will differ with each society and age, with each world view. Furthermore, science rarely proves a truth; it provides evidence of structure and process that supports an argument, or disproves a contrary position. However, I will produce a map, but I ask the reader not to interpret it as an accurate depiction of the terrain.

Sir Macfarlane Burnet may have been the first to give the immune response the formal framework of self-nonself discrimination, building it on the foundation of Paul Ehrlich's principle of *horror autotoxicus*. Burnet expanded the function of immunity from defense against microbial invaders and diseased or degenerated tissue to the lofty concept of guardian of structural and chemical self-integrity. However, as I indicated in the previous comments, close inspection yields too many mechanistic exceptions and paradoxes to rigidly accept this simple view, and Burnet was obliged to put quotation marks around the word self and speak of a " 'self' pattern." For over fifty years, immunology has pursued a biological and biochemical definition of self, which is turning into a mirage always just out of reach. Some alternatives and modifications of this teleology have been proposed.

Pasteur, Metchnikoff, and Ehrlich regarded immunity as a derivative of nutritive metabolic mechanisms, and Metchnikoff went further to postulate that the neurological networks of vertebrates advancing to consciousness support the immune functions of the animal. Walter Pierpaoli has suggested that fundamentally the purpose of the immune system is to ensure reproduction, thus not only protecting the individual, but future generations of selves as well. He views the association and mutual rising of immunological and reproductive physiology as an economical, efficient measure regulated by circadian rhythm. He also notes the ontogenic linkage of the thymus, hypothalamus, and pineal gland. With mounting evidence that the neurological and immunological mesh is strong, sharing chemical agents and receptors, J. Edwin Baclock proposed that the immune system serves as a sensor of internal environment as the eye and ear monitor the exterior. Immunity has therefore a surveillance function, which Burnet discussed earlier with reference to cancer cells.

Many would have problems accepting notions that recognize interdependency but still attempt separations. Clearly, mutually arising, co-evolving organs and systems can not be entirely segregated. We are dealing with organisms and communities of organisms that are defined by their environment and are linked with the continuum of earlier generations. To break the whole into so-called components for study—be it an individual organism, a society, or even the organism-like planetary system that J. E. Lovelock and Lynn Margulis have called Gaia—the parts must be treated as synergistically interdependent.

The immunological puzzle seems to be a variation on the holistic-reductionist conflict found in microbiology between the ecology school of Sergei Winogradsky, whose research on soil bacteria and fungi demonstrated a vast network of symbiotic interactions, and Robert Koch, who pioneered the principles of isolation and purification. Neither approach alone suffices to describe life. However, the reductive approach is by definition the more simple and also the easier of the two. It has dominated scientific thinking for many decades. Some immunologists have likened the immunological network to the neural system, fighting to maintain a Cartesian separation between them despite the increasing evidence of union and common origin. As Richard Gershon noted, just because an immunological response can occur in vitro without a neural influence, it does not exclude one, and in vivo it can be subjected to neural influence and be modified. A balance of approaches hence is needed.

Alastair J. Cunningham seemed to understand this when he wrote that the nervous, endocrine, and immune systems help maintain homeostasis or functional equilibrium, a Taoist principle. Self is not treated apart from environment; environment is integral to self. I am particularly in accord with his observation that the exchanges between organism and environment, internal as well as external, involve, besides energy, the transmission of information. Such data comprise sets of patterns, such as particular arrays of neuronal firing. In comparing the neurological and immunological systems, Cunningham found that both are information processors, adaptive to environmental stimuli, and dependent on memory or previously encountered elements. Both also show tolerance or habituation. An evolutional argument in support of this union was provided by Jesse Roth and colleagues, who, looking at the evolution of neuropeptides, hormones, and their receptors, pointed out that certain molecules resembling these messenger or regulator chemicals of intercellular communication may be found in bacteria, protozoa, and plants. They suggested that the interactions of organs and systems in vertebrates developed phylogenetically from these metabolic seeds.

Therefore, I accept distinct functions of thought, sensation, movement, digestion, excretion, respiration, and reproduction. However, I also subscribe to the psychophysiconeuroendocrinoimmunological (at the very least) regulatory network of the organism, with the psychological element being an expansive and deep, mysterious sink that transcends the conceptions of self, time, and place. Patterns—from molecular conglomerations of fuzzy atoms, through variations of cellular behavior, to unique eigen states of networks and systems—would in part be the basis of feelings, thoughts, perceptions, and consciousness, which, being distinct sets themselves, feed information back down and through the integral tiers of systems. Self and nonself, the two sides of the immunological coin, would thereby emerge from patterns, or sets of arrangements or of aggregates, the interacting networks being pattern analyzers. However, since these patterns are ephemeral, intangible, and memory dependent, cosmos and cognition rest on process.

Process is key to the evolving paradigm, replacing the materialistic and positivistic concept of independent, fixed structure. Furthermore, patterns also exist as oscillations and vibrations, whether atoms or physiological rhythms, with characteristics of phase, amplitude, and frequency. Such patterns can be regulated by nonlinear resonance and its entrainment effect, which synchronize, for instance the beating of chicken heart muscle cells in culture and the flashes of Asian fireflies on a bush.

Acknowledgment of the fundamental denominator of process is fairly new to modern Western scientific philosophy and psychology, championed especially by Alfred North Whitehead, but it is at the very core of Eastern experimentally based, introspective religio-philosophies. For example, to live Zen, a term referring to meditation, is to simultaneously function freely without psychological attachments within the relative and the absolute, the world of phenomena and that pre-thinking state of no-thing-ness, the interval between the quanta of ever arising and recognized patterns vainly described by the Perennial Philosophy. Again, the key is function and process, not name, not form, not value. The moment a person opens the mouth to provide an answer the truth is lost. Science, however, must orbit the world of manifestation and suffer the limitations of words and consensus. It would be nice to believe, however, that the progress of scientific thought and practice offers gradually closer approximations of fundamental existence or its developmental origins. By such increasingly higher spiral orbits—undergoing cycles of reductive and holistic frameworks—science could not only tolerate, but actually incorporate the formless, wordless reality that is beyond its manipulative grasp. In turn, theologicians and religio-philosophers would no longer be antagonistic to scientific pursuits and understandings, other than some opposed ethical positions on applications and technology. The psychobiological disciplines, with significant contributions by psychoneuroimmunology, are today the pioneering probes that are exploring the boundaries of these nether lands. Psychophysics will next join the expedition, and together doubtlessly create someday a powerful philosophical paradigm to launch the next scientific investigation, to lay new milestones along the waterways of immunology.

For further information:

Ader, R. (editor). 1981. *Psychoneuroimmunology.* Academic Press, New York. 661 p.

Bunge, M. 1980. *The Mind-Body Problem. A Psychobiological Approach.* Pergamon Press, Oxford. 250 p.

Comfort, A. 1984. *Reality & Empathy. Physics, Mind, and Science in the 21st Century.* State University of New York Press, Albany. 272 p.

Davies, P. C.W. and J. R. Brown. 1986. *The Ghost in the Atom.* Cambridge University Press, Cambridge. 157 p.

Gleick, J. 1987. Chaos. *Making a New Science.* Viking, New York. 352 p.

Hayward, J. W. 1987. *Shifting Worlds, Changing Minds.* New Science Library/Shambhala, Boston. 310 p.

Hoffmann, G. W. (editor). *Paradoxes in Immunology.* CRC Press, Boca Raton, FL. 368 p.

Jantsch, E. 1980. *The Self-Organizing Universe. Scientific and Human Implications of the Emerging Paradigm of Evolution.* Pergamon Press, Oxford. 343 p.

Whitehead, A. N. 1978. *Process and Reality* (Corrected edition). (D. R. Griffin and D. W. Sherburne, editors). Macmillan Company, 413 p.

Index

Page numbers appearing in bold indicate primary references.

Self-nonself, 4, 5, 43, 45, 61, 139, 158, 170, 182, 183, 186–188, 220, 232, 242, 313, 318–320
Semple, David, 8, 34
Serum sickness, 44, 53–56
Sewall, Henry, 2, 7, 10, 11, 12, 32, 51
Shakespeare, William, 7, 217
Shaw, George Bernard, 174, 279
Shiva theory, 166–169
Shreffler, Donald, 252
Side-chain theory, 80, 85, 156, 157, 166, 168, 169, 186, 187, 221
Simonsen, Morton, 143
Sloan-Kettering Institute, 300
Smallpox eradicated, 16, 17
Smith, Theobald, 8, 31, 32
Smith, Wilson, 205
Snell, George, 233, 261, **282, 283**
Southhampton University, 241
Stanford University, 144, 178
Stanley, Wendall, 185
State Bacteriological Laboratory (Stockholm), 289
State Serum Institute (Copenhagen), 82, 189
State Serum Institute (Steglitz), 78
State University of New York (Brooklyn), 144
State University of New York (Buffalo), 68, 107
State University of New York (Purchase), 291
Stent, Gunther, 304
Sternberg, George, 170
Stetson, Rufus, 225, 227
Stoll, Arthur, 205
Sturli, Adriano, 221, 266
Svedberg, The, 76, 95
Sydney University, 131
Synergism, 117, 118, **134, 135, 144–147,** 157, 175, 190, 191, 232, 242, 309

T cell, 44, 45, 47, 60, 61, 64, 117, 118, [terminology] 130, 132, 134, 135, **138, 139,** 143, 144, 147, 151, 153, 154, 167, 171, 175, 191, 192, 196, 213, 241, 242, 245, 251, 253, 256
  cytotoxic, 118, [terminology] 138, 143, 151, 152, 232, 245, 246, 248, 252, 253
  helper, 118, [terminology] 138, **148–149,** 190, 198, 232, 246, 252
  receptor, 139, 143, 147, 192, 196, 219, 253
  suppressor, 118, [terminology] 138, 139, 189, 190, 241, 242
Talmage, David, 187
Tan, Eng, 256
Taylor, R., 147
Tchistovitch, Theodore, 266
Technology,
  elegance, 297
  limits, 299, 300, 309
  influence on theory and philosophy, 160, 259
Template (instructional) theory, 157, 178, 179, 182, 185
Thomas, Lewis, 213
Thuillier, Louis, 27
Thymus, 117, 129, 130, 132–143, 145–148, 150, 171, 245, 253, 310, 318
Tillet, William, 39, 40
Tiselius, Arne, 76, 95, 96, 256, 261

Tizzoni, Guido, 14
Tokyo Medical School, 13
Tolerance, 45, [terminology] 67–68, 72, 88, **138, 139,** 142, 143, 182, 188, 191, 219, 224, 240–244, 246, 248
Tomasi, Thomas, Jr., 76, 107, 108, 111
Topley, W. W. C., 229
Toussaint, H., 19
Toxoid, 75, [terminology] 78, 80, 167, 168
Transfer factor, 196
Transfusion, 218, 222, 224, 247–251
Transplantation, 60, 117, 130, 132, 143, 170, 218, 219, 232, 233, 236–247, *see also* Histocompatibility
Traube, Moritz, 162
Trefouet, Jacques, 112
Trefouet, Therese, 112
Trinity College (Dublin), 34
Triplett, R. Faser, 135, 150
Trophoblast, 224, 232
Tyzzer, Ernest, 233

United States Army Epidemiology Board, 39
United States Department of Agriculture, 31, 32, 229
University College (London), 147, 205, 232, 237, 241
University of Adelaide, 182
University of Berlin, 12, 120, 161, 198
University of Bern, 208
University of Birmingham, 237
University of Breslau, 58, 78, 198
University of Brussels, 201
University of Budapest, 279
University of Buffalo, 68
University of California (Berkeley), 83
University of California (San Diego), 178
University of California (San Francisco), 161
University of Cologne, 148
University of Colorado, 135
University of Copenhagen, 189
University of Edinburgh, 244
University of Frankfurt, 68, 147, 189
University of Freiburg, 305
University of Geneva, 189
University of Glasgow, 208
University of Göttingen, 46, 161
University of Graz, 53, 54, 263
University of Heidelberg, 68
University of Hong Kong, 300
University of Illinois, 272, 294, 300
University of Konigsberg, 198
University of Lausanne, 51
University of Leiden, 189
University of Leipzig, 58, 78
University of Liverpool, 99
University of London, 70, 131, 181
University of Manchester, 277
University of Maryland, 277
University of Massachusetts
University of Melbourne, 181, 182
University of Michigan, 10, 229
University of Minnesota, 131
University of Montana, 289
University of Munich, 263